Genetic Testing *for* Cancer

Genetic Testing *for* Cancer

Psychological Approaches for Helping Patients and Families

Andrea Farkas Patenaude

Foreword by
Francis S. Collins

American Psychological Association • *Washington, DC*

Published by
American Psychological Association
750 First Street, NE
Washington, DC 20002
www.apa.org

To order
APA Order Department
P.O. Box 92984
Washington, DC 20090-2984
Tel: (800) 374-2721
Direct: (202) 336-5510
Fax: (202) 336-5502
TDD/TTY: (202) 336-6123
Online: www.apa.org/books/
E-mail: order@apa.org

In the U.K., Europe, Africa, and the Middle East, copies may be ordered from
American Psychological Association
3 Henrietta Street
Covent Garden, London
WC2E 8LU England

Typeset in Goudy by World Composition Services, Inc., Sterling, VA

Printer: Edwards Brothers, Ann Arbor, MI
Cover Designer: Naylor Design, Washington, DC
Technical/Production Editor: Gail B. Munroe

The opinions and statements published are the responsibility of the authors, and such opinions and statements do not necessarily represent the policies of the American Psychological Association.

Library of Congress Cataloging-in-Publication Data

Patenaude, Andrea Farkas.
    Genetic testing for cancer : psychological approaches for helping patients and families / Andrea Farkas Patenaude.—1st ed.
       p. cm.
    Includes bibliographical references and index.
    ISBN 1-59147-110-9
    1. Cancer—Genetic aspects—Psychological aspects. 2. Genetic screening—Psychological aspects. 3. Genetic counseling. I. Title.

RC268.4.P38 2004
616.99′4042—dc22   2004000359

British Library Cataloguing-in-Publication Data
A CIP record is available from the British Library.

Printed in the United States of America
First Edition

CONTENTS

FOREWORD

Nature or nurture?—perhaps the central question of biology, psychology, and life itself. Today, for the first time in humanity's history, we are gathering the tools necessary to answer that question. Indeed, although we do not yet have the ability to provide all of the details, we already know the short answer: It is neither nature alone nor nurture alone, nor even the two contributing independently, but the two interwoven in a complex and finely tuned fashion that make people who they are. This book joins two disciplines that have too often been viewed as disparate—genomics and psychology—that will need to work together to achieve a detailed understanding of these complex interactions.

With the essential completion of the human genome sequence in April 2003, the Human Genome Project successfully met all of its goals, and thus celebrated its end—ahead of schedule and under budget. It is important that this significant international achievement of sequencing the human genome did not represent the conclusion of the genomic era but the foundation for its true beginning. Now, at the start of that era, we can see today the outlines of what is to come. Despite the occasional over-the-top projections of "gene hype," there is much "gene hope" to point to. We already have abundant and convincing evidence that, along with other scientific, technological, and social advances, genomics will, indeed, bring major changes to our understanding of biology, to the health and well-being of us all, and to a number of important aspects of society. Those changes will represent the real genomics revolution—for as impressive an achievement as is sequencing the human genome, what is the benefit of knowing the sequence unless we can use that knowledge to improve human health and well-being?

As in much of her other work, in this book Andrea Farkas Patenaude has been a pioneer, performing an important service to both the psychology and the genomics communities by impressively bridging the gap that has too long divided them. Without better understanding of the genetic factors that influence both psychological well-being and psychopathology, and how they interact with environmental factors to do so, mental health professionals will not be able to serve their clients optimally. And, without better understanding of how individuals, families, and cultural groups view the influence of genetic factors on health and well-being, and how that understanding translates to changes in attitudes and behaviors, the vision of genomics as radically changing health care, and thus health, will never be fully realized.

There are at least three major areas in which psychologists and other mental health professionals will make key contributions to the "genomics revolution." First, they are necessary members of the transdisciplinary research teams needed to understand how genetic factors and nongenetic factors interact to lead to various forms of psychological well-being and pathology. Second, they are necessary to determining the individual, family, and cultural dynamics that influence how people learn, integrate, and use knowledge about genetics. Third, they will be important leaders and contributors to societal dialogue and decision making related to such charged issues as the relationship of genetics to concepts of identity, race, and ethnicity.

This is an exciting time of promise in understanding the causes, both genetic and nongenetic, of human health and disease. For that promise to become a reality, however, will take genomically literate psychologists and other mental health professionals and also experts in genomics who are well versed in the complexities of the mind–body interaction. The image of genetics and psychology as "worlds in collision" must give way to a collaborative spirit of "worlds in collusion." This book is a well-timed landmark in achieving that important goal. Welcome to our shared genomic era.

Francis S. Collins, MD, PhD
Director, National Human Genome
Research Institute, the National
Institutes of Health, Washington, DC

PREFACE

This book grew out of my belief that the work of psychologists would be affected by the ongoing revolution in human genetics. The focus of genetic research has moved from its base in the work of the monk Gregor Mendel to the high-speed, well-publicized, international effort to decipher the human genome. The Human Genome Project is less visual as a scientific achievement than a moon landing but will, I believe, be of far greater ultimate relevance to most people. The Human Genome Project reached its goal in April 2003, coinciding with the 50th anniversary of Watson and Crick's discovery of the double-helix structure of DNA. Publication of the complete sequence of the human genetic code signified both the end of this tremendous effort and the beginning of an exciting period of applying, extending, and translating the knowledge gained.

It is an amazing feat, the sequencing of the "code" for a human being. It took 12 1/2 years, $2.7 billion, and the work of hundreds of scientists in a dozen or so countries. The final product was not patented but was made freely available on the Internet to all, thanks in particular to the vision of the director of the project, Francis S. Collins. Although the effort involved sophisticated sequencing machines and the brilliance of many minds, it also required simple persistence in many forms. Several years ago, on a visit to the National Institutes of Health laboratory of Larry Brody, head of the Molecular Pathogenesis Section, some students and I observed the state-of-the-art sequencing equipment, but it was the corridor outside that quickly drew our attention. The walls had been covered with a continuous roll of paper tacked up at eye height. On the paper, drawn in pencil, was the in-progress sequence map of chromosome 7. Parts yet to be deciphered remained empty, but other parts, in a variety of handwritings, showed what was known. Chromosome 7 turned corners and snaked down the hall, the lab notes of a monumental project, remarkable as much for its final achievement as for teamwork through which its goals were achieved.

Now that the human genetic code is known, researchers are attempting to discover how it translates into signals that usually trigger normal development but, when altered by mutations, may initiate a cascade of events resulting in cancer or other diseases. Once specific genes are found and cloned, researchers may be able to develop genetic tests to determine whether there are mutations that predispose an individual to greater risk of developing a disease or syndrome. In the future, we will learn more about how genes interact, with either other genes or environmental factors, to protect the individual or initiate disease processes. The potential of genetic medicine is vast. Genetic testing to detect hereditary disease susceptibility offers many challenges for individuals who consider and undergo testing, for their families, for medical and psychological clinicians, and for researchers.

A remarkable aspect of the Human Genome Project was the decision to support and fund a simultaneous study of the ethical, legal, and social implications (ELSI) of the genetic advances that would result from the effort. The ELSI Program of what is now called the National Human Genome Research Institute has received 3% to 5% of the budget of the Human Genome Project since its inception more than 10 years ago. It has involved social scientists (anthropologists, psychologists, sociologists), ethicists, lawyers, and physicians in assessments of the ways genetics is changing medicine, law, privacy, families, and society. Psychological studies, such as those assessing distress associated with the use of genetic testing or studies of the psychological impact of changing ideas about race or identity that result from newly available genetic information, have been considered germane and fundable because they relate to the individual, family, and social impacts of modern genetic research. It was through funding from the ELSI Program that I came to work—or, more accurately, to work again—in the area of genetics.

My first foray into genetics was when I was a summer student in Bar Harbor, Maine, at the Jackson Laboratory, an internationally known center for the study of mouse genetics. Its JAX mice have been used in laboratories all over the world to create models of human diseases. These genetically identical mice enable scientists to conduct studies in cancer, obesity, diabetes, and many other diseases. My summer project, conducted under a lab scientist, was a study of mice that were the carriers of a type of anemia that was fatal if a mouse was unlucky enough to inherit a deleterious mutation from both parents. My job was to investigate whether the carrier mice had any physical abnormalities in their blood as a result of their genetic burden. It was a heady experience at age 15 to be given lab space and a small mouse colony, to be tutored by a senior scientist, to hear daily lectures from the geneticists who worked at or visited the lab, and to be expected by the end of the summer to write up the results of my project. By the end of that summer, I was sure I wanted to be a geneticist.

Later experiences, especially confrontations with the physical sciences, convinced me otherwise. I found my true calling was to psychology—specifically, to clinical psychology and the as yet unnamed field of health psychology. Some aspects of my work at the Children's Hospital in Boston, where I was first an intern and then a staff psychologist, involved genetic diseases. I wrote my dissertation on children with cystic fibrosis and their families, but when I moved into working clinically with cancer patients at the Dana–Farber Cancer Institute, I felt I had largely left the world of genetics behind.

My work had little or nothing to do with genetics until I was approached by Fred Li, an epidemiologist and oncologist, who asked me if I might be interested in working on a research project studying the impact of genetic testing on at-risk individuals from families with Li–Fraumeni syndrome (LFS). Li–Fraumeni syndrome is a rare, devastating, cancer susceptibility syndrome conveying high risk for cancer to both children (40% childhood cancer risk) and adults (90% lifetime risk). In 1990, Stephen Friend had found that mutations in the *p53* gene were responsible for the majority of LFS cases. As a result, it was possible to offer genetic testing to currently healthy members of families with LFS and inform them of whether they carried the mutation that had wreaked havoc in the lives of other family members. The ELSI Program was offering funding for projects evaluating the impact of this kind of testing. Oncologist Judy Garber and I applied for and then began a project that ultimately assessed and interviewed 32 members of families with LFS from across the United States who had chosen to undergo genetic counseling and, in most cases, genetic testing. Soon after our project began, another important cancer susceptibility gene was identified, the *BRCA1* gene, and Judy Garber and I began a similar study of men and women from families with known *BRCA1* mutations in their families. The ELSI Program organized research groups like ours that were receiving ELSI funding into a Cancer Genetics Study Consortium to encourage sharing of observations and research findings. We all learned a great deal from one another. From these efforts and similar ones in other countries, a new area of research was formed: the psychosocial study of cancer genetics.

This book introduces this new field of study to psychotherapists and counselors, to seasoned researchers from other fields, to medical and genetics clinicians, and to young investigators and students. My aim is to share what researchers have learned about how individuals with concerns related to hereditary cancer risk react to and cope with genetic information and how they make choices related to their health and lifestyle. The book incorporates clinical examples, drawn from my own work or that of my colleagues. It attempts to showcase this exciting, growing field in the hope that there will soon be more knowledgeable clinical psychologists and other mental health professionals to whom patients with genetic concerns about cancer can be referred. I hope it will also catalyze research interest to ensure that there will be sufficient investigators to study the important psychosocial questions that arise as the field of genetics changes medical diagnosis and treatment.

My clinical work in close association with genetic counselors, geneticists, oncologists, and high-risk patients, together with the writing of this book, has completed, in a gratifying manner, the circle of my interests. It has been exhilarating to find important links between psychology and genetics and to think of the even greater array of connections to come. I hope this book will transfer to the reader some of my enthusiasm and excitement about the critical importance of psychological factors in the full realization of the fruits of the Human Genome Project.

ACKNOWLEDGMENTS

A book comes into being through the direct and indirect influences of many people. Along with my own DNA, I received from my parents, Joseph and Sophie Farkas, a deep, nearly mystical sense of the magic that books can convey. My brother, Walden, was a writer long before I ever thought of writing a book. In our extended family, the joy that my Great-Aunt Anna got from the shelf of psychology books her sons and daughter-in-law authored made it clear that book writing was considered an admirable activity on both sides of our family. One of those sons, Dr. Irwin Sarason, and his wife, Dr. Barbara Sarason, have further modeled for me the pleasures and challenges of a life in psychology.

To write a psychological book, one must first become a psychologist. Many were the influences on that process. To name only a few, I am especially indebted to my thesis advisor, the late Dr. Donald Grummon, my internship director and later boss, the late Dr. Joseph Lord, and to Dr. Lucy Ferguson, Dr. Al Rabin, the late Dr. John Shlien, Dr. Ruth-Jean Eisenbud, the late Dr. Paul Russell, Dr. Lane Gerber, and the late Dr. Marion Winterbottom.

My interest in cancer gave me the opportunity to learn from many talented clinicians including Drs. Joel Rappeport, Jimmy Holland, Hal Churchill, Barbara Sourkes, Gerry Koocher, Mary Jo Kupst, Leah Baider, William Beardslee, Ron Brown, Susan Linn, Joanna Breyer, Kathy Hewett, Joshua Wootton, James Bowman, Joseph Fitzpatrick, Stan Berman, and Howard Kunin, among others.

I was fortunate to be invited into the world of cancer genetics by Dr. Frederick P. Li and to have been tutored by Dr. Judy Garber and Kathy

Schneider. Kathy Schneider also reviewed parts of this manuscript, for which I am particularly grateful. I have also learned a great deal from other insightful colleagues in this field, including Drs. Martin Richards, Wylie Burke, Sapna Syngal, Charis Eng, David Malkin, Nicole Alby, Francis Collins, Alan Guttmacher, Elizabeth Thomson, Michel Dorval, Eric Juengst, Caryn Lerman, Nancy Press, Sally Vernon, Suzanne Miller, Robert Croyle, Deborah Bowen, Ann-Marie Codori, and June Peters, Kathy Calzone, Stephanie Kieffer, Anu Chittenden, Kelly Branda, Elaine Hiller, Kristen Shannon, and many others.

This book grew out of my involvement with the American Psychological Association (APA) Advisory Committee on Genetic Issues. My thanks for that enriching experience to Drs. Carol Goodheart, Alice Chang, Jo Linder-Crow, Sandra Haber, Jill Reich, Richard Mc Carty, Ray Fowler, Dick Suinn, Martin Seligman, Pat DeLeon, Norine Johnson, and others who supported that effort.

APA Books has been a kind and patient publisher. Gary VandenBos was behind this idea from the start. Susan Reynolds never lost hope that this book would come to fruition (at least not that she let on!). Kristine Enderle has been an attentive and flexible development editor. Gail Munroe has been patient, kind, and persistent in overseeing all the final details of bringing this book through production.

Important support for the completion of this work came from the Harvard Medical School's 50th Anniversary Scholars in Medicine Fund. My thanks to Elinor Shore, Drs. Rosalind and Stuart Orkin, Dr. Mary Clark, Sara Kiarsis, and Dr. William Beardslee.

Kerrie-Anne DeFelice was a welcome partner in the delivery of each of the chapters in this book through her administrative assistance. Michelle Cox, Martha Mahoney, and Karen Eldridge have also provided extremely helpful support.

Vanessa O'Connor's cheerful and efficient efforts helped me to find time to do this work.

I am thankful for the continuing encouragement that came from Marilyn Zweifach and Don Rossmoore, Ken and Margaret Mallory, Karen Zelan, Madeleine Fraggos, Bill and Kristen Mitchell, Jim Lazarus and Susan Gershonhorn, Annie Wiesschhoff, Sara Campbell and Ken Maloney, Susan Liberman and David Rogovin, and Stephanie and Lester Adelman.

Drs. Michael Muto, Ursula Matalonis, and Brian Walsh contributed in truly essential ways and with great sensitivity and kindness to the fulfillment of this goal.

My profound thanks to the patients I have seen with genetic concerns who have candidly shared their fears and hopes and have taught me so very much.

Finally, this book is dedicated with love to my husband, Leonard Patenaude and our daughter, Madeleine Elizabeth Patenaude, with deepest thanks for their constant, caring support despite the time this work took from our joint endeavors and the clutter and, at times, anxiety that this project created. I am endlessly grateful to them for the unique joys of family life, which sustain and nurture me.

Genetic Testing *for* Cancer

INTRODUCTION

THE GENETIC REVOLUTION: WHERE ARE WE?

Sally poured herself a cup of coffee and took her aunt's letter to the sunroom. The letter had arrived five days earlier, but until now Sally hadn't been ready to read it. Two months earlier, her aunt had called and told her she was going to be tested for a breast and ovarian cancer gene. She suggested that Sally should think about whether she wanted to know the results when they were available. Even hearing that much had upset Sally. It brought back a lot of memories. Sally's mother had died of breast cancer when she was 15. It had been a horrible time. Years of therapy hadn't erased the horror of watching her mother get weaker and weaker and then finally succumbing to the disease, just when Sally needed her most. About six years later, her mother's younger sister, Aunt Marilyn, developed ovarian cancer. She had surgery and chemotherapy and has been fine ever since. Whenever Sally had told doctors about the history of cancer in her family, of two young sisters who had cancer, they had reassured her that the two cancers were not related and that she shouldn't worry so much. She should do all the usual kinds of screening. While her risk was definitely higher because her mother had cancer, it was still not that high. Then she had started to hear about a gene that gave women a higher chance of getting both breast and ovarian cancer. Sally remembered where she was—standing in a supermarket line—when she first read about the gene. It had given her cold chills. She had gone home and called her aunt, her sister, and her cousin. She had called her doctor and asked what to do. At that point, there wasn't anything she could do. The test for the gene wasn't available yet. Her family wasn't in any of the research programs that were going on, so they would have to wait. Sally gradually put thoughts about genes and cancer and tests in the back of her mind. She had too many other things to think about. She had three teenagers; that could erase almost anything from one's mind. Then her aunt's call brought it all back. Now the results must be here, or her aunt wouldn't have written to her.

Right after her aunt had told her she was going to get tested, Sally had a moment of thinking, "Why do I want to know this?" It hadn't lasted long. She knew that she needed to know, both for herself and for her kids. Yet she couldn't imagine what it would be like to learn that her aunt had this "bad gene" (that was how she thought about it) and then to think about being tested herself. She had lived in the shadow of her mother's cancer for so long. She had gotten used to how that felt. Before she had her kids, she had worried a lot about whether having kids would bring on breast cancer, but that was a long time ago. She had been fine, so she had forgotten about it. That was her style— not to dwell on things. But she knew that if her aunt had the "bad gene," she wouldn't be able to put it out of her mind so easily. Sally anticipated that it would be a big deal to get this information, so she had asked her aunt to send the result to her when she got it rather than telephoning her. She was afraid that she wouldn't be able to handle a phone call out of the blue with this powerful information. Yet, it had taken her all these days to feel ready to open the letter. She didn't quite know what to hope for. If her aunt didn't have the gene, it would mean that there was no good explanation for why the two sisters had gotten sick so young. If her aunt did have the gene, then she could be tested to see if she had the same mutation in her genes. Just the thought of this brought back the chills. If she did have it, her kids could be tested when they were 18 or older. "Could be." Would that be a good thing? Would it change anything for the better? Or would it just make her feel petrified for herself and her children and maybe make her feel like a bad parent for passing on such terrible things to her children? Did she want to know that much about what the likelihood of getting cancer herself—maybe more than a 50% chance? It was all in the envelope on her lap.

To whom could she talk about all this? They had changed insurance recently, and Sally now went to an HMO. She had an internist and a gynecologist, but she didn't feel close to either of them. She had been healthy and saw each of them for about 15 minutes a year. The internist never quite seemed to remember who she was. The gynecologist had recommended some special ultrasound but had said how hard it was, even with the ultrasound, to detect ovarian cancer until it was too late. That had helped Sally to put off making an appointment for such an unpleasant test. She had a mammogram; her insurance allowed it even though she was under 50 because of her family history, but she thought that was unpleasant enough. She didn't want to think about all of this because she felt very healthy and well. But what if her aunt's test had been positive? Who would she talk to? Sally thought of going back to her old therapist, but would she understand what all this gene stuff was about, or would Sally wind up having to explain it all to her? Suddenly, she felt very alone. She hadn't even told her husband about the letter. She knew it would upset him, and she wanted to absorb the news first. She took a deep breath and slit open her aunt's letter.

This scenario is fiction, but similar situations are unfolding in increasing numbers in families that have been heavily affected by cancer. Newspapers and magazines report the triumphs, frustrations, and conflicts of scientists involved in the Genetic Revolution. Scientists and doctors cautiously explain that new information about genetics will ultimately change medicine and allow us to save lives, but that it will take time before current research can be translated into medical progress. When we look at it through Sally's eyes, we can see the complex emotions that may arise when genetic information becomes available. We see the ambivalence about the possibility that, after all these years, medicine might have an answer to the question, "Why did this happen in our family?" and a partial answer to the other big question, "Am I going to get cancer, too?"

Some people with some family histories will be affected a lot sooner than others by the Genetic Revolution. Individuals from families where breast, ovarian, or colon cancer has occurred at young ages or where too many family members have developed certain types of cancers are already facing many of these questions. People in hereditary cancer families where genetic testing is available must decide what they want to know about inherited cancer predisposition. They must find the right doctors, get enough information to decide if they want testing, and deal with the anxiety that can surround such actions. If they do proceed with testing, they must decide with whom to share their decision, how to cope with the anxiety of waiting for the result, and, ultimately, how to live with the information they receive. All of these challenges stir up emotions and may evoke intrapersonal distress or familial conflict.

These challenges demand increased sophistication on the part of the physicians, nurses, genetic counselors, psychologists, social workers, psychiatrists, and other professionals who will see these potential patients. All professionals who deal with genetic information should not underestimate the emotional impact of that information on their patients. Although empathy for patients' experiences is important in all areas of medical and psychological care, this is an area where it is doubly important. It not only may affect what the patients feel but also may influence the use that patients make of the genetic knowledge they gain. The true test of whether genetic information actually generates the revolution in medicine that has been predicted rests, in large measure, on the psychological factors that determine the meanings people give to it and the plans they make based on their new knowledge. This includes the impact of the genetic information on people's self-esteem, their sense of the future, their sense of efficacy and control, their communication with their family members, and their health behaviors.

The concepts relevant to understanding the psychological issues in cancer genetics are not new: anxiety, depression, denial, adaptation, and resilience. It is their application at this crossroads between medicine and psychology that deserves explanation. It is as important that mental health and other medical professionals understand the psychological issues in cancer genetics as it is important that the patients understand the genetics of cancer.

THE GENETIC REVOLUTION

For centuries, physicians have been observing and recording the fact that, within some families, particular diseases occur at unusual rates. Galen (A.D. 131–203) described familial malignancies. Napoleon's family apparently had a predisposition to stomach cancer. In 1866, Paul Broca described the family of Madame Z where numerous relatives died of breast cancer or related metastases (Offit, 1998). However, it was only in the last quarter of the twentieth century that we developed the tools to search for the genetic signals that were the cause of these clusters. Advances in molecular biology and biotechnology have given us the ability to decode the sequence of DNA in the 30,000 or so human genes (International Human Genome Sequencing Consortium, 2001). The goal of the Human Genome Project, initiated in 1990, was to identify all the genes on the 23 human chromosomes. In February 2001, a draft sequence showing 94% of the human genome was published (International Human Genome Sequencing Consortium, 2001). The full genome sequence was completed by the 50th anniversary of the discovery of the double helix structure of DNA by Watson and Crick in April 2003. Yet, as we stand on the threshold of the 21st century, scientists have identified only a relatively small number of disease genes, and we are still far from understanding the complexity of how these genes operate. Genetic testing is in place for Huntington's disease; breast, ovarian, and colon cancer syndromes; cystic fibrosis; and a few other diseases. In absolute terms, the number of individuals currently directly affected by these genetic advances is relatively small. So, why is there so much talk about a revolution in medicine as large as that occasioned by the discovery of X rays?

One reason is that we are all the carriers of altered genes. Monique Mansoura and Francis Collins, Director of the National Human Genome Research Institute, have written (1998)

> All of us carry an estimated five to fifty significant genetic alterations. Genetic disease should not be thought of as the unfortunate fate of relatively few individuals who have been affected by rare inherited disorders. With our rapidly expanding understanding of the role of genes in common disorders, such as many forms of cancer, heart disease, diabetes, and mental illness, it seems more likely that in the future virtually all of our lives will be touched by the genetic revolution. (p. 334)

WHAT IS NEW ABOUT THE NEW GENETICS?

What is new about the New Genetics are the methods it uses and the extent of its impact. Taking the latter first, it is clear that genetic discoveries will have far greater impact on general medical treatment than genetics has had to date.

> Inaccurate beliefs about genetics persist, including the view that in the past it had no effect on the practice of medicine and that today it is pervasive. In fact, for decades knowledge of genetics has had a large role in the health care of a few patients and a small role in the health care of many. We have recently entered a transition period in which specific genetic knowledge is critical to the delivery of effective health care for everyone. (Guttmacher & Collins, 2002, p. 1512)

Harold Varmus, former NIH Director and President of the Memorial Sloan-Kettering Cancer Center, (2002) similarly says

> Medical genetics, once a tool for diagnosing a handful of relatively rare diseases inherited in simple mendelian fashion, has expanded into new territories: the prediction of a healthy person's risk of even common diseases such as cancer and cardiovascular disease; the analysis of patterns of gene expression as an adjunct to conventional diagnostic methods, such as histopathology; and the evaluation of multigenic diseases and responses to environmental agents and drugs . . . But the full potential of a DNA-based transformation of medicine will be realized only gradually, over the course of decades, as we try to understand the content of genomes and, most important, the physiological consequences of variations in their sequence. (p. 1526)

As for the methods of the new genetics, the map of the human genome gives scientists an amazing resource. It is available to all on the Internet at http://www.ncbi.nlm.nih.gov/genome/seq/. From the Human Genome Project we have come to new knowledge about genetics, some of it quite surprising. For example, there is the fact that any two humans share in common 99.9% of their DNA sequences (Guttmacher & Collins, 2002). This leaves, however, about 3 million locations or base pairs where we are not all the same, where the differences that constitute our unique qualities are initiated.

> However, it is not the base-perfect genome sequence, but rather the variants of this sequence, that will affect medical practice. DNA-sequence variants are estimated to occur in 1 of every 300 to 500 base-pairs in the human genome. These sequence variants give rise to the tremendous diversity we recognize in, for example, human physical traits, susceptibility to disease, and responses to treatments. (Drazen, 2000, p. 57)

The Human Genome Project sequences form a map. We know that genes are not fixed, independent elements, but that there are often important interactions between genes and between genes and the environment. From the map of the human genome, we know where to find a particular gene, but we certainly do not have all of the answers we seek about genetics and disease. We can look for some specific genetic mutations in some patients that can tell us some things about that patient's risk for certain diseases. We cannot yet survey all of the genes of a particular patient to understand broadly what his or her risks and strengths are in terms of their genetic makeup, but it is within the realm of possibility that we will be able to do that before long. With increasingly specific knowledge of the genetic basis for or contribution to many common diseases, it is likely that our approach to diagnosis and treatment will turn to genetic analysis, rather than waiting for symptoms to appear and be evaluated. Treatments, too, will increasingly focus on gene therapy, fixing or replacing what is "broken" in that person's genome.

As Drazen (2000) explains,

> . . . until now (except for conditions that follow a simple mendelian pattern of inheritance and phenotypic expression), we have been able to ascertain only a loose relation between the presence of a disease in a family and the presenting condition of a patient under evaluation. As the genetics of common and complex disorders, such as obesity, hypertension, stroke, emphysema, and schizophrenia are dissected and reported, the results of genetic blood-test panels in which the DNA-sequence variants at the loci of interest are treated as risk factors will become available on an overnight basis. These panels should help physicians refine differential diagnoses and provide a scientific basis for the individualization of medical therapy. (p. 57)

This is the promise of the New Genetics. But while we celebrate the completion of the genome, it is important to realize that until we understand the function of the genes, the specific ways in which they alter proteins, alone and in interaction, we will remain limited in what we can alter or "fix," despite our new knowledge of the location of genes. We have perhaps come to, as some have suggested, "the end of the beginning" of this new era of genetic medicine.

THE THERAPEUTIC GAP

Knowing which mutations predispose carriers to illness is not equivalent to being able to treat or cure the resulting disease. This has been referred to as the "therapeutic gap," a wide discrepancy between the achievement of scientific and medical goals (Holtzman & Watson, 1997). Excitement about the scientific advances of the Human Genome Project has led to monumental press coverage, much of it including overly optimistic views of the time needed to translate these scientific advances into practical improvements in medical care or prevention. This reporting unrealistically raises the hopes of individuals suffering from a given disease and of family members at risk for the same condition. Especially when the diseases are ones that carry a high fear burden, such as breast, colon, or prostate cancer, these raised hopes often result in frantic and frustrating searches for information about tests or treatments that are not yet available. Questions arise, often years before they can be answered, about when genetic testing will be available, who will be eligible for it, how much it will cost, where it will be available, and what it can reveal. The anxiety that is raised also resurrects memories of past illness and deaths in these families.

As we consider the experience of members of high-risk families who learn of a possible test that might provide long-awaited answers to questions about the risk of cancer in several generations of family members, we begin to understand the close connection between genetics and psychology. The availability of new, powerful, genetic information, despite the potential it carries for reducing the terrible disease burden the family has borne in the past, is itself a stressor that must be adapted to. Psychological factors govern the use people make of genetic information. If the fruits of the Human Genome Project are to be realized, the individual must be able to incorporate new, relevant genetic information (filtering out nonrelevant information), find doctors and genetic counselors trained to deliver accurate genetic information and to offer recommendations for risk reduction, and be willing to follow those recommendations (Baum, Friedman, & Zakowski, 1997). For the at-risk individual, excitement is mixed with ambivalence and other emotions related to a lifetime of illness and, possibly, loss. Hope is mixed with fear about how genetic information might affect the individual's emotional balance or change family relationships. He or she may well worry that having this new knowledge could lead to the eruption of old issues or new points of contention among relatives, without necessarily resolving the prevailing medical questions.

WHAT GENETIC COUNSELING AND TESTING OFFER—AND WHAT THEY CAN'T PROVIDE

It is usually through genetic counseling that individuals in high-risk families begin to define their risks for disease and their eligibility for genetic testing. Genetic counseling is a "communication process which deals with the human problems associated with the occurrence, or risk of occurrence of a genetic disorder in a family" (Ad Hoc Committee on Genetic Counseling, 1975, p. 240). There is nearly uniform agreement among professionals that genetic testing should be preceded by genetic counseling, so that the potential risks and benefits of the testing for that individual can be discussed and weighed against the individual's motivations and expectations (National Cancer Institute PDQ Cancer Genetics Summary, 2002).

The aims of genetic counseling are to impart information to family members about the medical facts concerning the genetic disease or diseases in question and information about inheritance patterns and risks of carrying the disease. Genetic counselors also inform family members about the options available for dealing with their risk of the disease if they are found to carry a disease-predisposing mutation. They help clients make appropriate choices about genetic testing. They also inform their clients about the potential emotional effects of learning individual genetic risk status and discuss potential family effects. Genetic counselors are trained to recognize signs of unusual emotional distress in their clients and to make appropriate referrals for further psychological assessment or treatment.

Ideally, genetic counseling is carried out over several sessions, so that there is time for discussion of all the areas of importance, time to contemplate the options, and time between sessions to discuss the options with other family members. As testing moves into the arena of the primary care provider, counseling tends to become abbreviated. Chen et al. (2002) reported that on average women being tested for breast cancer genes had 30 minutes of counseling prior to having their blood drawn for testing. This trend raises many questions about the adequacy of the information provided and about the absence of time to consider the individual's motivations, personal beliefs, and misconceptions. At least theoretically, this absence of sufficient time to make careful decisions and to prepare for the impact of receiving genetic information makes it more likely that after receiving results, individuals will experience adverse emotional reactions and become distressed. Some may find their way to a therapist, seeking help for the resolution of the conflicts and anxieties aroused by getting risk information. They may have belatedly realized they did not want or were not prepared to receive the information or may have encountered difficulty in dealing with the information within the context of their family. If individuals affected by such news are already in psychotherapeutic treatment, they are very likely to bring to their therapeutic sessions concerns about the raised hopes and possibilities of genetic information and about the continuing frustration, helplessness, and sense of personal inferiority about the unfair burdens of genetic illness. If not already in treatment, the likelihood that the individual distressed about inherited disease predisposition will see a therapist for these conflicts is considerably greater if his or her genetic counselor has a close connection with a mental health provider and can assist with a referral as soon as the problems are identified. When that is not the case, it can be years before the cause of the upset is clarified and the need for help is acted on. The distress of the tested individual may, in turn, affect the views of other family members about the advisability of being tested or of receiving personalized risk information, with potential health consequences. Chapter 4 deals in more detail with the content of typical genetic counseling sessions and with information about locating appropriately trained genetic counselors. It also discusses the potential value of consultation between mental health providers and genetic counselors, physicians, or nurses offering genetic services.

WHAT PEOPLE WANT TO KNOW FROM GENETIC COUNSELING AND TESTING

When seeking genetic consultation the central question at-risk individuals have is, "Do I carry the gene that caused people in my family to become ill?" Genetic testing can, in some cases, provide an answer to that question. Genetic testing is accomplished through the analysis of a small amount of blood to determine whether the individual carries the mutation associated with the genetic disease in their family. It is most useful when the mutation in the family has already been found in a member of the family who has the disease. When there is a known deleterious mutation in the patient's family, scientists or technicians can search only that section of the gene in which the known mutation is found to see if a similar change or mutation has occurred in the gene of the currently healthy relative. When it is not known whether there is a familial mutation, genetic testing of healthy family members may not give answers that are definitive (see the following sections and chaps. 2 and 3 for further explanation).

The second question most people seeking genetic consultation have is about what their risk is for developing the disease in question if they do carry a predisposing mutation. The concept of *penetrance* is a central one in understanding this question. Penetrance is defined as, "an all-or-none phenomenon that refers to the clinical expression, or lack of it, in the mutant gene" (Gelehrter, Collins, & Ginsburg, 1998, p. 27). Penetrance, in other words, describes the likelihood that carriers of the particular mutation or DNA sequence alteration will actually develop the disease for which they carry a hereditary predisposition. Penetrance is, however, a statistical concept, conveying a probability; it does not convey any information about the likelihood that a particular individual will develop cancer, Parkinson's disease, etc. The latter is, of course, the information that is truly desired—the knowledge in an individual case of whether the person is going to develop the illness and when (i.e., "Will I get cancer if I carry the genetic mutation in my family?"). We discuss, in future chapters, the penetrance of particular genetic mutations related to breast and colon cancer and some other conditions. We also discuss the ways in which variations in the penetrance of genes may change the utility of genetic testing for different people, may alter recommendations for medical treatment or screening and risk-reducing techniques, and may change the emotional climate in families in which these issues are pertinent.

It is often said that genetic testing is valuable because it gets rid of the uncertainty about whether an individual is at risk for a genetic condition that runs in his or her family. However, it would be more accurate to say that genetic testing initiates an "uncertainty trade." In most cases, genetic test results leave some level of uncertainty about either the individual's genetic status or disease risk. (See chap. 2 for the implications for the future of an individual with a detected mutation.) When there is not a known mutation in the family, testing that finds the absence of a mutation in a healthy family member could mean one of two things: (a) the person does not, in fact, have a deleterious mutation or (b) the mutation has simply not been found with the techniques currently available. It is only when there is a known mutation in a family member with the disease, and that same mutation is not found in the blood of another family member who is healthy, that the negative result can be said to be a true negative. In some other cases, where there is not an identified familial mutation and the whole gene is sequenced, mutations or polymorphisms may be found, but their significance in causing or predisposing the individual to disease may be unknown. Such a finding is said to be a polymorphism "of indeterminate significance." Individuals testing truly negative for the cancer-predisposing mutation in their family still face the general population risk for cancer and are advised to continue to follow whatever screening recommendations apply for the average individual. They cannot be assured that they will not get cancer, only that they do not have an increased risk of cancer due to hereditary factors. Individuals testing positive are likely to be at risk for several cancers, although it is also possible that they may never get any cancer. (This window of hope, even if it is only in some cases a 10% likelihood of not getting cancer, is very important to those found to be mutation carriers.) Mutation carriers do not know when the cancer or cancers will occur and how severe they are likely to be. In addition, as genetic knowledge advances, mutations have been found that result in increased predisposition for a number of different cancers. So, advancing knowledge may lead to a lengthening list of risks associated with the genetic mutation carriers are found to have. Thus, in a fair percentage of cases (varying with the quality of the techniques and completeness of the mutation knowledge available), individuals seeking genetic counseling or testing may be frustrated to find that they do not get an answer from their genetic testing that definitively answers all their questions about their hereditary cancer risk.

Andree Lehmann (1997), a French psychoanalyst, offered an interesting description of the role of psychological factors in genetic consultation. She wrote that genetic consultation offers, "new, objective, and scientific knowledge from outside" the person, but that it arouses within the person, "old, subjective, and irrational knowledge" (p. 383) of personal griefs, angers, and confusions about the connections between family and illness. The issues aroused by genetic testing are powerful ones that strike at the core of family and individual identity. Stiefel, Lehmann, and Guex (1977) compared genetic testing and psychoanalysis. Both, they said, are processes that are threatening in their power to give an individual information about themselves. Both deal with and affect our relationships to others, especially family members. In contrast, however, psychoanalysis is a lengthy process whereas genetic testing is relatively quick, with results often available in two to six weeks. Genetic information can be given to an individual, whereas the individual must slowly acquire the awareness that comes from psychoanalysis. There is another person involved in both processes. However, in psychoanalysis, the relationship to the analyst is key and is, itself, a focus of the process. In genetic counseling, the counselor plays a more educational role, although surely the sensitivity of the counselor in presenting genetic information and in inquiring about the reactions and relationships of family members plays an important role in determining the psychological impact of the experience.

Genetic testing represents the translation of scientific findings to a clinical level where individuals can be apprised of whether they carry a particular genetic mutation associated in their family or ethnic group with the development of disease. We discuss in chapter 3 the specifics of how testing is conducted. We consider the potential medical and psychological benefits of testing as well as the stresses and threats to family interrelationships that the introduction of genetic testing may engender in high-risk families.

HOW WILL INCREASING GENETIC KNOWLEDGE CHANGE SOCIETY?

Genetic advances will ultimately influence the diagnosis and treatment of most major diseases. However, changes will come much faster in some areas of medicine than in others. This book focuses on the psychological impact of advances in cancer genetics because this is the area in which genetics is currently having the greatest influence on the diagnosis and treatment of common diseases. Genetic testing is now available for a few forms of cancer, most notably breast and ovarian cancer, colon cancer, and some cancer syndromes. Prostate cancer may be the next area in which the knowledge of inherited predisposition makes genetic testing possible. In this book, I discuss in detail the implications of genetic risk information and test results for patients' cancer risks, their self-esteem, and their family interactions.

The genetics of the 21st century promises not only to affect our health behaviors (medical care and what we individually do to take care of ourselves) but also to change many of our social attitudes and policies. In the last decade of the 20th century, the nature versus nurture controversy has emphasized nurture, aspects of behavior that we control and that are conditioned by experience. New educational tracks were developed for individuals interested in defining a broader concept of health, which included physical, emotional, and spiritual aspects. Health psychology developed as a specialty aimed at helping individuals change their behaviors in ways that are thought to have important implications for stress reduction and disease prevention. Maximal endorsement of a "healthy lifestyle" has been identified as enhancing the likelihood of living a long, disease-free life. Personal responsibility for health has been emphasized, leading, in some cases, to self-blame when cancer or other illness occurred or was not responsive to treatment. Psychology sections of bookstores are packed with self-help volumes. Exercise machines and health club memberships are subsidized by employers or by health insurers. Lean cuisine replaced the meat and potatoes and bacon and eggs recommended as part of the American diet in the prior decades.

Increasing awareness of genetic factors in disease will again alter the balance of how health and disease are perceived. There is some fear that emphasis on genetic factors will lead to feelings of helplessness or futility about the possibility of altering the likelihood of becoming ill. Some people found to be carriers of mutations that carry high risks for disease might abandon efforts to maintain or adopt a healthier lifestyle. Some worry that, on a larger scale, misguided understanding of genetics could lead to reduced appropriation of funding for improvement of the environment or removal of toxic hazards. Others are concerned that people will be held responsible to a greater degree for the conditions such as obesity, cancer, or diabetes that they develop. Might insurers or employers argue that if people can know in advance through genetic analysis what their disease predispositions are and do not heed medical recommendations for risk reduction, that the occurrence of disease is, therefore, self-inflicted and not something they should pay for?

Concern exists also about society's protection of genetic information and the allocation of and access to genetic resources, as well as about possible discrimination on the basis of hereditary risk. There are also, of course, utopian views of the elimination of major diseases, like cancer, through gene therapy or other techniques that could exploit knowledge of genetic factors to cure or prevent illness. It is clear that the New Genetics is a catalyst for change in medicine, in psychology, and in society. This book hopefully brings together much of what is currently known about cancer genetics and about how informing people about their familial and individual risk for cancer affects their lives. Social change is never without its costs, even when the changes ultimately improve people's lives. When people are put in situations requiring adaptation and vulnerability, there is a role for those whose work involves enhancing self-efficacy, helping people evaluate risk, aiding decision making, assessing reaction, reducing stress, encouraging resilience and communication within families, and facilitating adoption of healthy behaviors. The New Genetics provides many opportunities to psychologists and others for such work. Mental health professionals with knowledge of this new and exciting area who wish to rise with the tide will find an array of fascinating challenges ahead.

REFERENCES

Ad Hoc Committee on Genetic Counseling. (1975). Genetic counseling. *American Journal of Human Genetics, 27,* 240–242.

Baum, A., Friedman, A. L., & Zakowski, S. G. (1997). Stress and genetic testing for disease risk. *Health Psychology, 16,* 8–19.

Chen, W., Garber, J. E., Higham, S., Schneider, K., Davis, K., Deffenbaugh, A., et al. (2002). BRCA1/2 genetic testing in the community setting: A study of 646 women. *Journal of Clinical Oncology, 20,* 4485–4492.

Drazen, J. M. (2000). Looking forward to serving you every week. *New England Journal of Medicine, 343,* 57–58.

Gelehrter, T. D., Collins, F. S., & Ginsburg, D. (1998). *Principles of medical genetics* (2nd ed.). Hagerstown, MD: Lippincott Williams & Wilkins.

Guttmacher, A. E., & Collins, F. S. (2002). Genomic medicine—a primer. *New England Journal of Medicine, 347,* 1512–1520.

Holtzman, N. A., & Watson, M. S. (Eds.). (1997, September). *Promoting safe and effective genetic testing in the United States. Final Report of the Task Force on Genetic Testing.* Bethesda, MD: National Human Genome Research Institute.

International Human Genome Sequencing Consortium. (2001). Initial sequencing and analysis of the human genome. *Nature, 409,* 860–921.

Lehmann, A. (1997). Aspects psychologiques du conseil genetique [Psychological aspects of genetic counseling]. In J.-Y. Bignon (Eds.), *Oncogenetique: Vers une medecine de presumption/prediction* (pp. 383–395). Cachan, France: Lavoisier.

Mansoura, M. K., & Collins, F. S. (1998). Medical implications of the genetic revolution. *Journal of Health Care, Law, and Policy, 1,* 329–352.

National Cancer Institute Physician Data Query. (2002). *Elements of cancer genetics risk assessment and counseling.* Retrieved March 16, 2002, from http://cancer.gov/cancerinfo/pdq/genetics/risk-assessment-and-counseling

Offit, K. (1998). *Clinical cancer genetics: Risk counseling and management.* New York: Wiley-Liss.

Stiefel, F., Lehmann, A., & Guex, P. (1997). Genetic detection: The need for psychosocial support in modern cancer prevention. *Supportive Care in Cancer, 5,* 461–465.

Varmus, H. (2002). Getting ready for gene-based medicine. *New England Journal of Medicine, 347,* 1526–1527.

1

GENES AND CANCER:
THE BASICS

Understanding patients' concerns about inherited cancer risk, recognizing overestimation of risk, and identifying unnecessary or premature worries can be crucial to providing psychological help to patients with family histories of hereditary cancer or positive genetic test results. Many health professionals, including physicians, would benefit from a review of basic genetics and updates on recent advances (Korf, 2000). Continuing education courses and training programs are being developed to give primary care physicians, nurses, and other specialists the genetic knowledge to serve their current and future patients effectively. The National Human Genome Research Institute (NHGRI) has an online glossary of genetic terms (http://www.genome.gov/page.cfm?pageID=10002096), as do many other sites (see the Additional Resources included at the end of this book).

This chapter first reviews the statistics of cancer incidence and mortality to help the reader focus on the societal impact of cancer and, thus, the importance of changes in cancer diagnosis or treatment related to genetics. We then discuss basic genetic concepts central to understanding the likely medical consequences of an inherited mutation in that gene. Finally, we offer a description of hereditary predispositions conveyed by the currently identified cancer genes.

CANCER: AN OVERVIEW

This book is about the psychological issues that commonly arise in families with hereditary cancer predispositions and the psychological and ethical concerns individuals confront when undergoing genetic counseling or testing. I offer a brief discussion about cancer generally to place our discussion about hereditary cancer and its psychological implications in the context of the larger disease.

Despite progress in cancer diagnosis and treatment, one in four deaths in the United States is due to cancer (Jemal et al., 2004). American women have about a one in three (38%) lifetime probability of developing some form of cancer, and American men have about a one in two (45%) lifetime cancer risk (Jemal et al., 2004). Figure 1.1 (top) shows the distributions of cancers for both men and women. Cancer can be considered a disease of aging because most cancers occur after age 60. One factor that first brought attention to hereditary forms of cancer was the fact that these cancers tend to occur at a much earlier age (during the 30s and 40s, or even younger) than sporadic (i.e., nonhereditary) cancers.

More than half a million Americans die of cancer annually (Jemal et al., 2004). Slightly more than half of these deaths result from four cancers: for men, lung and bronchus, colorectal, and prostate cancers; for women, lung and bronchus, breast, and colorectal cancers. Figure 1.1 (bottom) shows the distribution of U.S. cancer deaths for men and women. Although there have been reductions in death rates among men for lung and prostate cancer and for women in breast cancer (see Figure 1.2) since the mid-1990s, the absolute number of deaths from cancer has increased because of the aging of the U.S. population. There are also variations in incidence and death rates by race. In African Americans, cancer is more often diagnosed at later stages and is more likely to be fatal than similar cancers diagnosed in Caucasians (Jemal et al., 2004).

Cancer is not a single disease, but a family of many diseases, jointly characterized by unregulated cell growth that ultimately interferes with bodily function and is potentially fatal, if unchecked. Scientists are learning more and more about the differences between various types of cancer and also about the differentiation between tumors of the same cancer type that have different characteristics, such as HER-2 positive and negative breast cancer (Bilous et al., 2003). These forms of cancer may behave very differently and thus require different treatments and carry different prognoses. On the other hand, researchers are also finding unexpected links between various cancers. Through the study of inherited cancer predispositions, etiological connections between cancers, such as breast and ovarian cancer or between colon and endometrial (lining of the uterus) cancer, have been found. These links may provide important clues to the basic defects that

Estimated New Cases

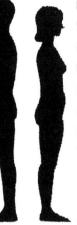

Prostate (33%)	Breast (32%)
Lung and Bronchus (14%)	Lung and Bronchus (12%)
Colon and Rectum (11%)	Colon and Rectum (11%)
Urinary Bladder (6%)	Uterine Corpus (6%)
Melanoma of the Skin (4%)	Ovary (4%)
Non-Hodgkin Lymohoma (4%)	Non-Hodgkin Lymphoma (4%)
Kidney (3%)	Melanoma of the Skin (3%)
Oral Cavity (3%)	Thyroid (3%)
Leukemia (3%)	Pancreas (2%)
Pancreas (2%)	Urinary Bladder (2%)
All Other Sites (17%)	All Other Sites (20%)

Estimated Deaths

Lung and Bronchus (31%)	Lung and Bronchus (25%)
Prostate (10%)	Breast (15%)
Colon and Rectum (10%)	Colon and Rectum (11%)
Pancreas (5%)	Pancreas (6%)
Non-Hodgkin Lymphoma (4%)	Ovary (5%)
Leukemia (4%)	Non-Hodgkin Lymphoma (4%)
Esophagus (4%)	Leukemia (4%)
Liver (3%)	Uterine Corpus (3%)
Urinary Bladder (3%)	Brain (2%)
Kidney (3%)	Multiple Myeloma (2%)
All Other Sites (22%)	All Other Sites (23%)

Figure 1.1. (top) Estimated new cases of cancer in the United States, 2003; (bottom) Estimated deaths from cancer in the United States, 2003. From "Cancer Statistics, 2003," by A. Jemal, T. Murray, A. Samuels, A. Ghafoor, E. Ward, and M. J. Thun, 2003, *CA: Cancer, A Journal for Clinicians, 53,* p. 9. Copyright 2003 by Lippincott Williams & Wilkins. Reprinted with permission.

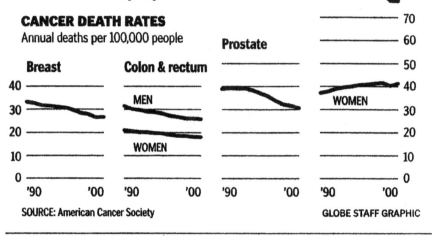

Downward trends

Treatment and screening advances have caused a decade-long drop in the number of Americans killed by the "big four" cancers that cause the majority of US cancer deaths.

CANCER DEATH RATES
Annual deaths per 100,000 people

Breast

Colon & rectum

Prostate

Lung & bronchus

SOURCE: American Cancer Society

GLOBE STAFF GRAPHIC

Figure 1.2. Decline in cancer deaths from 1990–2000. From "Advances Begin to Tame Cancer," by R. Mishra, July 6, 2003, *Boston Globe.* Copyright 2003 by Globe Newspaper Co. Reprinted with permission.

initiate a cascade of cancerous events. This information may be of use not only in understanding and treating individuals from families already heavily affected by cancer but also for those who develop cancer without a significant family history. This is one of the reasons the study of hereditary cancers is considered so important, despite the little-recognized fact that only about 5% to 10% of cancers are due to inherited mutations.

Major research efforts are directed at trying to ascertain who is at increased risk for various cancers. This question is important because knowledge of those more likely to develop cancer can inform questions about its etiology. More immediately, knowledge of the factors that increase cancer risk is useful to determine which screening practices should be recommended to whom and for evaluating whether those at increased risk benefit from more intensive screening. In fact, there are only a few clearly established acquired risk factors for most cancers. Acquired risks either occur in the environment of the individual, such as radiation, or are related to life history and lifestyle, such as one's weight or the age at which a woman has her first live birth. Tables 1.1, 1.2, and 1.3 list known or suspected acquired risks for breast, colon, and ovarian cancer. This is a challenging and changing

TABLE 1.1
Known and Suspected Risk Factors for Breast Cancer

Age >40 years
Alcohol intake (>3 drinks per week)
Benign breast disease (atypical hyperplasia)
Delayed childbearing (>30 years at 1st birth)
Early menarche (<14 years)
Estrogen replacement therapy
Family history of breast or ovarian cancer
Female gender
Hormone use (estrogen replacement therapy)
Nulliparity (no biological children)
Late menopause (>55 years)
Obesity
Previous malignant disease
Proliferative breast disease
Radiation to breasts

Note. From *Counseling About Cancer: Strategies for Genetic Counseling* (p. 15), by K. Schneider, 2002, New York: Wiley-Liss. Copyright 2002 by Wiley-Liss, a subsidiary of John Wiley & Sons. Reprinted with permission.

TABLE 1.2
Known and Suspected Risk Factors for Colon Cancer

Age >50
Alcohol
Cigarettes
Colorectal polyps (adenomatous polyps)
Chronic disease of the bowel (Crohn's disease, inflammatory bowel disease, ulcerative colitis)
Family history of colon or other related cancers
High fat intake (>40% total intake)
High red meat intake
Low fiber intake
Obesity
Radiation to pelvic area
Ulcerative colitis

Note. From *Counseling About Cancer: Strategies for Genetic Counseling* (p. 15), by K. Schneider, 2002, New York: Wiley-Liss. Copyright 2002 by Wiley-Liss, a subsidiary of John Wiley & Sons. Reprinted with permission.

body of knowledge and an area in which some seemingly counterintuitive findings can sometimes arise, such as the finding that *BRCA1* carriers who were smokers were somewhat less likely to develop breast cancer (Brunet et al., 1998). There is certainly much ongoing research, including that now being carried out in the fields of complementary and alternative medicine, to try to discover which individual or environmental factors cause or impede cancer development. We are still early in the process of understanding

TABLE 1.3
Known and Suspected Risk Factors for Ovarian Cancer

Daily talcum powder use (due to asbestos particles)
Delayed childbearing
Family history of ovarian, breast, or colon cancer
High lactose intake (dietary galactose)
Infertility
Nulliparity/low parity

Note. From *Counseling About Cancer: Strategies for Genetic Counseling* (p. 16), by K. Schneider, 2002, New York: Wiley-Liss. Copyright 2002 by Wiley-Liss, a subsidiary of John Wiley & Sons. Reprinted with permission.

the mechanisms by which associations between personal characteristics or environmental exposures lead to the development of cancers, however.

The identification of risk levels is tied to recommendations for cancer screening, with those individuals thought to be at increased risk being given recommendations for earlier, different, or more intensive screening. The American Cancer Society publishes screening recommendations for many types of cancer (Smith, Cokkinides, & Eyre, 2003), and the National Cancer

TABLE 1.4
American Cancer Society Recommendations for the Early Detection of Cancer in Average-Risk, Asymptomatic People

Cancer Site	Population	Test or Procedure	Frequency
Breast	Women, age 20+	Breast Self-examination Clinical breast examination	Monthly, starting at age 20 Every 3 years, ages 20–39 Annual, starting at age 40[a]
		Mammography	Annual, starting at age 40
Colorectal	Men and women, age 50+	Fecal occult blood test (FOBT)[b] *or*	Annual, starting at age 50
		Flexible sigmoidoscopy	Every 5 years, starting at age 50
		or Fecal occult blood test (FOBT)[b] and flexible sigmoidoscopy[c]	Annual FOBT and flexible sigmoidoscopy every 5 years, starting at age 50
		or Double contrast barium enema (DCBE)	DCBE every 5 years, starting at age 50
		or Colonoscopy	Colonoscopy every 10 years, starting at age 50
Prostate	Men, age 50+	Digital rectal examination (DRE) and prostate specific antigen test (PSA)	The PSA test and the DRE should be offered annually, starting at age 50, for men who have a life expectancy of at least 10 years[d]

(continued)

TABLE 1.4
American Cancer Society Recommendations for the Early Detection of Cancer in Average-Risk, Asymptomatic People *(Continued)*

Cancer Site	Population	Test or Procedure	Frequency
Cervix	Women	Pap test	Cervical cancer screening should begin approximately 3 years after a woman begins having vaginal intercourse, but no later than 21 years of age. Screening should be done every year with conventional Pap tests or every 2 years using liquid-based Pap tests. At or after age 30, women who have had 3 normal test results in a row may get screened every 2 to 3 years. Women 70 years of age and older who have had 3 or more normal Pap tests and no abnormal Pap tests in the last 10 years, and women who have had a total hysterectomy, may choose to stop cervical cancer screening.
Cancer-related checkup	Men and women, age 20+		On the occasion of a periodic health examination, the cancer-related checkup should include examination for cancers of the thyroid, testicles, ovaries, lymph nodes, oral cavity, and skin, as well as health counseling about tobacco, sun exposure, diet and nutrition, risk factors, sexual practices, and environmental and occupational exposures.

Note. From "American Cancer Society Guidelines for the Early Detection of Cancer, 2003," by R. Smith, V. Cokkinides, and H. J. Eyre, 2003, *CA: Cancer, a Journal for Clinicians, 53*, p. 29. Copyright 2003 by Lippincott Williams & Wilkins. Reprinted with permission.
[a]Beginning at age 40, annual clinical breast examination should be performed prior to mammography.
[b]FOBT as it is sometimes done in physicians' offices, with the single stool sample collected on the fingertip during a digital rectal examination, is not an adequate substitute for the recommended at-home procedure of collecting two samples from three consecutive specimens. Toilet bowl FOBT tests also are not recommended. In comparison with guaiac-based tests for the detection of occult blood, immunochemical tests are more patient-friendly and are likely to be equal or better in sensitivity and specificity. There is no justification for repeating FOBT in response to an initial positive finding.
[c]Flexible sigmoidoscopy together with FOBT is preferred compared with FOBT or flexible sigmoidoscopy alone.
[d]Information should be provided to men about the benefits and limitations of testing so that an informed decision about testing can be made with the clinician's assistance.

Institute Screening Board follows and interprets the research on screening efficacy (http://cancer.gov/cancerinfo/screening) for health professionals, patients, and the general public. Table 1.4 shows current recommendations from the American Cancer Society for average-risk, healthy individuals.

The shifting sands of scientific knowledge about cancer prevention make it difficult for men and women who are trying to take steps to minimize their cancer risks. This has recently been apparent in the about-face of medical recommendations on hormone replacement therapy for women in the general population on the basis of new data showing increased breast cancer risk and fewer cardiovascular benefits than previously thought (Weiss et al., 2002). Even without definitive evidence of links between risk factors and cancer etiology, however, many people develop personal strategies to try to maximize their sense that they are doing whatever possible to prevent cancer. This may include optimizing lifestyle factors through weight reduction, smoking cessation, or exercise and complying with screening recommendations. Others find compliance with recommended screening schedules or lifestyle recommendations difficult or impossible. Health psychologists have important roles in aiding individuals to set realistic expectations and to overcome barriers to "healthier" living.

A flip side of the emphasis on self-assessment and personal health responsibility, however, is the self-blame that some cancer patients experience following a diagnosis. These patients retrospectively feel that their failure to "eat right" or exercise sufficiently has led to their getting cancer, often ignoring the fact that the links between risk factors and cancer etiology remain largely unproven, with the exception of the role of smoking in causing approximately 30% of all lung cancer (Schneider, 2002). Indeed, some patients are so guilty about what they conceive of as their own contribution to developing cancer that they express relief when informed that they are carriers of a hereditary, cancer-predisposing mutation because they may then attribute their cancer to heredity, which they feel is not their "fault."

Heredity is a risk factor that is not acquired, that is, hereditary risk is inborn. Hereditary risks are said to be present in the "germline," in the genetic makeup with which one is born. Almost everyone who has a relative with cancer worries whether that cancer is an indication of an inherited predisposition that could place them at increased risk as well. Internists routinely inquire about family history, often with a special emphasis on cancer, which furthers the notion that much of cancer is hereditary. In addition, the genetic aspects of cancer, especially genetic testing for breast and colon cancer, have received much media attention. In fact, close relatives of those with cancer often face somewhat increased risks for the same cancer, although the relative risks are not typically large, except in cases in which there is a Mendelian mutation present in the family. (I consider these cases in chap. 2.)

Considerable confusion exists among the general population and even among many health professionals about the extent of the role hereditary factors play in cancer. The extensive media coverage on genetics has led many to conclude that heredity must be a common cause of cancer when, in fact, heredity accounts for only 5% to 10% of most cancers. Some additional cancers occur in a pattern that appears to be "familial," that is, the cancers occur in a family more often than expected, but not in a pattern consistent with Mendelian inheritance.

Overestimation of cancer risk, especially breast cancer risk, is common among both those who do and those who do not have hereditary or familial risks (Iglehart et al., 1998; Offit, 1998). Many women, for example, are not

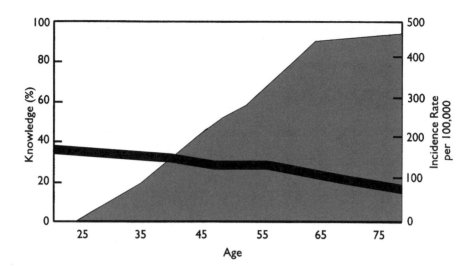

Figure 1.3. Breast cancer rates and age of onset. The incidence of breast cancer increases steadily with age (shaded area) from about 100 cases per 100,000 at age 35 to about 500 cases per 100,000 by age 75. Knowledge of the association of breast cancer risk with age (dark line) decreases by 35% of those surveyed around age 30 to 16% by age 75. From *Clinical Cancer Genetics* (p. 68.), by K. Offit, 1998, New York: Wiley-Liss. Copyright 1998 by Wiley-Liss, a subsidiary of John Wiley & Sons. Reprinted with permission.

fully aware that age is the most important risk factor for breast cancer, and they begin to worry about developing breast cancer decades before they turn 60, the age at which the rates increase sharply. (See Figure 1.3 for age-related breast cancer risks and data on age-related risk.) Although heightened risk perception may serve the useful function of providing motivation for recommended screening, such as mammography or colonoscopies when age standards dictate that it is appropriate, it may also cause extreme distress or even cancer phobia. Some women, for example, have gone as far as having their breasts removed prophylactically in the absence of significant family history of breast cancer because surgery was the only way, they believed, to tame their constant worry about developing breast cancer.

For those who are at increased hereditary risk because of an inherited mutation in a known cancer susceptibility gene, it is especially difficult to know how important other risk factors are for cancer prevention. Scientific controversy about the role of risk factors for cancer etiology remains among the general population, but there is even less known about how or whether these risk factors play a role in the initiation of cancers when a hereditary susceptibility is present. There are recommendations about the nature and timing of screening procedures for those at increased hereditary risk (Burke et al., 1997), but most of these are based on expert opinion because there is, as yet, no proof of the efficacy of most of these practices in reducing cancer incidence or mortality in this population. Welch and Burke (1998) caution that clinicians must moderate their advice to patients who are concerned about hereditary predisposition to illness, given the tendency to overestimate disease risk and the unproven benefit of surveillance strategies.

In summary, although there is much progress in cancer diagnosis and treatment, it remains a deadly disease. Studies of the 5% to 10% of patients whose cancer is clearly caused by inherited mutations will likely aid future progress toward cancer cures and prevention, albeit more slowly and with more clinical dilemmas for patients and health professionals along the way than might be hoped.

BASIC GENETIC CONCEPTS

The goal of educating mental health professionals about genetics is not to give them the level of understanding and training to make them first-line providers of genetic counseling. (A few psychologists have gone through training to become genetic counselors, but most do not want or need this level of genetics preparation.) Instead, the goal is to understand enough about patients' concerns to help patients with their worries, their decisions, and their family communication and concerns that are centrally or peripherally related to cancer genes or other hereditary predispositions. To determine whether referral to a genetic counselor or geneticist is warranted may require a basic appreciation of what information patients need to make relevant decisions and how a genetic counselor goes about trying to answer those questions.

Many people have global ideas about genetics but might have trouble actually defining basic terms. Following are definitions of important, basic genetics terms.

What Is DNA?

Deoxyribonucleic acid (DNA) is the chemical inside the nucleus of a cell that carries the genetic instructions. The DNA is arranged in the double helix formation, looking like a twisted ladder (see Figure 1.4). Watson and Crick's contribution was to identify that DNA has the structure of a double helix, which can explain how genetic material is carried and reproduced. DNA is composed of a sugar molecule, a phosphate molecule, and the nucleotide bases that form the rungs of the ladder. These nucleic acid bases are the chemicals adenine, thymine, guanine, and cytosine, which are symbolized by the letters A, T, G, and C. In base pairing, adenine always pairs with thymine, and guanine always pairs with cytosine. Two bases form

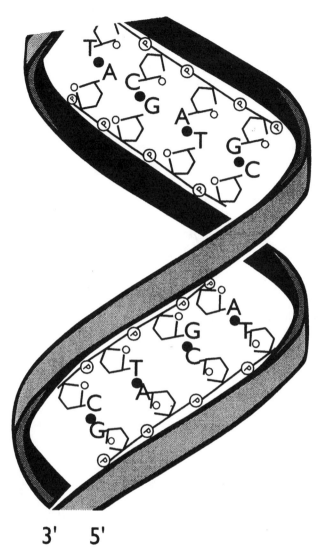

3'   5'

Figure 1.4. Structure of DNA. The DNA molecule is composed of two nucleotide chains arranged in a double helix. The double helix is held together by hydrogen bonds between complementary bases A–T and G–C. The bases at the center are attached to the backbone of the molecule, consisting of sugar and phosphate molecules. From *Clinical Cancer Genetics* (p. 41), by K. Offit, 1998, New York: Wiley-Liss. Copyright 1998 by Wiley-Liss, a subsidiary of John Wiley & Sons. Reprinted with permission.

a "rung of the DNA." The order of the nucleic bases, symbolized by the letters A, T, G, and C, is the genetic code. A change in even one letter (i.e., one chemical) can make changes in the proteins, which cause the person to develop cancer or other serious conditions.

What Is a Gene?

A gene is the basic unit of heredity. It is passed from parent to child. It is composed of DNA. Codes in the DNA control the making of specific proteins, which is how the physical changes controlled by genetic factors come into being. Some characteristics, like eye color, are controlled by one gene. Others are due to interactions between genes or interactions between genes and environmental factors. It is now believed that there are about 30,000 to 35,000 genes in the human genome, the total set of human genes (International Human Genome Sequencing Consortium, 2001). The Human Genome Project has now completed both the physical mapping of the location of the genes and the sequencing or decoding of all of the genes in the human genome. This will be of use in beginning to understand how genes work to cause or to prevent disease. To do genetic testing and look for disease-predisposing mutations, one must know the exact sequence of the gene. Figure 1.5 illustrates the different levels of description of a gene and its sequence.

There are three major kinds of cancer-causing genes that are important in clinical medicine. These are the oncogenes, the tumor suppressor genes, and the DNA-repair genes. (Cavenee & White, 1995). Oncogenes are genes

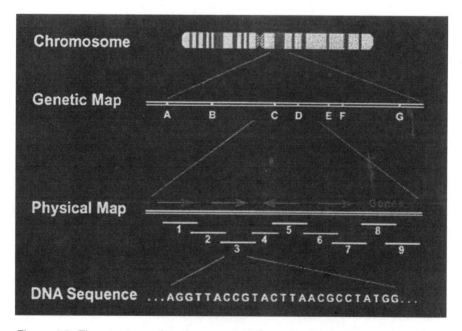

Figure 1.5. The structure of a chromosome. From the National Human Genome Research Institute: http://history.nih.gov/exhibits/genetics/sect5.htm

TABLE 1.5
Three Classes of Cancer Predisposition Genes

Gene	Syndrome
Tumor suppressor genes associated with cancer predisposition	
APC	Familial adenomatous polyposis
VHL	von Hippel–Lindau syndrome
WT1	Wilms's tumor syndromes
RB1	Hereditary retinoblastoma
NF1	Neurofibromatosis 1
NF2	Neurofibromatosis 2
p53	Li–Fraumeni syndrome
p16/CDK4	Hereditary melanoma syndromes
PTCH	Nevoid basal cell carcinoma syndrome
MEN1	Multiple endocrine neoplasia 1
BRCA1	Breast ovarian cancer syndrome
BRCA2	Breast ovarian cancer syndrome
DNA damage response genes associated with cancer predisposition	
hMSH2	Hereditary nonpolyposis colon cancer
hMLH1	Hereditary nonpolyposis colon cancer
hPMS1	Hereditary nonpolyposis colon cancer
hPMS2	Hereditary nonpolyposis colon cancer
ATM	Ataxia telangiectasia
XPA,C,D,F	Xeroderma pigmentosum
BLM	Bloom syndrome
Oncogenes associated with cancer predisposition	
RET	Multiple endocrine neoplasia 2, familial medullary thyroid cancer
MET	Familial papillary renal carcinoma syndrome

Note. From *Clinical Cancer Genetics* (p. 68), by K. Offit, 1998, New York: Wiley-Liss. Copyright 1998 by Wiley-Liss, a subsidiary of John Wiley & Sons. Reprinted with permission.

whose usual functions are related to normal growth and development but that cause cancer when they become mutated or otherwise overactive. Tumor suppressor genes normally regulate cell growth but cause cancer if they are inactivated. Mismatch-repair genes normally fix problems in the DNA but can cause cancer, like the tumor suppressor genes, if they become inactivated (Offit, 1998). Table 1.5 gives examples of the classification of major cancer predisposition genes.

What Is a Chromosome?

Chromosomes are the "packages" of genes that are found in the nucleus of a cell. We have 23 pairs of chromosomes, for a total of 46. Chromosome pairs 1 through 22 are numbered to identify them. The 23rd pair of chromosomes is the sex chromosomes, one X and one Y in a male and two Xs in

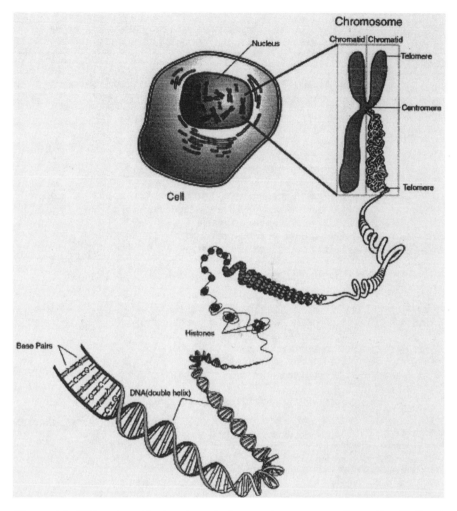

Figure 1.6. Different methods of analyzing a chromosome. From the National Institutes of Health: http://www.genome.gov/Pages/Hyperion//DIR/VIP/Glossary/Illustration/chromosome.shtml

a female. Each chromosome is said to have two arms. One, which is usually the shorter, is referred to as *p* as in *petit* and is the arm above the centromere, the central structure of the chromosome. The other, usually the long arm, is referred to as *q* (only because it is the next letter in the alphabet) and is the arm below the centromere (see Figure 1.6). Disease genes are identified by their location. *BRCA1*, for example is located at 17q21. *BRCA1* is on the long arm of the 17th chromosome at the 21st band (a structural marking) in the chromosome. *BRCA2* is at 13q12 (i.e., on chromosome 13, on the long arm, at the 12th band).

Before genes are found, their presence or absence can be approximated by a process called *linkage*. Linkage uses the fact that the unidentified gene is known to be near a known gene or marker on a particular chromosome. By looking for the known gene, a numerical estimate can be derived about the likelihood that the individual does or does not also have a mutation in the disease gene in question. Determining the risk of carrying a deleterious mutation by linkage is less accurate than results achieved by genetic testing.

What Is a Mutation?

Mutations are alterations in the structure of the DNA composing a gene. Some mutations make no appreciable difference. But other changes in the DNA cause deleterious disruptions in the way the gene codes the protein (or proteins) it makes, resulting in disease.

We have learned a great deal about the various types of mutations or variants that exist (Guttmacher & Collins, 2002) and about how at least some of them relate to disease etiology. Missense mutations, nonsense mutations (stop codon), and frame-shift mutations are all forms of what is known as point mutations. These are changes in a single DNA base in a sequence, and they explain the mechanism by which changes in the gene occur. Figure 1.7 illustrates by analogy the sorts of disruptive changes that different kinds of point mutations make in the structure of a gene.

It is also possible to look at the product of those changed sequences and categorize mutations by what impact they have. Some are "silent," that is, they have little effect on the phenotype, the way the organism appears or "works," because the resulting sequence still codes for the same or a similar amino acid. Some mutations actually decrease the disease risk of the person who carries them, as in a mutation in a gene referred to as CCR5, which conveys resistance to HIV infections (Guttmacher & Collins, 2002). The mutations with which we are most frequently concerned, however, are those that do cause disease through either a loss of function that alters the functional activity of a protein or a gain in function that causes the protein to take on a toxic function.

The names given to mutations are a function of the nature of the mutation and its location. For example, one of the three mutations of *BRCA1* that are common to the Ashkenazi Jewish population is the 187delAG mutation. This means that the mutation is found at the 187th nucleotide where a deletion (hence, "del") of adenine (A) and guanine (G) occurs. If there is an insertion of extra nucleotides, the term "ins" would replace the "del" term, as in mutation 926ins11.

Germline mutations are those that are inherited, that is, that are carried with the genetic material one inherits from one's parents. Hereditary cancers are caused by germline mutations. Mutations can occur after conception that are not inherited, but "sporadic." Mutations of this sort are implicated in cancers that are not hereditary.

How Can the Message Go Wrong?

There are several ways the genetic code can be altered. Sometimes <u>genes</u> are deleted or in the wrong place on a <u>chromosome,</u> or pieces of genes are swapped between chromosomes. As a result, the gene may not work or may turn on in the wrong part of the body.

"Point mutations" alter the genetic code by changing the letters in the <u>codons</u> -- the three-symbol genetic words that specify which <u>protein</u> to make. This can change the protein.

Original message: SAM AND TOM ATE THE HAM

What it does	Kind of point mutation	Example of altered protein
Frameshift mutation	Message starts in the wrong place	AMA NDT OMA TET HEH AMS
Stop codon	Prevents part of the protein from being made	SAM AND TOM
Missense mutation	Causes an amino acid substitution	SAM AND TOM ATE THE DAM
mRNA splicing mutation	Portion of message is left out, leading to a shortened protein	SAM THE HAM

Figure 1.7. Examples of different kinds of errors that can occur in the genetic code because of mutations. From the National Institutes of Health: http://history.nih.gov/exhibits/genetics/sect1a.htm

CHARACTERISTICS OF GENES

It is important to know whether a cancer gene is autosomal dominant or autosomal recessive and to know the penetrance of the gene.

Dominant or Recessive?

The terms "dominant" and "recessive" refer to the patterns of inheritance by which characteristics of individuals are passed on to succeeding generations. When a gene is recessive, both parents must pass on a characteristic or predisposition to their child for the child to express it. When only one parent must pass on a gene for the child to have the characteristic or predisposition expressed, the gene is described as autosomal dominant.

Recessive conditions are more difficult to recognize; the disease may not appear in subsequent generations, may seem to skip generations, or may seem to appear spontaneously because carriers do not show any signs of the condition. There may be many generations in which no person inherits two recessive genes, one from each parent. When a disease caused by a recessive gene does occur, however, it means that both parents of that individual carry at least one of the altered genes. This raises the likelihood that several siblings in the same generation may inherit two mutated genes and develop the disease. Such a circumstance is often referred to as horizontal transmission, meaning transmission to several members of the same generation. When a condition is dominant, it is more visible because anyone inheriting even one mutated allele inherits at least a predisposition to the condition (alleles are alternate forms of the same gene; one allele is inherited from each parent for each gene in the genome). It is more typical to see conditions caused by dominant genes in multiple generations of the same family. This is sometimes referred to as vertical transmission, that is, occurring through consecutive generations of a family.

Most of the common cancer predisposition genes are autosomal dominant. If one parent carries the mutation that conveys predisposition to cancer in their family, then each of the children has a 50% chance of inheriting the dominant mutation. Inheriting this mutation in a dominant cancer-predisposition gene means that the child has an increased lifetime risk of developing cancer and that each of his or her children will also have a 50% chance of inheriting the mutation. The 50% risk of passing on the deleterious mutation is independent, meaning that in each pregnancy the chances are still 50–50 that the child will inherit the mutation. Whether previous children inherited the mutation or not has no bearing on whether a specific child inherits it, a concept that is frequently misunderstood. When siblings undergo cancer genetic testing, they often think that if one of them has the mutation, this lowers the chance that the other sibling will have it (or vice versa). In fact, the risk is identical for each sibling, and the odds one will have it are not at all influenced by whether the brother or sister has the mutation.

If a gene is recessive, inheriting just one mutated allele from a parent does not usually affect the individual because he or she will also have inherited one normal allele from the other parent. That normal allele will predominate and determine the expression of the characteristic or predisposition governed by that gene. If two parents each carry one recessive allele and one normal allele, then their child has a 25% chance of inheriting the altered characteristic or predisposition. Cystic fibrosis is an example of a disease that is caused by a recessive gene. Recessive genes can result in patterns in which the disease or other phenotype appear to "skip" generations. This is because members of the "skipped" generation were heterozygotes, that is, they inherited one normal allele and one recessive, disease-predisposing allele. Thus, they will not develop the disease but will be carriers of the deleterious mutation.

Penetrance

Penetrance refers to the likelihood that carrying a mutation in a particular gene will result in the development of the characteristic or disease that the gene governs. A penetrance of 100% in a disease gene means that everyone who carries that mutation will develop the condition with which it is associated. This is the case, for example, with Huntington's disease, a progressive, neurological, genetic disease caused by mutations in a single gene, the *HD* gene. Everyone who inherits a mutation in his or her *HD* gene develops Huntington's disease. Thus, for people to learn through genetic testing that they carry the *HD* mutation is equivalent to having a crystal ball that tells them with certainty that they will get Huntington's disease if they live long enough. (Disease onset is typically in the 40s). Given that there are no current treatments or preventive measures that can be taken in the face of certain knowledge that one will develop Huntington's disease, about 90% of the individuals at risk for Huntington's disease have chosen not to undergo genetic testing (Harper, Lim, Craufurd, & the UK Huntington's Disease Prediction Consortium, 2000).

Anything less than 100% penetrance is referred to as incomplete penetrance. A penetrance of, say, 85% for a cancer predisposition gene indicates that not everyone who inherits the mutation develops the disease; about 15% of mutation carriers will never develop cancer. This makes the psychological set for these mutation carriers and at-risk individuals considerably different from that of individuals at risk for Huntington's disease. Although 85% is a high lifetime risk of getting cancer, at least for those whose personalities tend toward optimism, the door remains open that they will be among the fortunate 15% who do not develop cancer despite their mutation status. Increasingly successful cancer treatments and the possibility of preventive or risk-reducing options may further reduce fears about finding out one's positive mutation status through genetic testing.

Penetrance estimates may also be the basis for deciding which steps to take to reduce the risk of cancer and how far a provider should go to disseminate cancer risk information through a patient's family. The penetrance of an inherited, cancer-predisposing mutation also affects the degree of emotional distress that the mutation carrier may experience. It is different to have the population risk of 1 in 9 (or 11%) risk of breast cancer versus an 85% risk associated with some cancer predisposition genes. Not only the woman, but also her physicians may view her options very differently depending on the penetrance of the cancer predisposition gene for which she carries a mutation. Surgeons are not likely to perform prophylactic mastectomies (removal of healthy breasts) on a 35-year-old woman with standard risk of breast cancer or colectomies (colon removal) on a teenage boy with an average risk of colon cancer. Patients with general population cancer risk requesting such services might well be referred for psychological services. Most breast oncology surgeons would at least suggest consideration of prophylactic mastectomy to a 35-year-old woman with a familial *BRCA1* mutation, however, and would strongly recommend colon removal for a young man with familial adenomatous polyposis (FAP), a hereditary colon cancer (see chap. 2, this volume). The penetrance of these genes suggests high likelihood that the individual will develop cancer at an unusually early age, making risk-reducing surgery an important option to consider.

A number of factors should be taken into consideration by people who carry a cancer-predisposing mutation and are trying to determine whether they will get cancer and when it might occur. First, at least for some genes, penetrance rates vary according to the group in which they are measured. For example, *BRCA1* was first studied in very high-risk breast–ovarian cancer families, defined as families with four or more first-degree relatives who had breast or ovarian cancer. In those families, the penetrance of the *BRCA1* mutation in causing breast cancer was found to be 85% (Ford, Easton, Bishop, Narod, & Goldgar, 1994). A few years later, the penetrance of *BRCA1* was studied in a group of Ashkenazi Jewish women. Particular genetic mutations in *BRCA1* were found much more commonly in that group than in the general population. The penetrance for breast cancer among these Ashkenazi Jewish *BRCA1* carriers was 56% (Struewing et al., 1997), however, not the 85% found earlier in the more diverse high-risk group. The penetrance of *BRCA1* in causing breast cancer is thus usually given as a range, 56% to 85%. The penetrance figure that is most relevant to an individual depends on how closely their family approximates the group in which the gene penetrance was measured. So a genetics professional working with an Ashkenazi Jewish woman without a striking family history might conclude that her risk is more likely 56% of getting breast cancer in her lifetime. It is not always clear which is the most relevant penetrance estimate, but a genetics professional can help a concerned individual evaluate her family history in light of the increasing knowledge about penetrance in various groups of differing ethnicity or other factors.

*   *   *

Case Example. A 70-year-old Ashkenazi Jewish man from a very high risk breast-ovarian family was found upon genetic testing to be positive for a *BRCA1* mutation known to be associated with high rates of breast cancer among his female relatives. He was advised that his result meant that his married daughter was at 50% risk to have inherited this mutation from him and that, if she had the mutation, she had about an 85% lifetime risk of developing breast cancer. She was tested shortly thereafter and found to also be mutation positive. Given that she had young children and was quite frightened of breast cancer, she chose to have prophylactic mastectomies, given the high likelihood that she would develop breast cancer. Some months after her surgery, the Struewing et al. (1997) paper was released, which said that the penetrance of *BRCA1* mutations among Ashkenazi Jews was 56%. The father called the testing program upset and angry. He felt that he had been deceived by having been given the 85% breast cancer risk at the time of his testing. He said that perhaps if his daughter had thought she had only a 56% risk, closer to 50–50, that perhaps she would not have chosen to have her breasts removed prophylactically. He expressed guilt for having passed on to his daughter the mutation that led her to make this drastic choice. He was able to have a discussion with the medical oncologist who informed him that, in the case of his family, the 85% risk was actually appropriate because they were a very high-risk family, like the ones in which 85% penetrance had been studied. Although this was not exactly "good" news, it reduced his current distress. He could stop worrying that he and the genetic counselors had imparted incorrect information to his daughter and could know, therefore, that her decision had been founded on the "right" risk statistics. The broader issues of his guilt for passing on the mutation might have been addressed in psychological consultation had he chosen to pursue such treatment.

* * *

Individuals seeking genetic information are looking for increased certainty about their risks. In that context, it is sometimes difficult to accept that, even after genetic testing becomes possible, the interpretation of the test results and their power to predict the likelihood of disease is subject to change with increasing scientific knowledge. Scientific advancement is often a successive approximation to a right answer. There are critical transition moments, such as the point at which a new gene is identified, but the translation of that finding into clinical medicine is a lengthy process. Genetic information given to patients by knowledgeable genetics professionals reflects the latest solid evidence available, which, little by little, fills in the picture of how a particular gene or mutation "works." Some patients need help in understanding that genetic information, such as that about penetrance, is changeable as evidence from different populations accumulates.

Particularly when major decisions about risk-reducing surgery or chemoprevention or treatment of life-threatening illness are in the balance, the wish for definitive data on which to base the decision is understandable. Patients with known or possible genetic predisposition for cancer feel under the "gun" of time, especially since many hereditary cancers occur in early adulthood. To take steps to prevent cancer, to act "in time," may require acting when not all of the facts are known. Some individuals are more comfortable than others with this idea. It is particularly important to explore these issues of emerging and changeable knowledge with patients contemplating major life decisions, such as prophylactic surgery. This issue may often not receive sufficient emphasis in discussions with primary care physicians or in briefer forms of genetic counseling. Given the pressure to convey a large body of complex, genetic information in a short time period in these settings particularly, discussion of the changing nature of genetic information is sometimes omitted. Patients seeking certainty may find it hard to hear or remember caveats about the possibility that some of the information they receive may change in the future. And, on the other hand, patients may have to make decisions based on current, incomplete knowledge. Later information may show them to have erred in estimating their own risk, as, for instance, in the case of a woman at high risk of breast cancer who opted to have prophylactic mastectomies prior to the possibility of BRCA1/2 testing and who was later found not to be a mutation carrier. Many women in this circumstance have coped with this knowledge by reminding themselves of the years of decreased worry they experienced because of the surgery they chose to have. Others who are more troubled by the discrepancy between their earlier perceptions and fears and the ultimate reality that they faced only population risk of breast cancer might benefit from psychological help. Treatment might focus, at least in part, on helping the woman to accept that she made the best decision she could with imperfect information under conditions of stress.

WHAT IS GENOMICS?

Genomics is a new term used to describe the study of the functions and interactions of all the genes in the genome. Genomics is a broad field that takes into consideration the interactions among genes and among genes and the environment. Genomics will play an increasing role in health care (Guttmacher & Collins, 2002).

Pharmacogenomics refers to the new field that promises to improve our understanding of why drugs work much more effectively in some people than in others. Pharmacogenomics involves studies of the genetic characteristics of individuals that govern the efficacy of medications and the likelihood that the individual develops adverse side effects from the medicine. Many people believe that pharmacogenomics is the area in which the fruits of the Human Genome Project will most rapidly affect treatment of the general population. In many cases, physicians' choice of medicines and dosages may one day depend on an assessment of the particular genetic characteristics of the patient. Understanding of these characteristics could, for example, be useful in determining which type and dosage of chemotherapy a patient with cancer will receive. Patients may benefit from experiencing fewer side effects and from not having to "try" successive medications to determine which one is most effective for them.

With this basic information about cancer and cancer genetics reviewed, the next chapter explores more specifically what is known about the major cancer predisposition genes. It considers the medical and psychological implications that genetic testing brings to the fore among individuals who think they may have an inherited cancer predisposition.

REFERENCES

Bilous, M., Dowsett, M., Hanna, W., Isola, J., Lebeau, A., Moreno A., et al. (2003). Current perspectives on HER2 testing: A review of national testing guidelines. *Modern Pathology*, 16, 173–182.

Brunet, J. S., Ghadirian, P., Rebbeck, T. R., Lerman, C., Garber, J. E., Tonin, P. N., et al. (1998). Effect of smoking on breast cancer in carriers of mutant *BRCA1* or *BRCA2* genes. *Journal of the National Cancer Institute*, 90, 761–766.

Burke, W., Daly, M., Garber, J., Botkin, J., Kahn, M.J. E., Lynch, P., et al. (1997). Recommendations for follow-up care of individuals with an inherited predisposition to cancer II: BRCA1 and BRCA2. *Journal of the American Medical Association*, 277, 997–1003.

Cavenee, W. K., & White, R. L. (1995). The genetic basis of cancer. *Scientific American*, 272, 68–76.

Ford, D., Easton, D. F., Bishop, D. T., Narod, S. A., & Goldgar, D. E., for the Breast Cancer Linkage Consortium. (1994). Risks of cancer in *BRCA1*-mutation-carriers. *Lancet*, 343, 692–695.

Guttmacher, A. E., & Collins, F. S. (2002). Genomic medicine—a primer. *New England Journal of Medicine*, 347, 1512–1520.

Harper, P., Lim, C., & Craufurd, D., for the UK Huntington's Disease Prediction Consortium. (2000). Ten years of presymptomatic testing for Huntington's disease: The experience of the UK Huntington's Disease Prediction Consortium. *Journal of Medical Genetics*, 37, 567–571.

Iglehart, J. D., Miron, A., Rimer, B. A., Winer, E. P., Berry, D., & Shildkraut, J. M. (1998). Overestimation of hereditary breast cancer risk. *Annals of Surgery*, 228, 375–384.

International Human Genome Sequencing Consortium. (2001). Initial sequencing and analysis of the human genome. *Nature, 409,* 860–921.

Jemal, A., Murray, T., Samuels, A., Ghafoor, A., Ward, E., & Thun, M. J. (2003). Cancer statistics, 2003. *CA: A Cancer Journal for Clinicians, 53,* 5–26.

Jemal, S., Tiwari, R. C., Murray, T., Ghafoor, A., Samuels, A., Ward, E., Feuer, E. J., & Thun, M. J. (2004). Cancer statistics, 2004. *CA: Cancer Journal for Clinicians, 54,* 8–29.

Korf, B. R. (2000). Medical education in the "post-genomic" era. *Postgraduate Medicine, 108,* 15–18.

Offit, K. (1998). *Clinical cancer genetics: Risk counseling and management.* New York: Wiley-Liss.

Schneider, K. (2002). *Counseling about cancer: Strategies for genetic counseling* (2nd ed.). New York: Wiley-Liss.

Smith, R. A., Cokkinides, V., & Eyre, H. J. (2003). American Cancer Society guidelines for the early detection of cancer, 2003. *CA: A Cancer Journal for Clinicians, 53,* 27–43.

Struewing, J. P., Hartge, P., Wacholder, S., Baker, S. M., Berlin, M., McAdams, M., et al. (1997). The risk of cancer associated with specific mutations of BRCA1 and BRCA2 among Ashkenazi Jews. *New England Journal of Medicine, 336,* 1401–1408.

Weiss, L. K., Burkman, R. B., Cushing-Haugen, K. L., Voigt. L. F., Simon, M. S., Daling, J. R., et al. (2002). Hormone replacement therapy regimens and breast cancer risk. *Obstetrics and Gynecology, 100,* 1148–1158.

Welch, H. G., & Burke, W. (1998). Uncertainties in genetic testing for chronic disease. *Journal of the American Medical Association, 280,* 1525–1527.

2

CANCER GENES AND CANCER RISK

[Psychological] Clinicians need not become medical experts, but they
must obtain sufficient background to understand the choices, treatments,
and experiences of the adult with a chronic condition.

(Goodheart, 1998)

The discovery since the early 1990s of genes that greatly raise the risk
for certain types of cancer in mutation carriers brought the work of the
Human Genome Project to public attention. For many, this initiated the
genetic revolution in medicine. Because the predictive potential of this
information has outpaced development of therapeutic or preventive options
for mutation carriers, these discoveries also highlighted the ethical and
emotional dilemmas that accompany the availability of genetic information.
To understand the human conflicts and uncertainties that members of high-
risk cancer families face, one must have at least a basic understanding of
the kinds of information about inherited cancer risk that is provided to
those who seek cancer genetic counseling. This chapter reviews the major
cancer genes and the information currently available for mutation carriers
about the risks they face as a result of their inherited cancer predisposition.

GENES FOR BREAST AND OVARIAN CANCER

What Genes Are There?

BRCA1 and BRCA2 were the first major cancer genes to be found
that conveyed predisposition to common cancers or cancer syndromes
that were not extremely rare. In the search for BRCA1, an international

consortium shared clinical and genetic data on families in which four or more women had had early-onset breast or ovarian cancer (defined as diagnosis under 45 age years of age). The race of nearly Olympic proportions ended in 1994 when Miki et al. (1994) published the cloning of BRCA1 in Science. The BRCA1 gene, located on chromosome 17q21, is a large gene, composed of 5,592 nucleotides that cover 100,000 base pairs of DNA.

The cloning of BRCA1 was of major importance because it meant that cancer genetic testing could be initiated with the potential to inform some at-risk individuals about their susceptibility for breast or ovarian cancer. Prior research had indicated that interest in testing to learn about individualized genetic risk was high (more than 75% of those at risk; Lerman, Daly, Masny, & Balshem, 1994; Lerman, Seay, Balshem, & Audrain, 1995). It was clear, however, that BRCA1 did not account for all of the hereditary breast cancer in identified high-risk families. In 1995, BRCA2 was cloned (Wooster et al., 1995). Located on chromosome 13q12-13, it is also a large gene, composed of 11,385 nucleotides spread over 70,000 base pairs.

Myriad Genetics Laboratories, Inc. was granted the U.S. patent for full gene analysis of BRCA1/2, and they do most, but not all, of the BRCA1/2 testing in this country. There have been challenges to the Myriad patent in Canada and in Europe.

Over 2,000 mutations have been found in BRCA1 and BRCA2, many, but not all, of which are associated with the presence of breast or ovarian cancer (Open Access On-Line Breast Cancer Mutation Database, n.d.). This multiplicity of cancer-predisposing mutations in BRCA1 and BRCA2 has important implications for exactly what genetic testing can tell us. If a single mutation had uniquely been found to cause these cancers, then anyone wanting to know whether she was at increased hereditary risk could have his or her DNA examined to determine the presence or absence of that mutation. However, this is not the case. On BRCA1 and BRCA2 there are many disease-producing mutations and many other chromosomal alterations whose significance is unclear with regard to cancer risk. Although BRCA1 and BRCA2 mutations do not tend to occur in sporadic (nonhereditary) cases of breast or ovarian cancers, the array of mutations in both genes that produce breast or ovarian cancers means genetic testing is most informative when it is known which gene and which mutation on that gene is associated with the occurrence of cancer in that family. This can be determined if an individual in the family who has already been diagnosed with breast or ovarian cancer is willing to undergo genetic testing to look for the presence of a particular mutation in BRCA1 or BRCA2. If a mutation is found in either of these genes, it can then be assumed that this is the mutation responsible for the development of cancer in that person and that this mutation indicates increased hereditary cancer risk in other family members. If the person tests negative for a known familial mutation, he or she is not at increased hereditary risk for cancer. Knowing which mutation to look for among the 70,000–100,000 base pairs on the genes opens the door for individuals in the family who have not had cancer to be tested and to receive clear information about whether they carry the deleterious mutation in question. Their test result will tell them definitively whether they are at increased hereditary risk for breast or ovarian cancer.

It is unfortunate that it is not always possible to test an individual in each family who has had cancer to determine the location of a familial mutation. This greatly limits the individuals who can be assured of a definitive answer about their mutation status from BRCA1/2 testing. In many families with significant family histories of breast or ovarian cancer, there are no living family members who have had breast or ovarian cancer. In other families, the relative with cancer may be unwilling to be tested for a variety of reasons (e.g., cost; the person does not want to know, is too ill, or fears loss of insurance; estrangement within the family). Because families are so dispersed and many have experienced an early death of a mother or other female relative, the relative seeking testing may be unknown or barely connected to the person whose testing could provide the "address" of the familial mutation. This situation can create great tension within some families (see chap. 7, "A Family Matter"). The healthy or unaffected person wishing to know his or her own genetic test result is largely dependent on another family member whose wishes may be based on accurate knowledge of the pros and cons of testing but may also be based on no information at all. Without the relative's willingness to be tested, the individual wishing to know his or her status is limited in the information he or she can gain from the test results. Full sequencing of BRCA1 or BRCA2 genes (at a cost of more than $2,000) may indicate the presence of a mutation that is known to predispose to breast and ovarian cancer, and this would constitute a positive test result. If a mutation was not found, the test result could not be considered a definitive negative because the hereditary predisposition may be due to a mutation that was overlooked, a breast and ovarian cancer gene that has yet to be found, or another unrecognized variant.

In many families, the genetic testing of a person with cancer is not a difficult decision. In these families, the women who have had breast or ovarian cancer are in close communication with and concerned about the risk to their relatives. They want, for their own sake and that of their family, to know whether they carry a mutation responsible for their cancer. Testing of the proband (the person in the family who is the identified case) occurs without family disruption and leads, if he or she is mutation-positive, rapidly to the testing of other at-risk relatives wanting to know their own status.

There is an alternative for people in some families without a known mutation. If they happen to be members of an ethnic group in which one or more mutations associated with cancer development have been found with high frequency, they can be tested to see if they carry any of those mutations. *Founder effect* is the term used to describe the high frequency of certain genetic mutations among members of a group who can trace their ancestry to a small, isolated group of ancestors. Through intermarriage within the group, the frequency of the mutation proliferates. Founder effects for *BRCA1* or *BRCA2* have been found among Ashkenazi Jews (Oddoux et al., 1996; Struewing et al., 1995a), Icelanders (Thorlacius et al., 1996), and French Canadians (Simard et al., 1994), among others. In the United States, Ashkenazi Jewish individuals can be tested for the two *BRCA1* mutations (187delAG and 5382insC) and one *BRCA2* mutation (6174delT) that are thought to be due to founder effects and responsible for increased rates of hereditary breast and ovarian cancers among members of this group. This panel testing costs $415, much less than the $2,975 of full sequencing of *BRCA1/2* (Myriad Laboratories, Inc., personal communication, March 15, 2004). A positive result found by testing for this panel of mutations carries the same implications of high personal cancer risk as would a positive result in a person with a known familial mutation. Testing negative for the common mutations in this panel does not convey the same reassurance as a negative test for an identified familial mutation, however. A negative finding on a panel test of a few mutations leaves open the possibility that the relatives who had cancer had a mutation other than that known to be common within their ethnic group. It is estimated that 10% of the *BRCA1/2* mutations that occur in Ashkenazi Jewish people, for example, are not founder mutations (National Cancer Institute Physicians Data Query, 2002). Therefore, testing negative for the panel mutations is considered indeterminate.

Although *BRCA1* and *BRCA2* are thought to account for up to 80% of cancer in high-risk breast and ovarian cancer families (Eeles, 2000), there must be at least one more major cancer predisposition gene yet to be found to account for the high rates of breast and ovarian cancer in families who do not have *BRCA1* or *BRCA2* mutations. Individuals who are not found to have *BRCA1* or *BRCA2* mutations may later have the option of being tested for a *BRCA3*, *BRCAX*, or other gene found to contribute to cancer in these families.

Increased hereditary risk for breast cancer is associated with a number of other rare hereditary syndromes or conditions. Cowden's syndrome, a very rare condition (there are only about 200 known patients), conveys an approximately 30% risk of breast cancer, typically in younger than average women (i.e., below age 50; Greene, 1997). It is known to be due to the autosomal dominant gene *PTEN* (Eng, 2000). Ataxis telangiectasia (AT) is a hereditary neurological and immunological disease (Schneider, 2002; Swift et al., 1991). Female relatives of patients with ataxia-telangiectasia were found in some studies to have a fivefold increased rate of developing breast cancer, although this finding has not been confirmed. Because 1% of the female U.S. population is heterozygous for ataxia-telangiectasia, its role in the development of breast cancer is of particular concern (Easton, 1994). Current recommendations are that mothers of children with the disease should begin their mammograms early, around age 30 (Schneider, 2002).

As more genes are found and more sensitive technologies developed, people who initially received indeterminate or negative results may receive new interpretations of those results or may be offered the opportunity to be retested. Repeated testing for cancer genes can arouse considerable emotion and reaction. Even following thorough genetic counseling about the independence of risk for each mutation (there are rare reports of individuals who have been found to have mutations in both *BRCA1* and *BRCA2*; Ganguly et al., 2001), some people feel that "good luck" on the prior testing increases their chances of not being carriers of the mutations for which they are subsequently tested. Others find repeated negative testing frustrating, leaving them without any genetic explanation for the rates of cancer in their family. Some people decide that they do not wish to put themselves through the ups and downs of repeated testing and prefer living with uncertainty about their genetic status.

Considering the Options

When individuals who are considering genetic testing are asked what would be different if they knew their carrier status for a deleterious mutation, the question often leads to an important discussion of the limited options for screening, surveillance, and risk reduction. Most of the options are not dependent on actual knowledge of gene status. A woman with a significant family history may opt for chemoprevention, prophylactic surgery, or a careful screening program, whether or not she knows her gene status. Although she may believe that her motivation would be greater for certain options if she were to know her status, the anxiety about repeated testing may be more than she is willing to endure. She might use psychotherapy to help her decide whether she wishes to pursue some of the more extreme risk-reducing options, such as prophylactic oophorectomy (removal of healthy ovaries to try to prevent disease) or prophylactic mastectomy. Therapy can also help her consider that options may change over time as new efficacy data and treatments become available and to decide whether she is the kind of person who can adapt well to a position of "watchful waiting." Psychotherapy might also help assuage the guilt or remorse reported by some women who do not want to pursue all available options. Therapy may also help some accept that, for them, having all possible genetic information could be deleterious to their emotional stability and well-being.

What Kinds of Cancer Risk Do These Genes Convey?

BRCA1 and BRCA2 primarily convey increased risk for breast and ovarian cancers, but they are also associated with more moderate increases in risk for several other types of cancer (discussed later in this chapter). The extent of the cancer risk is assessed by attempting to determine the penetrance of the gene, that is, the degree of correlation between the presence of the gene (genotype) and the presence of the characteristic (phenotype), in this case, cancer. Measures of penetrance can vary in different populations, depending on how the sample was acquired. The earliest studies of BRCA1 and BRCA2 penetrance were conducted among families affected by repeated generations of early-onset breast and ovarian cancers because these were the families that were most likely to have hereditary etiology. Subsequent studies have included families with less dramatic cancer histories that have shown somewhat lower lifetime rates of cancer, resulting in lower estimates of cancer risk for mutation carriers.

The lifetime risk of breast cancer for female BRCA1 and BRCA2 mutation carriers ranges from 56% (Struewing et al., 1997) to 85% (Ford, Easton, Bishop, Narod, & Goldgar, for the Breast Cancer Linkage Consortium, 1994). Most often, breast cancer of hereditary etiology occurs at earlier than usual ages (i.e., under age 50). The risk of a second cancer in the other (contralateral) breast in cases of hereditary etiology is greatly increased. Among men, breast cancer occurs in approximately 6% of male BRCA2 carriers but occurs less commonly in male BRCA1 mutation carriers (Struewing, et al., 1995a).

The risk for ovarian cancer in BRCA1 mutation carriers ranges from 27% (Ford et al., 1998) to 60% (Easton, Ford, Bishop, & the Breast Cancer Linkage Consortium, 1995). The risk of ovarian cancer with BRCA2 mutations is estimated to be between 20% and 27% (Breast Cancer Linkage Consortium, 1999; Ford et al., 1998).

BRCA1 conveys about a 6% risk of colon cancer for mutation carriers (Ford et al., 1994), although the age of onset is approximately the same as for sporadic colon cancer. Colon cancer risk for BRCA2 mutation carriers may be increased, but to what extent it is not yet clear (Eeles, 2000). Prostate cancer risk is about 8% in BRCA1 mutation carriers (Ford & Easton, 1995) and between 6% and 14% in BRCA2 (Breast Cancer Linkage Consortium, 1999), but age of onset is not earlier than in typical population cases. Pancreatic cancer risk appears increased to 7% in BRCA2 mutation carriers (Ozcelik et al., 1997).

Patients learning that a mutation in their BRCA1 or BRCA2 genes can increase their risk for cancers other than those that have occurred in their family are likely to be distressed. Women from families with breast cancer are often unaware that if they are found to be mutation carriers, they may be at increased risk for ovarian cancer as well. The shock may be especially great for women who have survived their initial diagnosis of breast cancer and are coming for genetic counseling or testing, primarily for the purpose of providing genetic information to their children. Learning that they may be at increased risk for ovarian cancer and that it may be advisable to consider prophylactic removal of their ovaries may arouse fear as they anticipate the possibility of experiencing a second cancer. The realization that somewhat increased risk for colon and possibly pancreatic cancer is associated with *BRCA1/2* raises issues for men who are considering testing or who have been found to be carriers. Many of these men come to genetic counseling or testing with the goal of providing information that may be of use to their daughters. Awareness of the colon and possible pancreatic risks and of an increased (if still low) risk of male breast cancer with *BRCA2* may come as a shock to a man who has lived in a family in which concern has always focused on female relatives and their risk for breast and ovarian cancers.

Questions have been raised about whether there are any differences in the survival of breast or ovarian cancer patients who are *BRCA1/2* mutation carriers. The data remain unclear. Several studies suggested better prognostic features of the cancer and longer survival for ovarian cancer patients who carried *BRCA1* mutations, but a Swedish study found that this advantage was not sustained over time (Johannsson, Ranstam, Borg, & Olsson, 1998). Studies of survival after breast cancer for *BRCA1* or *BRCA2* mutation carriers have also shown contradictory results. Several showed no difference in survival between mutation carriers and others with no known mutation (Lee et al., 1999; Verhoog et al., 1998). One French study of survival in *BRCA1*-positive breast cancer patients found that these patients had tumors with poorer prognostic characteristics and reduced survival compared with non-*BRCA1* patients (Stoppa-Lyonnet et al., 2000).

Every woman with a mother or sister who has had breast or ovarian cancer worries that she is at increased risk for developing the same disease. When a young woman is diagnosed with breast cancer, she is likely to worry additionally that she is a carrier of a cancer predisposition gene, given that early age of onset is a hallmark of hereditary cancers. Genetic counseling can be useful to such women in helping to determine how likely it is that hereditary factors are relevant to the etiology of their cancer.

The risk to first-degree relatives (mothers, sisters, or daughters) of a breast or ovarian cancer patient varies with the rest of the family history, particularly the age of onset of the cancer and the age of the woman in question, but the risk is typically much less than the level of women's fears. About 5% to 10% of women in the general population have a mother or sister with breast cancer (National Cancer Institute Physicians Data Query, 2002). Overall the lifetime risk of breast cancer for women with affected first-degree relatives is about twice the population risk of 8% to 9%, but this could be lower or higher depending on the specifics of the family history. If the woman is under age 50 and the breast cancer in her first-degree relative was diagnosed before that relative was 50 (indicating a slightly higher risk of a hereditary breast cancer predisposition), then her risk may be somewhat higher. Many of these daughters and sisters feel that cancer is inevitable, that their risk is 100%, and that their developing cancer is only a matter of time. Personal risk statistics developed during genetic counseling may help them to realize that, although they cannot be reassured completely, their assumption of inevitability is emotionally based, rather than statistically based. Psychological support and help with both intellectual and emotional differentiation of the woman from her mother or sister may help to reduce soaring anxiety, which may be unrealistic.

Similarly, early age of onset, even when a young woman has a first-degree relative with breast cancer, does not convey as high a likelihood of being a BRCA1 or BRCA2 carrier as is commonly assumed. Data have been published about risks in an unselected population sample showing that the risk of being a BRCA1 or BRCA2 carrier for young women (under age 35) diagnosed with breast cancer is 9.2%. Even young women diagnosed with breast cancer before age 45 who also have a first-degree relative with breast cancer have only a 12% chance of being a BRCA1/2 carrier (Malone et al., 2000). Although these women have much to deal with related to their cancer diagnoses, realization that their risk of having an inherited mutation in BRCA1/2 is not so high (in the range of the population risk of breast cancer) may help them avoid panic about an immediate need to undergo genetic testing or to have prophylactic surgery. Young women (under age 50) who are diagnosed with breast cancer reportedly experience greater psychological distress than older patients (Bloom, Stewart, Johnston, & Banks, 1998; Dunn & Steginga, 2000). Concern about developing cancer in the other breast because of a woman's hereditary risk, her risk for other cancers, or the risk to her offspring are likely contributors to such distress. Additional fears include not living to raise young children, which may lead women to accept more drastic options for prevention (see chap. 6 on prophylactic surgery).

Similarly, for ovarian cancer, the risk of developing cancer if one has a first-degree relative who had ovarian cancer is increased from the general population risk of 1%; overall, however, the risk remains low. The lifetime risk of developing ovarian cancer among women with a first-degree relative who had the disease is about 5%; the risk to women with several relatives with ovarian cancer is about 7.2% (Stratton et al., 1998).

Widespread publicity about cancer genes and about breast cancer in general has led many people to overestimate the frequency of BRCA1 or

BRCA2 mutations in the general population and to overestimate one's personal risk of being a carrier of breast cancer (see Risk Perception in chap. 5). Although there are steps that can be taken to achieve greater certainty about one's personal risk, awareness of the low level of the mutations in the general population may help individuals to make decisions with less attendant anxiety.

Recommendations to Prevent Cancer for BRCA1/2 Mutation Carriers

Knowledge of cancer risk is medically useful only if that knowledge alters some action or behavior that can prevent the disease or reduce its impact. In 1997, the Cancer Genetics Studies Consortium published guidelines for individuals found to be BRCA1/2 mutation carriers (see Table 2.1; Burke et al., 1997). The authors of these recommendations made clear that they were based on expert opinion in the absence of data about the extent to which following them would reduce the incidence or impact of cancer for mutation carriers. In general, the guidelines recommend starting breast screening (breast self- and clinical examinations, mammography) at earlier than usual ages, 25 to 35 years of age. Others have suggested that surveillance should start five years before the age at which the first case of breast cancer in the family was diagnosed. Ovarian surveillance (transvaginal ultrasound and CA-125 blood tests), which is of notably poor predictive value as a population screen, is nonetheless recommended for mutation carriers, also beginning at ages 25 to 35. Physicians are advised to inform patients about the option of prophylactic surgery. (At the time of the 1997 recommendations, there were no data on the efficacy of prophylactic surgery; however, as discussed in chap. 6, subsequent supporting data have been published.) The recommendations stated that there is no evidence about the impact of lifestyle modifications (dietary restrictions, low alcohol intake, etc.) for BRCA1/2 carriers. The recommendations for prostate and colon cancer screening for carriers primarily encourages utilization of recommended population screening tools (i.e., rectal exam and PSA [prostate specific antigen] tests for prostate cancer; fecal occult blood tests and sigmoidoscopy [examination of part of the colon using an endoscope to visualize the interior of the organ] for colon cancer) that are typically begun at age 50 for both those at increased hereditary risk and members of the general public.

More recently, chemopreventive measures have been introduced that offer potential risk-reducing benefit for those at increased risk of breast cancer. In 1998, a prospective, randomized, double-blind study found that taking the antiestrogen drug tamoxifen for four years was associated with a 49% reduction in breast cancer among women at increased risk for breast cancer, with and without a family history of breast cancer (Fisher et al.,

TABLE 2.1

Options for Surveillance for Carriers of *BRCA1* and *BRCA2* Mutations

Intervention	Provisional Recommendation	Quality of Evidence*	Cautionary Issues
Breast cancer			
Breast self-examination	Education regarding monthly self-examination	Expert opinion only	Benefit not proven
Clinician breast examination	Annually or semiannually, beginning at age 25–35 years	Expert opinion only	Benefit not proven
Mammography	Annually, beginning at age 25–35 years	Expert opinion only (I Randomized trial, average-risk women aged 50–69 years)	Risks and benefits not established for women under age 50 years
Ovarian cancer			
Transvaginal ultrasound with color Doppler and CA-125 level	Annually or semiannually, beginning at age 25–35 years	Expert opinion only	Benefit not proven; level of ovarian cancer risk estimated to be lower in *BRCA2* mutation carriers
Prostate cancer			
Prostate cancer surveillance (*BRCA1* mutation carriers only)	Inform regarding options for screening involving rectal examination and prostate specific antigen level, annually, beginning at age 50 years	Expert opinion only	Benefit not proven; many agencies do not recommend screening due to uncertainty of benefit from early detection
Colon cancer			
Colon cancer surveillance	Follow recommendations for general population: fecal occult blood test annually and flexible sigmoidoscopy every 3–5 years, beginning at age 50 years	Evidence from average risk populations: I randomized trial (fecal occult blood test); II-2 case control study (sigmoidoscopy)	Relevance of population-based data uncertain

Note. From "Recommendations for Follow-Up Care for Individuals With an Inherited Predisposition to Cancer. II. *BRCA1* and *BRCA2*," by W. Burke et al., 1997, *Journal of the American Medical Association, 277,* p. 996. Copyright 1997 by the American Medical Association. All rights reserved. Reprinted with permission.

1998). Some additional risk for endometrial cancer and stroke was found in women over age 50 who took tamoxifen. Raloxifene, a drug originally developed for osteoporosis treatment, was also subsequently shown to reduce breast cancer risk in postmenopausal high-risk women (Chlebowski et al., 2002). A study comparing the effects of these two drugs in preventing cancer among high-risk women, and specifically among *BRCA1/2* mutation carriers, is underway (Study of Tamoxifen and Raloxifene—STAR trial; Vogel, Costantino, Wickerham, Cronin, & Wolmark, 2002). In several decision-analysis studies comparing prophylactic surgery and use of tamoxifen or raloxifene in mutation carriers, quality-of-life measures indicated that chemoprevention might be more acceptable than surgery, especially for younger women at high genetic risk (Grann et al., 2000), and that the two risk-reducing options might therefore prevent an equal number of breast cancers (Eisinger et al., 2001) despite a greater theoretical advantage to prophylactic surgery.

Studies in both the United States and the United Kingdom have looked at the emotional and psychosexual impact of these chemopreventive medications. Overall, few adverse effects have been found in group means on psychological symptom inventories, although considerable individual variation in anxiety was noted (Day et al., 1999; Fallowfield et al., 2001). Some women feel anxious about taking any medication without long-term data on its cancer risks. Others object to the side effects of tamoxifen treatment; women taking tamoxifen report menopause-like vasomotor and gynecologic symptoms that differed in nature but not intensity from symptoms reported by a matched placebo group (Fallowfield et al., 2001).

Many researchers are attempting to find a link between particular mutations in these genes and the phenotypic characteristics of the cancers that result from them (e.g., Gayther et al., 1995). For example, if a family with a *BRCA1* mutation has had largely ovarian cancer, is it because the particular mutation they have primarily conveys a risk for ovarian cancer and not breast cancer? This information will be valuable when it becomes available because it will inform at-risk individuals about the particular cancers for which they most need to consider surveillance or prevention options. Currently, in the absence of such information, mutation carriers have no option other than considering themselves at increased risk for all cancers related to *BRCA1/2*.

Although much has been learned from *BRCA1/2* genetic testing, significant work remains before the identification of carriers of *BRCA1/2* mutations can be said to have clear and consistent benefits in terms of disease prevention. This may be frustrating for those who had hoped genetic testing would provide immediate answers about the presence or absence of cancer predisposing mutations and the benefits of preventive or risk-reducing surgeries.

COLON CANCER

About 10% of colon cancer, or about 13,000 cases, are probably attributable to hereditary causes (Lynch & Lynch, 2000). There are two major forms of hereditary colon cancer, hereditary nonpolyposis colon cancer (HNPCC) and familial adenomatous polyposis (FAP).

Hereditary Nonpolyposis Colon Cancer

Hereditary nonpolyposis colon cancer is an autosomal dominant disorder characterized by early-onset (mid-40s) colon cancer and an increased risk for endometrial and ovarian cancer, as well as for other cancers, such as gastrointestinal and urinary tract, brain, and breast tumors (Lynch & Lynch, 2000; Syngal, Fox, Eng, Kolodner, & Garber, 2000). Some controversy exists regarding the definition of HNPCC, and a number of criteria exist to provide research uniformity for this syndrome (which may also be referred to as Lynch syndrome). Differences among the criteria relate primarily to the number of affected close relatives and the kinds of secondary cancers that merit inclusion (see Table 2.2 for a listing of HNPCC criteria). The original and modified Amsterdam I criteria identify only about 45% to 64% of families with hereditary mutations (Giardiello, Brensinger, & Petersen, 2001). Only 18% of individuals with a germline mutation meet Amsterdam II criteria (Syngal et al., 1999). The Bethesda Guidelines are thought to be the criteria that leave out the fewest families who are carriers of deleterious mutations likely to cause HNPCC, but none of the guidelines is perfect for the task of identifying families who have HNPCC. Likewise, none is an exclusion criterion; that is, families in which there is a suspicion of HNPCC cannot be ruled out or excluded from genetic counseling, testing, or careful surveillance because they do not meet the criteria.

What Genes Are Associated With HNPCC?

Six genes have been found to be associated with HNPCC. Two of these, *MSH2* and *MLH1*, are the most common and are the two for which commercial testing is currently available. The other genes include *MSH3*, *MSH6*, *PMS1*, and *PMS2*. All of the associated genes are members of a class called mismatch repair genes because of their role in DNA replication. They account for only about 40% to 60% of families meeting the criteria for HNPCC families; therefore, other genes with an etiological connection to HNPCC will undoubtedly be found.

As with breast cancer susceptibility genes, definitive testing for cancer is only available for individuals from families in which a mutation has been found in members who have had colorectal cancer. Because of the number

TABLE 2.2
Clinical Criteria for HNPCC

Name	Criteria
Amsterdam[a]	1. One or more cases of CRC diagnosed before age 50, 2. Two generations in which CRC has occurred, and 3. Three relatives with colorectal cancer (CRC), one or more of whom is a first-degree relative (FDR) of the other two
Modified Amsterdam[b]	1. Very small families with only two CRCs in FDRs if at least two generations have CRC and one or more of the cases is diagnosed age <55 years, *or* 2. Families with two FDRs affected with CRC and the presence of a third relative with an unusual early-onset neoplasm or endometrial cancer
Amsterdam II	Three or more relatives with an HNPCC-associated tumor, one of whom is a third-degree relative of the other two, involving at least two generations in which one or more of the cases is diagnosed age <50 years
Bethesda[b]	1. Subjects with cancer in families that fulfill Amsterdam criteria 2. Subjects with two HNPCC-related cancers, including synchronous and metachronous CRCs or associated extracolonic cancers 3. Subjects with CRC and an FDR with CRC and/or HNPCC-related extracolonic cancer and/or colorectal adenoma; one cancer diagnosed age <45 and the adenoma diagnosed age <40 years 4. Subjects with CRC or endometrial cancer diagnosed at age <45 years 5. Subjects with right-sided CRC with an undifferentiated pattern (solid/cribiform) on histopathology diagnosed age <45 years 6. Subjects with signet ring cell type CRC diagnosed age <45 years *or* 7. Subjects with adenomas diagnosed age <40 years

Note. HNPCC = hereditary nonpolyposis colon cancer. Adapted from "Sensitivity and Specificity of Clinical Criteria for Hereditary Non-Polyposis Colorectal Cancer Associated Mutations in *MSH2* and *MLH1*," by S. Syngal et al., 2000, p. 642. Copyright 2000 by the BMJ Publishing Group. Reprinted with permission.
[a]All criteria must be met.
[b]Meeting all features under any of the numbered criteria is sufficient.

of possible genes involved in HNPCC, the many mutations that have been found in the six identified cancer-predisposing genes, and the fact that there are other, as-yet-unidentified genes that predispose carriers to HNPCC, genetic testing for colorectal cancer genes is considerably more difficult to interpret than is testing for breast and ovarian cancer. It is also more difficult to determine who would be likely to benefit from genetic testing. Because full sequence genetic predisposition testing for colorectal cancer genes costs between $1,600 and $2,000 (according to Myriad Genetics Laboratories,

Inc., Salt Lake City, UT), it is important to target those for whom testing is likely to produce an interpretable result. Several techniques have been shown to aid in decision making about predictive testing and interpretation of test results. Microsatellite instability (MSI) testing and testing for the expression of protein products in the tumors of affected family members can aid researchers in identifying the gene to be tested and indicate when further investigation of a negative test is warranted (Ward et al., 2002). Microsatellites are repetitive elements in the DNA of a gene, which can involve substantial or minor increases in the repeat length of the DNA microsatellites that can result from mutations in mismatch repair genes. MSI testing can be helpful in deciding whether further investigation is needed when a genetic test result shows one of the more than 90 missense mutations that have been found in HNPCC. MSI is found in more than 90% of the colorectal cancers from patients with HNPCC. However, high-MSI tumors are also found in 15% of sporadic colon cancers and other tumors (Vasen, 2000). The functional significance of these mutations, that is, whether they result in genes with deleterious products, is unclear in many cases. The combined use of the Amsterdam or Bethesda criteria for HNPCC, MSI testing, and immunostaining, if possible, can improve recommendations for the use of genetic testing because no single indicator is fully reliable in determining who are likely to be carriers of HNPCC-causing mutations.

For Which Cancers Do These Genes Convey a Predisposition?

The lifetime cancer risk (all cancers) associated with mutations in the genes responsible for HNPCC is between 85% and 90% (Lynch & Lynch, 2000), and the risk of developing colon cancer is thought to be between 70% and 85% (Vasen, 2000). Risks appear to differ for men and women. Men in HNPCC families who have mutations in their mismatch repair genes are more likely to get colorectal cancer (74%) than women (30%; Dunlop et al., 1997). Women who are carriers are estimated to have an approximately 40% risk for endometrial (uterine lining) cancers and a 9% risk for ovarian cancer (Aarnio, Mecklin, Aaltonen, Nystrom-Lahti, & Jarvinen, 1995; Watson et al., 1994, 2001; Watson & Lynch, 1993). Overall cancer risk was 91% for men and 69% for women. Hereditary colon cancer occurs earlier (average age of 44 years) than sporadic colon cancer (average age of 64 years; Vasen et al., 1996). HNPCC mutation carriers have better survival rates than individuals with sporadic colon cancer (Gryfe et al., 2000).

Multiple primary cancers, a hallmark of hereditary cancers in general, is also indicative of HNPCC and serves as a sign physicians note in deciding whether a family history may be positive for HNPCC. Practitioners may be more likely to miss the diagnosis of HNPCC, however, if the case presenting to them is not colorectal cancer, but another associated cancer, such as ovarian cancer. For a physician to be able to gather a thorough family history, patients may be required to do extensive research among their relatives. Family history information presented by patients about gastrointestinal and other nonbreast tumors is less reliable than information presented about breast cancer (K. Schneider, personal communication, January 16, 2003).

What Measures Are Recommended for HNPCC Mutation Carriers to Prevent Cancer?

There are several reasons why it is important to recognize whether an individual is a member of an HNPCC family. These reasons include the following:

1. Because the age of onset for hereditary colon cancer is earlier than the age at which colon cancer occurs in the general population, knowing whether there is an inherited colon cancer mutation in the family may alter the age at which healthy people in the family begin screening for gastrointestinal polyps. Colonoscopic screening for such individuals is recommended every 1 to 2 years beginning at age 25, about 25 years earlier than the recommendation for the general population. (Colon cancer in the general population typically begins to occur in the mid-60s.)
2. Shorter intervals (1–2 years) between testing than the 5-year intervals recommended for members of the general population are also recommended for those who may be HNPCC mutation carriers (Burke et al., 1997).
3. More extensive ovarian and endometrial screening than usual may be recommended for at-risk women from HNPCC families. This includes recommendations for transvaginal ultrasound and endometrial biopsy (Brown, St. John, Macrae, & Aittomaki, 2001; Lynch & Lynch, 2000) despite the fact that there is no definitive data as yet to show that careful early surveillance reduces the mortality of gynecological cancer in HNPCC. In the future, increased knowledge about whether specific mutations lead to gynecologic instead of colorectal cancers in HNPCC-positive women might lead to targeting of interventions, emphasizing early, intensive screening for only the type of cancer for which the woman is most at risk (Brown et al., 2001).
4. When a member of an HNPCC family is diagnosed with colon cancer, treatment of the disease may differ from that which is generally advised. More aggressive surgery is likely to be recommended, including colectomy for colorectal cancer at the first cancer diagnosis rather than only removing the small

area of the colon where the tumor was found (Lynch & Lynch, 2000).

5. Prophylactic surgery may be considered by members of HNPCC families who find "watching and waiting" unacceptable. Prophylactic total or subtotal colectomy may be considered prior to the diagnosis of colorectal cancer, especially if a significant number of polyps are found during colonoscopy. After subtotal colectomy, a surgery that spares the rectum while removing the rest of the colon, patients must undergo screening endoscopic evaluation every six months because a 1% per year risk for rectal cancer remains. An important part of the decision about which surgery (total or subtotal colectomy) is recommended involves an assessment of the individual's ability to comply with the recommendation for rectal surveillance every six months. Psychological intervention may be useful at this juncture to help in making this important decision. Women in HNPCC families may consider having their uterus and ovaries removed prophylactically after they complete childbearing to reduce their risk of ovarian or endometrial cancer. Discussion with a knowledgeable psychologist about possible psychological consequences of the surgery and the timing of surgery can reduce patient burden.

6. Diagnosis of HNPCC and the genetic counseling that follows make possible informed discussions with other family members about the implications of one person's diagnosis or genetic test result for the cancer risk of relatives. Genetic testing may be helpful in determining which members of the family are and are not at increased hereditary risk for colon and other related cancers.

*   *   *

Case Example. Impact of Diagnosis of Hereditary: Cancer Syndrome in a Young Man. Rick, a college sophomore, was seen for a psychological consultation just a few days before his subtotal colectomy surgical date. About six months earlier his father, a man in his mid-50s, had been diagnosed with colon cancer. At the time, Rick and his father had been genetically tested, and both had tested positive for HNPCC. Several months later, Rick noticed blood in his own stools for several days running. He told his mother (with some embarrassment), who took him to see the doctor. Rick was found to have a large polyp in his colon that could not be removed during colonoscopy. Subtotal colectomy was recommended, and a surgery date was set. Rick later moved up the surgery date so that he could get on with what he had come to feel was a necessary and important step in his health care. In the psychological session, he described the rapid education he had received about colon cancer and his risk for getting it. He had come to feel strongly that surgery was a necessary and life-saving option for him—so much so that when an alternate approach was mentioned, he found himself unhappy about the possibility of not having surgery. He was realistically concerned about the impact surgery and its sequelae would have on his dating life and self-image. He disliked the scar he would have if they did the surgery traditionally but said that he was hoping they were able to do it laparoscopically. Rick was articulate in describing the rapid reorganization of his life and his concerns following news of his being HNPCC-positive and requiring surgery. Although a few weeks before his worries had focused on school and social life, he was now sharing concerns about cancer with his father and feeling somewhat out of sync with friends who had been supportive but whose lives focused on very different issues. Surgery was playing havoc with his academic program. He had to take a semester off from school and was thinking about how and when to reenter that environment. He did not appear resentful but rather grateful for the opportunity to prevent cancer, which would have far greater consequences. The experience also touched on other conflicts in his life. Taken together there seemed to be sufficient reason to recommend psychotherapy once surgery was complete.

Various dietary aids (aspirin, calcium, estrogen replacement for women, and folate) have been suggested to reduce the risk for colon cancer in the general population. So far there has been inadequate data as to the efficacy of these substances for the general population from national or international medical bodies. Individuals with hereditary colon cancer have often been excluded from the studies that do exist; there are no studies of the impact of these factors on the development of cancer in the HNPCC population (National Cancer Institute Physicians Data Query, 2004). The recommendations for early, regular screening and colectomy for mutation carriers are based on expert opinion; there have not been randomized, controlled studies of the efficacy of these interventions. One study of the efficacy of colon cancer screening in Finland did find that among the mutation carriers who chose to be screened, there were 62% fewer cancers and 65% fewer deaths; other factors associated with compliance may also play a role, however (Jarvinen et al., 2000).

Familial Adenomatous Polyposis

Which Genes Are Associated With FAP?

Familial adenomatous polyposis is a syndrome that occurs in the presence of inherited or de novo mutations in the *APC* gene (Kinzler et al., 1991). FAP affects approximately 1 person in 10,000 (Bisgaard, Fenger,

Bulow, Niebuhr, & Mohr, 1994). Its significance as a hereditary cancer syndrome is greater than its frequency might suggest because (a) the APC gene is 100% penetrant, meaning that anyone who inherits a deleterious mutation in APC will develop FAP; (b) there is a surgical treatment for FAP; and (c) FAP has an early age of onset, making this hereditary cancer syndrome one of the few for which genetic testing of children is advised as the standard of care.

FAP: Natural History and Associated Conditions

In FAP, polyps (hundreds or even thousands) form in the colon and rectum. Although not initially cancerous, these adenomatous polyps eventually become malignant. The polyps start to form in childhood; 15% of people with FAP have polyps by age 10, 75% by age 20, and 90% by age 30 (Lal & Gallinger, 2000). If left unattended, colorectal cancer typically develops in FAP family members by age 35, about 30 years earlier than cases occur in the general population (Herrerra, 1990). Once the number of polyps approaches 100, removal of part or all of the colon is typically recommended to prevent development of colon cancer.

A number of malignant and benign conditions are associated with FAP including cancers of the gastrointestinal tract, thyroid, liver, and brain. Desmoid tumors occur frequently and, although benign, can be fatal by virtue of their tendency to encompass surrounding organs. These dense connective-tissue tumors are responsible for 11% of the deaths caused by FAP (Lal & Gallinger, 2000). Dental abnormalities and skin cysts may occur. FAP is also associated with somewhat increased risks for thyroid and small bowel cancers, hepatoblastoma, and brain tumors (Herrerra, 1990). There are connections between particular mutations in APC and age of onset, number of polyps, and the kinds of associated conditions that occur. Because these are not one-to-one correlations, there may be mitigating genetic or environmental factors affecting the correlation between genotype and phenotype (Lal & Gallinger, 2000).

What Measures Are Recommended for FAP Mutation Carriers to Prevent Cancer?

Before the possibility of genetic testing, children and adults with a parent or sibling who had FAP (and were thus at 50% risk of carrying an APC mutation) would have annual flexible sigmoidoscopies beginning at about age 10 to determine whether they had any visible polyps. If polyps were found, a colonoscopy was performed and repeated once every year or two. When the number of polyps reached 100, surgical removal of the colon was recommended, often performed in late adolescence or early adulthood to try to prevent the development of cancer. It was known, theoretically, that half of those who underwent repeated screenings were not mutation carriers, but because it was not known which individuals, in fact, were, all were screened. Those who did not develop polyps into young adulthood were screened until they reached middle age because, in some individuals at risk for FAP, polyps do not form until then.

The costs, both financial and emotional, of such screening were great. With the advent of genetic testing, individuals from families suspected of having FAP can be tested to see whether they have one of the more than 300 mutations in APC that are known to occur. When the mutation is known, individuals testing negative are considered true negatives; for them, colon screening can be sharply reduced or curtailed until middle age. When a mutation is not identified within the family of the patient, genetic testing cannot provide a definitive answer about whether the person being tested carried the mutation causing FAP in their family. Individuals in such a circumstance would be encouraged to continue annual colonoscopies.

Screening for the noncolorectal conditions associated with FAP should continue in mutation carriers even after colectomy. Also, if parts of the colon are left intact, such as when a subtotal colectomy is done, patients are recommended to undergo endoscopic surveillance of the remaining tissue every six months (Giardiello et al., 2001).

OTHER HEREDITARY CANCER SYNDROMES

MEN2

Multiple endocrine neoplasia type 2 (MEN2) is an example of a cancer syndrome in which genetic testing offers a clear differentiation of those in need of treatment (surgical removal of the thyroid) and those who are spared a hereditary predisposition to cancer. MEN2 carriers have a 95% or higher lifetime risk of developing medullary thyroid cancer (Eng, 1996; O'Riordan et al., 1994) as well as risk for overstimulation of the adrenal glands caused by tumors called pheochromocytomas. Medullary thyroid cancer does not cause symptoms in its early stages and hence is often not found until it has metastasized, when it can be fatal. Surgical removal of the thyroid is relatively simple, and the consequences can be treated with medication. In some subtypes of MEN2, thyroid removal is recommended as early as 12 months of age (Van Heurn et al., 1999).

In 1993, direct mutation testing was introduced for the RET gene, an autosomal dominant gene responsible for MEN2. Genetic testing makes it possible for members of MEN2 families to discontinue the insufficiently sensitive biochemical testing that had previously been necessary from early childhood into the 30s to look for early indicators of thyroid cancer.

Although long-term psychological studies are not available, it is clear that determination of who needs thyroidectomy and who does not may not only save lives, but should also reduce the burden of repeated, imperfect biochemical screening of those not at risk. Short-term psychological findings suggest a need for intensive psychological and genetic counseling for patients prior to testing and a general reduction in distress after the immediate stress of testing subsides (Grosfeld et al., 1996). Parents are sometimes reluctant to act immediately on information provided by genetic testing and, to forgo the biochemical screening of their children on which they had previously relied (Grosfeld et al., 2000). Parental disagreement about which course of action to follow can generate familial distress. Identification of carriers at such early ages can lead to stigma and medicalization of the child, especially when other children in the family are found not to require special medical attention.

Psychological effects of MEN2 have been noted. Some children who test negative have reported feeling isolated within their family as attention is focused on mutation-positive siblings. Adults who test negative have felt guilty about relatives who are mutation carriers (Grosfeld et al., 1997). Children who are found to be carriers have suffered subsequent self-esteem losses. A case report describes trichotillomania (compulsive hair pulling), depression, and social withdrawal in a 13-year old girl who had a prophylactic thyroidectomy following genetic testing that showed she was a mutation carrier (Giarelli, 1999). Adults often do not share their concerns about MEN2 with friends, either before or after genetic testing. Communication within families about MEN2 often improves around the genetic testing of family members, although in some families there is a split between those who seek and those who avoid genetic testing (Grosfeld et al., 1996).

Li–Fraumeni Syndrome

Although there are recommended, surgical, risk-reducing treatments for FAP and MEN2, the diversity and unpredictability of tumors that can arise in patients with Li–Fraumeni syndrome (LFS) makes preventive action difficult. A rare autosomal dominant condition, LFS is characterized by the early appearance of cancers, typically including sarcoma, leukemia, breast cancer, brain tumors, and adrenocortical carcinoma (Li, Correa, & Fraumeni, 1991). Both adults and children are at risk. Lifetime cancer risk is 90% and the risk of developing cancer in childhood is about 40% (Williams & Strong, 1985). There is also a high rate of multiple primary cancers, that is, diagnosis of different types of cancer in the same individual (Hisada, Garber, Fung, Fraumeni, & Li, 1998). Mutation carriers have a 50% risk of passing the deleterious *p53* mutation to their offspring. Because these patients are known to be especially sensitive to radiation exposure, knowledge that a cancer patient is from an LFS family could alter treatment plans. Other than getting regular physicals and (for women) starting mammograms at earlier than usual ages, there are no specific recommendations for members of LFS families. These families often have devastating histories of cancer affecting multiple simultaneous generations. The death of several generations of parents at early ages has adverse financial effects as well.

Genetic testing for the *p53* mutations that have been found in the majority of LFS family members with cancer was instituted after the gene was cloned in 1991 (Malkin et al., 1991). For individuals deciding about whether to learn their *p53* status, the decision should be guided, at least in part, by the patient's psychological characteristics and anxiety about cancer risk; knowing one's hereditary risk status is not likely to alter screening to any great degree. On the other hand, testing can alleviate the fears of the 50% of noncarriers who may make different life decisions about reproduction, education, career, and so on after learning that they do not have a greatly magnified risk of cancer. The understandable ambivalence about knowing one's *p53* status is illustrated by the findings of a study of at-risk individuals from LFS families offered *p53* testing in a research program in which only 39% elected to undergo genetic testing (Patenaude et al., 1996).

Retinoblastoma

Rb1, the gene responsible for hereditary retinoblastoma, was the first gene found to convey a hereditary cancer predisposition. In most cases of hereditary retinoblastoma (a malignancy of the eye), cancer occurs in both eyes (bilaterally), an indication that the retinoblastoma has hereditary origins. Some inherited cases occur in only one eye (unilaterally), however. Genetic testing of these unilateral cases can clarify whether the disease is inherited. This differentiation has implications not only for the risk to the other eye, but also for the risk of developing other cancers. People with retinoblastoma also have a 50% likelihood of developing a second primary cancer (Desjardins, 1991). Children of hereditary retinoblastoma patients have a 50% risk of inheriting the deleterious mutation and thus a very high risk of developing retinoblastoma, whereas children of patients with sporadic retinoblastoma are not at increased risk.

INFORMATION ABOUT RARE CANCER SYNDROMES

There are many other syndromes that a patient might report in discussing his or her family history of cancer and related conditions. Information about rare syndromes or diseases can be obtained from the Genetic Alliance (http://www.geneticalliance.org) or the National Organization of Rare Diseases Foundation (http://www.rarediseases.org).

PROSTATE CANCER

Commercial genetic testing for prostate cancer genes is not yet a reality. A number of studies in the United States and abroad clearly indicate that there are familial patterns in the occurrence of prostate cancer (e.g., Matikainen et al., 2001; Steinberg, Carter, Beaty, Childs, & Walsh, 1990). Some suggest that there are one or more autosomal dominant genes, whereas others suggest X-linked inheritance, in which the predisposing gene is carried by mothers and transmitted only to their sons (Carter et al., 1992). Only one prostate cancer gene has been cloned to date (Tavtigian et al., 2001).

Age, race, and family history are the major risk factors for prostate cancer. It is estimated that 5% to 10% of prostate cancer is hereditary in origin. Having a brother or father with prostate cancer is thought to increase the risk to a male relative by 2 to 3 times the population risk (Stanford & Ostrander, 2001). This is especially true if the prostate cancer was diagnosed before the age of 55. African Americans have higher rates than Caucasian men, who, in turn, have higher rates of prostate cancer than Asian men (Whittemore et al., 1995). It is not known whether or how racial and hereditary predisposition interact.

As previously discussed in the section on breast cancer, there is an increased rate of prostate cancer among men with *BRCA1* or *BRCA2* mutations (Ford et al., 1994). There have also been reports of increased rates of prostate cancer among men with mutations in other cancer susceptibility genes, such as *p53* (Birch et al., 2001).

Screening tests for prostate cancer recommended for men over age 50 with general population risks (Littrup, Goodman, & Mettlin, 1993) include a PSA blood test and a digital rectal examination. Unfortunately, the specificity of the PSA test (about 75%) is not high (Offit, 1998), meaning that 25% of men with localized prostate cancer will have normal PSA values. Although there is much ongoing research aiming to try to improve the utility of PSA screening (e.g., Karazanashvili & Abrahamsson, 2003), to date there is no definitive proof of the efficacy of PSA screening for early detection of prostate cancer in men at increased hereditary risk for the disease. Men with family histories are nonetheless advised to begin PSA testing at an earlier age, age 40, than men in the general population (Offit, 1998). Although the psychological literature in this area is limited, studies suggest that men with a family history of prostate cancer do tend to undergo screening including a PSA test and digital rectal examination (Bock et al.,

2003) and that the men do not find screening to be psychologically distressing (Bratt, Emanuelsson, & Gronberg, 2003).

SUMMARY

Many people who are worried about their risk for cancer believe, in error, that definitive genetic testing is possible for everyone who wants to be tested. Useful testing is, in most cases, limited to those families in which a mutation can be pinpointed as occurring in one or more relatives who have developed cancer (usually, but not always, at early ages). This testing of an affected individual in the family provides the template or "address" against which others in the family can match up their own DNA to determine whether it has the same altered element or mutation. Only in this case can genetic testing provide the kind of yes-or-no answer that most people worried about hereditary cancer risk seek. When a negative test is found in this circumstance, people can be reasonably sure that they are not carriers. The risk of a false negative exists, but for commercially available genetic tests, the chance of this occurring is small. If there is concern about a false negative, measures such as repeating the test or doing the test in two laboratories may ensure the validity of the test.

The limits to the applications of genetic tests for cancer susceptibility may be critically important to share with patients who consider testing. Referral for genetic counseling is the surest way to help patients determine whether they are likely to find the answers they seek through genetic testing. It may be important as a first step to make sure patients understand that testing is not equally useful to all who might seek it. This can help them to understand the complexity of the task they are undertaking and the risk for personal disappointment if definitive testing proves to be impossible.

Another risk of genetic counseling and testing is that people seeking information about risk for one type of cancer may receive information about their risks not only for the type of cancer they are worried about but also for a variety of other cancers. Some may experience this as receiving more information than they wanted, others may experience it as overwhelming and paralyzing. Patients may feel it is difficult to stop the process of being informed about cancer risks once it is initiated. Other people with different personality characteristics welcome receiving as much information as possible about their risks and are grateful to learn anything that may prevent cancer in themselves or their relatives. Certainly some of the variance among reactions to genetic testing for cancer may have to do with personality differences between "monitors" who actively seek out health-related information and "blunters" who prefer not to focus on risks and uncertainty related to their health (Miller, 1996). People's reactions to risk notification for one or more cancers may also have to do with the manner in which the information is presented, the framing of the risks, and the degree to which the imminence of the threat is graded according to the age and gender of the individual. Another factor in how people hear information about their risk for cancer genes is their family situation, both their current families and the family cancer history that they carry. Having a young-adult daughter who may be at very high cancer risk in a family in which the mother has had breast or ovarian cancer and an aunt died from breast cancer at an early age may make the prospect of finding out the young woman's risk stressful for all family members. Learning about additional cancer risks for cancers the family had not previously experienced may feel like the proverbial straw that breaks the back of the family member's composure while awaiting results. On the other hand, a man with no children or with only young sons who is being tested for BRCA1 in a research endeavor may have relatively low levels of anxiety, possibly even after he realizes that he and his sons may have some increased cancer risk if he is shown to be a carrier.

Understanding that there are significant emotional, ethical, and legal implications of genetic testing for breast and ovarian cancer, the Ethical, Legal, and Social Implications Program of the Human Genome Project has provided funding for studies of the psychological and social ramifications of genetic testing for breast and ovarian cancer. These studies revealed, among other things, that ambivalence about being tested is far greater than expected among at-risk people. Only one quarter to one third of those eligible for BRCA1/2 testing accepted invitations for free testing in research programs studying the impact of genetic counseling and testing (Lerman et al., 1996; Patenaude et al., 1996).

Information about cancer predisposition genes is constantly changing. It is less than a decade since the discovery of major cancer predisposition genes. Even after all the major genes are identified, there will be new findings about the efficacy of preventive or risk-reducing options and about gene-environment interactions. It can be helpful to discuss with patients the changeable nature of cancer genetic information. Knowing that the scientific underpinnings of recommendations for mutation carriers may change over time might help some patients feel it is legitimate to wait to decide on a course of action, for example, to decide whether to undergo prophylactic surgery. This would be especially true if the evidence currently available is equivocal about what is helpful in their circumstance. Other patients may be eager to do something immediately and to follow any professional recommendations. They will be most comforted by the current recommendations that are backed by strong supporting evidence, such as the recommendation for prophylactic mastectomy for women at high or moderate risk of breast cancer. Others may use a psychotherapeutic consultation or ongoing psychotherapy to decide that, for them, doing nothing but surveillance in the short term is the preferred option, and a reasonable one. They may feel that until more definitive advice is available about the value of various risk-reducing options or until options are available with less burden to their quality of life, they would prefer to be screened at regular intervals by competent doctors.

Patients should be encouraged to check with medical professionals routinely about new data relevant to the decisions they face. The roles of psychotherapists with patients concerned about hereditary cancer are varied. They include supporting patients through the emotionally evocative process of gathering information about family history and helping them make decisions about whether to seek genetic counseling or testing. Whether or not patients seek genetic testing, high-risk individuals must decide which screening or risk-reduction options to accept and which to forgo. A therapist (and especially a therapist who is knowledgeable about the issues related to their dilemma) can help patients make decisions consistent with their personality style, their emotional and financial resources, and the availability of social support.

Individuals who are members of families affected by rare cancer syndromes may be particularly subject to frustration and fear related to their family experience. Many of these syndromes are unfamiliar to primary care providers and others. Often family members have been told that there is no relationship between the cancers or other conditions of various family members, only to learn later that they are all part of a hereditary cancer syndrome. Once the characteristics of the syndrome become clear to family members, many become experts on the syndrome, reading everything they can find and finding similarly affected people through rare-disease listservs or other support mechanisms. In turn, they often find themselves educating medical professionals with whom they come in contact about the syndrome. Others, such as teachers and therapists, also need education about the condition and its implications. It can be frustrating for patients to know more than the professionals who care for them about what the hereditary cancer syndrome in their family consists of and how it may affect family members.

REFERENCES

Aarnio, M., Mecklin, J. P., Aaltonen, L. A., Nystrom-Lahti, M., & Jarvinen, H. J. (1995). Life-time risk of different cancers in hereditary non-polyposis colorectal cancer (HNPCC) syndrome. *International Journal of Cancer, 64,* 430–433.

Birch, J. M., Alston, R. D., McNally, R. J., Evans, D. G., Kelsey, A. M., Harris, M., et al. (2001). Relative frequency and morphology of cancers in carriers of germline *Tp53* mutations. *Oncogene, 20,* 4621–4628.

Bisgaard, M. L., Fenger, K., Bulow, S., Niebuhr, E., & Mohr, J. (1994). Familial adenomatous polyposis (FAP): Frequency, penetrance, and mutation rate. *Human Mutation, 3,* 121–125.

Bloom, J. R., Stewart, S. L., Johnston, M., & Banks, P. (1998). Intrusiveness of illness and quality of life in young women with breast cancer. *Psycho-Oncology, 7,* 89–100.

Bock, C. H., Peyser, P. A., Gruber, S. B., Bonnell, S. E., Tedesco, K. L., & Cooney, K. A. (2003). Prostate cancer early detection practices among men with a family history of disease. *Urology, 62,* 470–475.

Bratt, O., Emanuelsson, M., & Gronberg, H. (2003). Psychological aspects of screening in families with hereditary prostate cancer. *Scandinavian Journal of Urology and Nephrology, 37,* 5–9.

Breast Cancer Linkage Consortium. (1999). Cancer risks in *BRCA2* mutation carriers. *Journal of the National Cancer Institute, 91,* 1310–1316.

Brown, G. J. E., St. John, D. J. B., Macrae, F. A., & Aittomaki, K. (2001). Cancer risk in young women at risk for hereditary surveillance in nonpolyposis colorectal cancer: Implications for gynecologic surveillance. *Gynecologic Oncology, 80,* 346–349.

Burke, W., Petersen, G., Lynch P., Botkin, J., Daly, M., Garber, J., et al., & the Cancer Genetics Studies Consortium. (1997). Recommendations for follow-up care of individuals with an inherited predisposition to cancer. *Journal of the American Medical Association, 277,* 915–919.

Carter, B. S., Beaty, T. H., Steinberg, G. D., Childs, B., & Walsh P. C. (1992). Mendelian inheritance of familial prostate cancer. *Proceedings of the National Academy of Science USA, 89,* 3367–3371.

Chlebowski, R. T., Col, N., Winer, E. P., Collyar, D. E., Cummings, S. R., Vogel, V. G., III, et al. (2002). American Society of Clinical Oncology technology assessment of pharmacologic interventions for breast cancer risk reduction including tamoxifen, raloxifene, and aromatase inhibition. *Journal of Clinical Oncology, 20,* 3328–3343.

Day, R., Ganz P. A., Constantino, J. P., Cronin, W. M., Wickerman, D. L., & Fisher, B. (1999). Health-related quality of life and tamoxifen in breast cancer prevention: A report from the National Surgical Adjuvant Breast and Bowel Project P-1 study. *Journal of Clinical Oncology, 17,* 2659–2669.

Desjardins, L., Haye, C., Schlienger, P., Laurent, M., Zucker, J. M., & Bouguila, H. (1991). Second non-ocular tumours in survivors of bilateral retinoblastoma: A 30-year follow-up. *Opthalmic Paediatrics & Genetics, 12,* 145–148.

Dunlop, M. G., Farrington, S. M., Carothers, A. D., Wyllie, A. H., Sharp, L., Burn, J., et al. (1997). Cancer risk associated with germline DNA mismatch repair gene mutations. *Human Molecular Genetics, 6,* 105–110.

Dunn, J., & Steginga, S. K. (2000). Young women's experience of breast cancer: Defining young and identifying concerns. *Psycho-Oncology, 9,* 137–146.

Easton, D. F. (1994). Cancer risks in AT heterozygotes. *International Journal of Radiation Biology, 66* (Suppl. 6), S177–S182.

Easton, D. F., Ford, D., Bishop, D. T., & the Breast Cancer Linkage Consortium. (1995). Breast and ovarian cancer incidence in BRCA1-mutation carriers. *American Journal of Human Genetics, 56*, 265–271.

Eeles, R. A. (2000). Screening for hereditary cancer and genetic testing, epitomized by breast cancer. *European Journal of Cancer, 35*, 1954–1962.

Eisinger, F., Charafef-Jauffret, E., Jacquemier, J., Birnbaum, D., Julian-Reynier, C., & Sobol, H. (2001). Tamoxifen and breast cancer risk in women harboring a BRCA1 germline mutation: Computed efficacy, effectiveness and impact. *International Journal of Oncology, 18*, 5–10.

Eng, C. (1996). Seminars in medicine of the Beth Israel Hospital, Boston. The RET proto-oncogene in multiple endocrine neoplasia type 2 and Hirschsprung's disease. *New England Journal of Medicine, 335*(13), 943–951.

Eng, C. (2000). Will the real Cowden syndrome please stand up: Revised diagnostic criteria. *Journal of Medical Genetics, 37*, 828–830.

Fallowfield, L., Flessig, A., Edwards, R., West, A., Powles, T. J., Howell, A., & Cuzick, J. (2001). Tamoxifen for the prevention of breast cancer: Psychosocial impact on women participating in two randomized controlled trials. *Journal of Clinical Oncology, 19*, 1885–1892.

Fisher, B., Constantino, J., Wickerham, D., Redmond, C., Kavanah, M., Cronin, W., et al. (1998). Tamoxifen for prevention of breast cancer: Report of the National Surgical Adjuvant Breast and Bowel Project P-1 Study. *Journal of the National Cancer Institute, 90*, 1371–1388.

Ford, D., & Easton, D. F. (1995). The genetics of breast and ovarian cancer. *British Journal of Cancer, 72*, 805–812.

Ford, D., Easton, D. F., Bishop, D. T., Narod, S. A., & Goldgar, D. E., for the Breast Cancer Linkage Consortium. (1994). Risks of cancer in BRCA1-mutation-carriers. *Lancet, 343*, 692–695.

Ford, D., Easton, D. F., Stratton, M., Narod, S., Goldgar, D., Devilee, P., et al. (1998). Genetic heterogeneity and penetrance analysis of the BRCA1 and BRCA2 genes in breast cancer families. *American Journal of Human Genetics, 62*, 676–689.

Ganguly, A., Citron, M., Gomilow, L., Citron, M., Godmilow, L., Ahrens, M., & Ganguly, T. (2001). Caucasian family with two independent mutations: 2594delC in BRCA1 and 5392AG in BRCA2 gene. *American Journal of Medical Genetics, 101*, 146–152.

Gayther, S. A., Warren, W., Mazoyer, S., Russell, P. A., Harrington, P. A., Chiano, M., et al. (1995). Germline mutations of the BRCA1 gene in breast and ovarian cancer families provide evidence for a genotype-phenotype correlation. *Nature Genetics, 11*, 428–433.

Giardiello, F. M., Brensinger, J. D., & Petersen, G. (2001). American Gastroenterology Association technical review on hereditary colorectal cancer and genetic testing. *Gastroenterology, 121*, 199–213.

Giarelli, E. (1999). Spiraling out of control: One case of pathologic anxiety as a response to a genetic risk of cancer. *Cancer Nursing, 22*, 327–339.

Goodheart, C. D. (1998). Psychological interventions in adult disease management. In G. Koocher, J. Norcross, & S. Hill (Eds.), *The psychologist's desk reference* (pp. 321–325). New York: Oxford University Press.

Grann, V. R., Jacobson, J. S., Whang, W., Hershman, D. L., Heitjan, D. F., Antman, K. H., & Neugut, A. I. (2000). Prevention with tamoxifen or other hormones versus prophylactic surgery in BRCA1/2-postive women with BRCA1/2 mutations. *Cancer Journal From Scientific American, 5,* 283–292.

Greene, M. (1997). Genetics of breast cancer. *Mayo Clinic Proceedings, 72,* 54–65.

Grosfeld, F. J. M., Beemer, F. A., Lips, C. J. M., Hendriks, K. S. W. H., & ten Kroode, H. E. J. (2000). Parents' responses to disclosure of genetic test results of their children. *American Journal of Medical Genetics, 94,* 316–323.

Grosfeld, F. J. M., Lips, C. J. M., Beemer, F. A., van Spikjer, H. G., Brouwers-Smalbraak, G. J., & ten Kroode, H. F. J. (1997). Psychological risks of genetically testing children for a hereditary cancer syndrome. *Patient Education and Counseling, 32,* 63–67.

Grosfeld, F. J. M., Lips, C. J. M., ten Kroode, H. F. J., Beemer, F. A., van Spijker, H. G., & Brouwers-Smalbraak, G. J. (1996). Psychosocial consequences of DNA analysis for MEN type 2. *Oncology, 10,* 141–157.

Gryfe, R., Kim, H. J., Hsieh, E. T. K., Aronson, M. D., Holowaty, E. J., Bull, S. B., et al. (2000). Tumor microsatellite instability and clinical outcome in young patients with colorectal cancer. *New England Journal of Medicine, 342,* 69–77.

Herrerra, L. (1990). *Familial adenomatous polyposis.* New York: Liss.

Hisada, M., Garber, J. E., Fung, C. Y., Fraumeni, J. F., & Li, F. P. (1998). Multiple primary cancers in families with Li–Fraumeni syndrome. *Journal of the National Cancer Institute, 90,* 606–611.

Jarvinen, H. J., Aarnio, M., Mustonen, H., Aktan-Collan, K., Aaltonen, L. A., Peltomaki, P., et al. (2000). Controlled 15-year trial on screening for colorectal cancers in families with heredity nonpolyposis colorectal cancer. *Gastroenterology, 118,* 829–834.

Johannsson, O. T., Ranstam, J., Borg, A., & Olsson, H. (1998). Survey of BRCA1 breast and ovarian cancer patients: A population-based study from southern Sweden. *Journal of Clinical Oncology, 16,* 397–404.

Karazanashvili, G., & Abrahamsson, P. A. (2003). Prostate specific antigen and human glandular kallikrein 2 in early detection of prostate cancer. *Journal of Urology, 169,* 445–457.

Kinzler, K. W., Nilbert, M. C., Su, L. K., Vogelstein, B., Bryan, T. M., Levy, D. B., et al. (1991). Identification of FAP locus genes from chromosome 5q21. *Science, 253,* 661–665.

Lal, G., & Gallinger, S. (2000). Familial adenomatous polyposis. *Seminars in Surgical Oncology, 18,* 314–323.

Lee, J. S., Wacholder, S., Struewing, J. P., McAdams, M., Pee, D., Brody, L. C., et al. (1999). Survival after breast cancer in Ashkenazi Jewish BRCA1 and BRCA2 mutation carriers. *Journal of the National Cancer Institute, 91,* 259–263.

Lerman, C., Daly, M., Masny, A., & Balshem, A. (1994). Attitudes about genetic testing for breast-ovarian cancer susceptibility. *Journal of Clinical Oncology, 12,* 843–850.

Lerman, C., Narod, S., Schulman, K., Hughes, C., Gomez-Caminero, A., Bonney, G., et al. (1996). *BRCA1* testing in families with hereditary breast-ovarian cancer. A prospective study of patient decision making and outcomes. *Journal of the American Medical Association, 275,* 1885–1892.

Lerman, C., Seay, J., Balshem, A., & Audrain, J. (1995). Interest in genetic testing among first-degree relatives of breast cancer patients. *American Journal of Medical Genetics, 57,* 385–392.

Li, F. P., Correa, P., & Fraumeni, J. F., Jr. (1991). Testing for germline *p53* mutations in cancer families. *Cancer, Epidemiology, Biomarkers, and Prevention, 1,* 91–94.

Littrup, P. J., Goodman, A. C., & Mettlin, C. J. (1993). The benefit and cost of prostate cancer early detection. *CA: Cancer Journal for Clinicians, 43,* 134–149.

Lynch, H. T., & Lynch, J. F. (2000). Hereditary nonpolyposis colorectal cancer. *Seminars in Surgical Oncology, 18,* 305–313.

Malkin, D., Li, F. P., Strong, L. C., Fraumeni, J. F., Nelson, C. E., Kim, D. H., et al. (1991). Germline *p53* mutations in a familial syndrome for breast cancer, sarcomas, and other neoplasms. *Science, 250,* 1233–1238.

Malone, K. E., Daling, J. R., Neal, C., Suter, N. M., O'Brien, C., Cushing-Haugen, K., et al. (2000). Frequency of *BRCA1/BRCA2* mutations in a population-based sample of young breast carcinoma cases. *Cancer, 88,* 1393–1402.

Matikainen, M. P., Pukkala, E., Schleutker, J., Tammela T. L., Koivisto, P., Sankila, R., et al. (2001). Relatives of prostate cancer patients have an increased risk of prostate and stomach cancers: A population-based cancer registry study in Finland. *Cancer Causes and Control, 12,* 223–230.

Miki, Y., Swensen, J., Shattuck-Eidens, D., Futreal, P. A., Harshman, K., Tavtigian, S., et al. (1994). A strong candidate for the breast and ovarian cancer susceptibility gene *BRCA1. Science, 266,* 66–71.

Miller, S. M. (1996). Monitoring and blunting of threatening information. In I. G. Sarason, G. R. Pierce, & B. R. Sarason (Eds.), *Cognitive interference: Theories, models and findings* (pp. 175–190). Hillsdale, NJ: Erlbaum.

National Cancer Institute. (2004). *Genetics of colorectal cancer (PDQ).* Retrieved February 2, 2004, from http://www.cancer.gov/cancerinfo/pdq/genetics/colorectal

National Cancer Institute Physicians Data Query. (2004). *Genetics of breast and ovarian cancer.* Retrieved January 14, 2002, from http://cancer.gov/cancerinfo/pdq/genetics/breast-and-ovarian

Oddoux, C., Streuwing, J. P., Clayton, C. M., Neuhausen, S., Brody, L. C., Kaback, M., et al. (1996). The carrier frequency of the *BRCA2* 617delT mutation among Ashkenazi Jewish individuals is approximately 1%. *Nature Genetics, 14,* 188–190.

Offit, K. (1998). *Clinical cancer genetics: Risk counseling and management*. New York: Wiley-Liss.

Open Access On-Line Breast Cancer Mutation Database. (n.d.). Retrieved June 6, 2002, from http://research.nhgri.nih.gov/bic/

O'Riordan, D. S., O'Brien, T., Weaver, A. L., Gharib, H., Hay, I. D., Grant, C. S., et al. (1994). Medullary thyroid carcinoma in multiple endocrine neoplasia types 2A and 2B. *Surgery, 116*, 1017–1023.

Ozcelik, H., Schmocker, B., DiNicola, N., Shi, X., Langer, B., Moore, M., et al. (1997). Germline *BRCA2* 6174delT mutations in Ashkenazi Jewish pancreatic cancer patients. *Nature Genetics, 16*, 17–18.

Patenaude, A. F., Schneider, K. A., Kieffer, S. A., Calzone, K. A., Stopfer, J. E., Basili, L. A., et al. (1996). Acceptance of invitations for *p53* and *BRCA1* predisposition testing: Factors influencing potential utilization of cancer genetic testing. *Psycho-Oncology, 5*, 241–250.

Schneider, K. (2002). *Counseling about cancer* (2nd ed.). New York: Wiley-Liss.

Simard, J., Tonin, P., Durocher, F., Morgan, K., Rommens, J., Gingras, S., et al. (1994). Common origins of *BRCA1* mutations in Canadian breast and ovarian cancer families. *Nature Genetics, 8*, 392–398.

Stanford, J. L., & Ostrander, E. A. (2001). Familial prostate cancer. *Epidemiology Review, 23*, 19–23.

Steinberg, G. D., Carter, B. S., Beaty, T. H., Childs, B., & Walsh, P. C. (1990). Family history and the risk of prostate cancer. *Prostate, 17*, 337–347.

Stoppa-Lyonnet, D., Ansquer, Y., Dreyfus, H., Gautier, C., Cauthier-Villars, M., Bourstyn, E., et al. (2000). Familial invasive breast cancers: Worse outcome related to *BRCA1* mutations. *Journal of Clinical Oncology, 18*, 4053–4059.

Stratton, J. F., Pharoah, P., Smith, S. K., Easton, D., & Ponder, B. A. (1998). A systematic review and meta-analysis of family history and ovarian cancer. *British Journal of Obstetrics and Gynecology, 105*, 493–499.

Struewing, J. P., Abveliovich, D., Peretz, T., Avishai, N., Kaback, M. M., Collins, F. S., et al. (1995a). The carrier frequency of the *BRCA1* 185delAG mutation is approximately 1 percent in Ashkenazi Jewish individuals. *Nature Genetics, 11*, 198–200.

Struewing, J. P., Brody, L. C., Erdos, M. R., Kase, R. G., Giambarresi, T. R., Smith, S. A., et al. (1995b). Detection of eight *BRCA1* mutations associated in 10 breast/ovarian cancer families, including 1 family with male breast cancer. *American Journal of Human Genetics, 57*, 1–7.

Struewing, J. P., Hartge, P., Wacholder, S., Baker, S. M., Berlin, M., McAdams, M., et al. (1997). The risk of cancer associated with specific mutations of *BRCA1* and *BRCA2* among Ashkenazi Jews. *New England Journal of Medicine, 336*, 1401–1408.

Swift, M., Morrell, D., Massey, R. B., & Chase, C. L. (1991). Incidence of cancer in 161 families affected with ataxia-telangiectasia. *New England Journal of Medicine, 325*, 1831–1836.

Syngal, S., Fox, E. A., Eng, C., Kolodner, R. D., & Garber, J. E. (2000). Sensitivity and specificity of clinical criteria for hereditary non-polyposis colorectal cancer associated mutations in MSH2 and MLH1. *Journal of Medical Genetics, 37,* 641–645.

Syngal, S., Fox, E. A., Li, F. P., Dovidio, M., Eng., C., Kolodner, R. D., & Garber, J. E. (1999). Interpretation of genetic test results for hereditary nonpolyposis colorectal cancer: Implications for clinical predisposition testing. *Journal of the American Medical Association, 282,* 247–253.

Tavtigian, S. V., Simard, J., Teng, D. H. F., Abtin, V., Baumgard, M., Beck, A., et al. (2001). A candidate prostate cancer susceptibility gene at chromosome 17p. *Nature Genetics, 27,* 172–180.

Thorlacius, S., Olafsdottir, G., Tryggvadottir, L., Neuhausen, S., Jonasson, J. G., Tavtigian, S. V., et al. (1996). A single BRCA2 mutation in male and female breast cancer families from Iceland with varied cancer phenotypes. *Nature Genetics, 13,* 117–119.

Van Heurn, L. W., Schaap, C., Sie, G., Haagen, A. A., Gerver, W. J., Freling, G., et al. (1999). Predictive DNA testing for multiple endocrine neoplasia 2: A therapeutic challenge of prophylactic thyroidectomy in very young children. *Journal of Pediatric Surgery, 34,* 568–571.

Vasen, H. F. (2000). Clinical diagnosis and management of hereditary colorectal cancer syndromes. *Journal of Clinical Oncology, 182* (Suppl. 21), 81S–92S.

Vasen, H. F., Wijnen, J. T., Menko, F. H., Kleibeuker, J. H., Taal, B. G., Griffioen, G., et al. (1996). Cancer risk in families with hereditary nonpolypsis colorectal cancer diagnosed by mutation analysis. *Gastroenterology, 110,* 1020–1027.

Verhoog, L. C., Brekelmans, C. T. M., Seynaeve, C., van den Bosch, L. M. C., Dahmen, G., van Geel, A. N., et al. (1998). Survival and tumour characteristics of breast-cancer patients with germline mutations of BRCA1. *Lancet, 351,* 316–321.

Vogel, V. G., Costantino, J. P., Wickerham, D. L., Cronin, W. M., & Wolmark, N. (2002). The study of tamoxifen and raloxifene: Preliminary enrollment data from a randomized breast cancer risk reduction trial. *Clinical Breast Cancer, 3,* 153–159.

Ward, R., Meldrum, C., Williams, R., Mokany, E., Scott, R., Turner, J., et al. (2002). Impact of microsatellite testing and mismatch repair protein expression on the clinical interpretation of genetic testing in hereditary non-polyposis colorectal cancer. *Journal of Cancer Research and Clinical Oncology, 128,* 403–411.

Watson, P., Butzow, R., Lynch, H. T., Jukka-Pekka, M., Jarvinen, H. J., Vasen, H. F., et al. (2001). The clinical features of ovarian cancer in hereditary nonpolyposis colorectal cancer. *Gynecologic Oncology, 82,* 223–228.

Watson, P., & Lynch, H. T. (1993) Extracolonic cancer in hereditary nonpolyposis colorectal cancer. *Cancer, 71,* 677–685.

Watson, P., Vasen, H. F., Mecklin, J. P., Jarvinen, H., & Lynch, H. T. (1994). The risk of endometrial cancer in hereditary nonpolyposis colorectal cancer. *American Journal of Medicine, 96,* 516–520.

Williams, W. R., & Strong, L. C. (1985). Genetic epidemiology of soft tissue sarcomas in children. In H. Mueller & W. Webers (Eds.), *Familial cancer* (pp. 151–153). Basel, Switzerland: Karger.

Whittemore, A. S., Wu, A. H., Kolonel, L. N., John, E. M., Gallagher, R. P., Howe, G. R., et al. (1995). Family history and prostate cancer risk in black, white, and Asian men in the United States and Canada. *American Journal of Epidemiology, 141,* 732–740.

Wooster, R., Bignell, G., Lancaster, J., Swift, S., Seal, S., Mangion, J., et al. (1995). Identification of the breast cancer susceptibility gene BRCA2. *Nature, 378,* 789–792.

3

GENETIC COUNSELING
FOR CANCER GENES

Genetic counseling is the translation center where genetic advances are transformed into risk estimates for at-risk populations, one individual at a time. Cancer genetic counseling is a subspecialty that requires an amalgam of skills and knowledge from the fields of genetics, oncology, and psychology. An increasing number of high-risk genetics clinics, at cancer centers and other hospitals, now offer genetic counseling for cancer predisposition. An oncologist or geneticist may be in charge of the clinic and may provide some of the medical information at the counseling session.

Cancer genetic counseling did not exist 15 years ago; today there are too few counselors to keep up with demand, and thus other professionals are stepping in to provide these services (Kieffer & Vockely, 1997). Specially trained oncology nurses are providing genetic counseling in many centers (Dimond, Calzone, Davis, & Jenkins, 1998), and primary care physicians (Watson, Shickle, Qureshi, Emery, & Austoker, 1999) are being offered training opportunities to help them appropriately refer patients or to provide counseling themselves. Serious questions surround the issues of how much counseling is necessary, who should provide it, and how those at risk for hereditary conditions will pay for counseling (Cummings, 2000).

An important role for mental health professionals working with a patient who is struggling with unresolved questions or fears related to hereditary cancer risk is to help him or her understand the benefits that cancer genetic counseling can provide and, if desired, help the patient locate appropriate services. Even knowing that not all genetic counselors are trained in the delivery of cancer genetic risk information can be helpful. With time and experience, a therapist may come to know and collaborate with local cancer genetic counselors who can facilitate patient referral when it is needed. Some patients may prefer to seek genetic counseling from their physician. Psychologists knowledgeable about cancer genetic counseling and testing can help patients formulate the questions they want genetic counselors to answer and find who can best provide such information.

WHO ARE GENETIC COUNSELORS?

The first graduating class of genetic counselors finished their training in 1971. Some of the oldest and best known genetic counseling programs in the United States are those at Sarah Lawrence College, Brandeis University, University of California at Berkeley and Irvine, University of Wisconsin, and Rutgers University, but there are about 25 genetic counseling training programs in the United States (National Society of Genetic Counselors, n.d.). Genetic counselors typically have a master's degree in genetic counseling, public health, or a related field. Certification as a genetic counselor occurs through a national board exam given by the American Board of Genetic Counseling every three years. In the United States, there are currently several thousand genetic counselors. To date, it has been a largely female profession, possibly because, before the advent of cancer genetics, the patients of genetic counselors were primarily pregnant women. The number of male counselors may well increase in the coming years, especially as genes related to cancers in men, such as prostate or testicular cancer, are found.

Basic coursework for genetic counselors includes the study of molecular and reproductive biology, human and medical genetics, counseling skills, and research methodology. Additional courses may be taken in psychology, health policy, biomedical law, and medical sociology (Brandeis University Genetic Counseling Program, 1998).

Genetic counselors do internships as well as coursework and are typically supervised by senior genetic counselors in hospitals or clinics. They work in close relationship to geneticists, oncologists, or surgeons, often seeing patients together or in sequence during the same visit. Some genetic counselors work in private practice, and others work for clinical laboratories that do genetic testing.

Genetic counselors receive training in interviewing and, depending on their program, may also receive some training in the theory and practice of psychotherapy. Some genetic counselors have a special interest in the more psychotherapeutic aspects of their work and go on to receive additional psychotherapy training in psychology or marriage and family counseling programs. There is a Psychotherapy and Expanded Counseling Skills Special Interest Group within the National Society of Genetic Counselors. There are also at least a few psychologists who have been trained as genetic counselors.

Seymour Kessler is a doctoral-level geneticist and San Francisco Bay– area psychologist who has worked closely with genetic counselors for many decades. He has written a number of classic articles (now compiled in a book) that focus on the elements of counseling skills for the genetic counselor (Kessler, 2000). A wonderful essay, "Empathy and Decency," of value to both psychologists and genetic counselors, offers examples of how profession-als can offer genuine support to patients in difficult moments without losing sight of professional boundaries. He says, "These strategies neither require much time nor complex skills. They merely give voice to the natural thought-fulness and sensitivity we all have within us, characteristics that attracted us to the helping professions to begin with" (p. 106).

Mental health professionals, genetic counselors, and genetic nurses often work in harmonious, close relationships as members of genetic counsel-ing testing programs or research projects. Genetic counselors share with psychologists and social workers the challenges of being nonmedical profes-sionals working in medical settings. Their roles are complementary and overlap to some extent, but they are sufficiently different, in most cases, that major boundary issues or professional jealousies do not arise.

HOW TO FIND A CANCER GENETIC COUNSELOR

Fewer than 500 genetic counselors are specialists in cancer genetic counseling. These counselors have undertaken special training or apprentice-ships working with oncologists involved in seeing patients at high risk for hereditary cancers. There is a subset of cancer genetic counselors within the National Association of Genetic Counselors (http://www.nsgc.org) who form the Familial Cancer Risk Counseling Special Issues Group. There are not official standards for providing cancer genetic testing.

In trying to ascertain if a particular genetic counselor has cancer genetic counseling experience it would be useful to ask about the types of cancer the counselor has provided cancer genetic counseling for and how many cases they have seen, whether there is an oncologist connected to the program and whether the oncologist consults directly to the patients. The National Cancer Institute maintains a directory of individuals and labora-tories that provide cancer genetic counseling, or cancer genetic testing. The URL for those interested in finding a counselor in their area is: http://www.cancer.gov/search/genetics_services/.

In addition, local oncology clinics or the nearest Comprehensive Cancer Center should be able to provide referral to local cancer genetics counselors. The National Society of Genetic Counselors also has a Web site to help individuals locate cancer genetic counselors. The Web site for that list is http://www.nsgc.org/resourcelink.asp.

Mindful that genetic counseling is provided by individuals with diverse training, we shall refer to "genetic counselors" below as a generic term to mean those people trained to provide cancer genetic counseling.

COMPONENTS OF CANCER GENETIC COUNSELING: WHAT TO EXPECT

Cancer genetic counseling typically involves a minimum of two visits. The first visit usually takes between one and two hours (Schneider & Marnane, 1997). The second visit is usually about an hour and, if testing has been done, may include the disclosure of genetic test results. Depending on the patient's familiarity with the genetic cancer predisposition in their family and the principles of genetics and on their psychological state, patients may wish to schedule a second pretesting session to review what was discussed in the first session and to clarify misconceptions before making a final decision about testing (Peters & Stopfer, 1996; Richards et al., 1995). Patients vary enormously in the pacing of their genetic counseling experience. Some are already convinced that they want testing and may feel that any counseling is an unnecessary hurdle. Others may take years between learning that they are appropriate testing candidates and making a decision about whether they want testing. No one should be pushed to move more quickly than they feel they can in confronting genetic information and the choices that the knowledge engenders. On the other hand, psychotherapeutic counseling may help people who feel tormented by the options and paralyzed by their own incapacity to decide what is best for them.

PREVISIT

When a potential patient calls a cancer genetic counselor, the counselor will usually ask a few questions about the patient's family history or reasons for seeking counseling. This is to establish that the counseling is appropriate and that the counselor's skills are in the area of genetic counseling in which help is sought. The counselor will explain the plan for the visits that will take place. Some counselors may ask the patient to complete a family history form prior to the first visit. The counselor may also suggest that the patient bring a spouse, close friend, or companion to the visit. For some patients with extensive family experience with cancer, walking into a cancer unit or cancer center may give rise to painful memories. This is often an unexpected reaction, and it may be useful to discuss this possibility with patients.

FIRST VISIT

The first visit provides the opportunity to accomplish the following:

1. Determine the autonomy of the individual's request (i.e., the absence of coercion from other family members).
2. Determine the questions the person wants answered.
3. Offer and explain a risk estimate, on the basis of a pedigree drawn by the counselor.
4. Discuss the individual's risk for one or more types of cancer.
5. Explain testing and screening options.
6. Discuss the "fit" between the individual's style and the options available.
7. Plan for future referrals, consultations, and, if desired, genetic testing.
8. Discuss the importance of genetic information to other family members.

Autonomy

Autonomy is the cornerstone of informed consent. Although it may seem obvious, the first issues to be determined in seeing patients for genetic counseling are why they are there and whether they truly wish to receive the information that genetic counseling provides. During the first visit, the genetic counselor assesses the autonomy of the patient's involvement. Because of the intertwined needs of family members with regard to genetic information, the potential for coercion is higher in genetic counseling and testing than in most other medical circumstances. In asking about motivations and goals for testing or in talking about possible emotional risks of testing, a seasoned genetic counselor can often recognize a reluctant participant. A counselor will be alerted by uncomfortable, repeated, or anxious references to children or nieces or nephews seeking information about the genetic status in a patient who has had cancer when the patient does not truly seem to want to know his or her own risk status. A reluctant patient might also be an elderly mother who does not wish to know her own mutation status but whose daughter wants to know where to look for a mutation or a 21-year-old single woman whose sisters have all tested positive for a cancer gene and who have pushed her to find out if she carries the deleterious mutation as well.

Such pressures are often difficult to resist. The older woman may feel that she should do this for her daughter but feels anxious about receiving what she suspects will be a positive genetic test because she thinks it will lead to unremitting anxiety and remorse. Her style has been not to think about these things for many years, but after her daughter talked to her about testing, she is having difficulty sleeping, and thoughts of cancer and guilt about her daughter's risks preoccupy her. Likewise, the young woman in the other family may feel that her older sisters are in a better position to deal with the information genetic counseling provides. They have their husbands and their children; they can think about having their ovaries prophylactically removed. She doesn't have a serious boyfriend, has to think about finishing school and finding a job, and doesn't want to be drawn into their world of doctors and fear. Nonetheless, they seemed so well intentioned and they made the appointment for her, so she felt she had to go. In reality, she does not want to deal with this now. There will be time for thinking this through when she is older and more settled. She sees her doctor for regular breast exams and is too young for mammograms, she thinks, so why do this? Nonetheless, some gnawing worry, memories of her mother's death, and her sisters' pushing led her to keep the counseling appointment.

A basic tenet of cancer genetic counseling is that a patient's decision should represent his or her own wishes. Although altruism does motivate many relatives to be tested, if the wish to help others is not consonant with one's own feelings about testing, there will likely be adverse effects. By questioning and observing the patient, genetic counselors hope to be able to pick up any resistance. In genetic testing research programs in which standard psychological measures are a part of the protocol, scores on such measures may help to inform the counselor about the level of distress a patient is experiencing and whether additional evaluation or referral is needed. An experienced counselor can help patients tease apart their feelings and fears and consider what broader range of options may be available to both the patient and to those who might be depending on the result. The counselor might suggest that the mother think about the issues before proceeding and return to talk again or suggest that the mother and daughter come in to talk together about the options. The counselor might discuss with the young, college-age woman that nothing additional is recommended in terms of cancer surveillance for a woman her age, even if she were found to be positive for a cancer predisposition gene; thus no strong contraindication exists to her putting off further counseling and testing for another five years. The counselor might remind her that counseling could inform her of her risk and the options for surveillance or risk reduction but would then encourage her to make her own choices. Discussion of the possibility that more will be known in five years about the effectiveness of the options for mutation carriers and that additional options might be available could also help the young woman in defending her decision to her sisters. The counselor might also remind her that although her sisters were all positive, her own risk remains 50–50, meaning she has an even chance of not having inherited the mutation found in her family.

Depending on how upset the individual is or how unclear his or her wishes are, the genetic counselor might recommend that the patient talk with a psychologist or other mental health provider. A psychotherapist can help patients sort out the various pressures and emotions they are experiencing and help them deal with feelings within the family that genetic testing has aroused. Alternatively, if the genetic counselor is unsure of whether the observed or described distress is sufficient to merit psychological referral, he or she might first consult with a mental health provider to discuss the case.

Family History Taking

It is likely that the patient has given at least some family cancer history to a physician or other specialist before coming for genetic counseling to establish the level of risk in the family. A genetic counselor is likely to take a more extensive and careful family history than those previously taken, asking in detail about the specific kinds of cancer that relatives have had, the age of the relative at diagnosis, and any special features (e.g., cancer in both breasts, or bilaterality). In addition, the counselor (especially if she or he is involved in a research program) may initiate efforts to verify the prior cancer diagnoses reported. This would involve getting permission from the patient for the counselor to receive medical record verification of the diagnoses. It could also involve direct contact between the counselor and some relatives, if they are willing to be contacted for questioning about the nature of their cancer. Sometimes patients initiate medical record searches for definitive information about relatives' cancer diagnoses. (Psychological considerations of such endeavors are discussed later in the chapter; see Hazards of Gathering Family History Information.)

Because some ethnic groups tend to have higher rates of adverse mutations, the discussion with the genetic counselor is likely to include questions about the cultural and geographic backgrounds of the patient's parents and his or her families. The counselor will try to ascertain whether the individual is from one of the ethnic groups in which common founder mutations have been identified, such as Ashkenazi Jews, Icelanders, and French Canadians (Hopper & Jenkins, 1999).

Prior gathering of family history can be useful preparation for a genetic counselor visit. Gathering this information may involve asking some difficult questions of a number of relatives. As detailed in chapter 7, "A Family

Matter," this process can be challenging, and the consequences can span a full range from disturbing the equilibrium in some families to cementing cohesion or bringing back estranged members in other families.

Pedigree

At the first visit, the genetic counselor will begin to draw a pedigree for the patient based on the information provided. A pedigree is a systematized drawing depicting the relationship of blood relatives within a family and their current status (alive or dead) that incorporates information about when and where diseases have occurred within the family. Using the pedigree and one or more of the models for estimating cancer risks, the genetic counselor will be able to produce an estimate of the level of hereditary cancer risk that the individual carries. The counselor is looking for patterns or clues within the pedigree that suggest the presence of hereditary factors in the cancers that have occurred. These include, for example, early age of onset, multiple primary cancers, and other combinations of indications for particular syndromes (see chap. 2, "Cancer Genes and Cancer Risk," for more specific indicators). No single factor indicates by itself the presence of a hereditary cancer predisposition in the family, but taken together this information can help the counselor make more informed predictions about whether there are indications for an inherited predisposition, which gene or genes might be involved, and the estimated risk that any particular individual carries a deleterious mutation. In some cases, additional information or verification of diagnoses may be needed from the medical records of relatives to complete the pedigree.

Although psychologists are not usually called on to draw pedigrees, when working with a population with genetic health risks, it is useful to understand how to read a pedigree because they are an important part of the discussions that occur in determining a patient's risk.

The Power of the Pedigree

Considering the wealth of information condensed into an extended family pedigree, it is not surprising that construction and review of a pedigree can elicit strong emotions. The visual representation of the path of disease through a family is often a vivid reminder of the power an inherited disease has to disrupt family life. Recognition of a pattern suggesting an inherited cause of illness is easier to interpret in some cases than in others in which, even with a pedigree, the pattern may not be obvious. For example, in families with breast and ovarian cancer that have mostly male offspring or small family size, the presence of a deleterious *BRCA1* or *BRCA2* mutation may be much more difficult to spot than in a large kindred (extended family) with many daughters who develop breast and ovarian cancer at early ages.

Well-constructed pedigrees often can help genetics professionals spot hereditary cancer syndromes quickly. To watch a seasoned genetic counselor or geneticist interpret a pedigree is as impressive as listening to a seasoned psychotherapist evaluate and diagnose a patient in a brief interview. In both instances, the value of the finished product is only as good as the knowledge and skill of the person asking the questions. In the case of the pedigree, the person constructing it must know which features of the cancer are associated with hereditary etiologies and which nonmalignant conditions are associated with hereditary cancer syndromes.

The accuracy of the family history provided also influences the value of a pedigree. In chapter 7, "A Family Matter," I discuss the extent to which information that patients provide can be assumed to be accurate.

Pedigrees reveal extremely private information. Out-of-wedlock births, abortions, miscarriages, diagnoses and age at diagnosis, consanguinity, and so forth can all be diagrammed into a pedigree and are included because they may have diagnostic implications. It is valuable to bear in mind that a pedigree drawn in a conversation with one person in the family may reveal previously unknown information to other relatives, sometimes leading to shock or distress. Learning that one's family, and especially one's parent's, circumstances were not what one had always thought can be upsetting in long-lasting ways. Family members who wish to share a pedigree with other relatives as part of sharing the medical information about inherited disease they have received should be encouraged to think carefully about how and when to introduce the topic and the pedigree and about whether it might contain information that might be unknown to some family members.

Pedigrees, like snapshots, reflect the family circumstance at the particular time it was composed. Time alters the accuracy and utility of the information in a pedigree. Constant updating is crucial. The additional diagnoses, deaths, births, and other information that are added to a pedigree may help elucidate whether a cancer syndrome is present in the family. Sequential pedigrees of a Li–Fraumeni syndrome family (see chap. 2 for discussion of this syndrome), for example, can illustrate the impossibility of knowing early on from the pedigree that the pattern of cancers fit the criteria for the syndrome (Garber, Goldstein, Kantor, Dreyfus, Fraumeni, & Li, 1991). Pedigrees from the latest period clearly show the unusual pattern of adult and childhood cancers that would have led easily to the diagnosis of Li–Fraumeni syndrome by a cancer geneticist or genetic counselor. In the middle stages of a family history, a pedigree might suggest the syndrome to highly experienced professionals, but its identification would not have been easy and might well have been missed. The continuing evolution of a pedigree as the family history reveals more of the telltale signs of a hereditary cancer syndrome explains, in part, why some families have been frustrated and have had to wait sometimes several generations before their familial condition was recognized.

Although the symbols and abbreviations of a pedigree initially seem like a complex foreign language, the symbols used are actually quite limited in number. Basic familiarity with the pedigree nomenclature is not so difficult to accomplish, and the ability to read a pedigree fosters communication and a sense of genetic competence. Although efforts to unify pedigree nomenclature (Bennett et al., 1995) continue, there are some differences in the ways that groups represent the families they see. If unfamiliar markings appear, the genetics professional can be asked to explain the markings to the patient or therapist.

Basic Symbols

Pedigrees use standard symbols to denote an individual's gender, whether the person is affected (has ever had cancer or other illnesses in question), and whether the person is alive at the time of the pedigree construction. Figure 3.1 shows symbols that have been identified as standards by the Pedigree Standardization Task Force of the National Society of Genetic Counselors. Figure 3.2 illustrates how individual pedigree symbols are joined to reveal the family cancer history of an individual. Figure 3.3 shows that a single pedigree can be used to describe the family history of several illnesses in a single drawing.

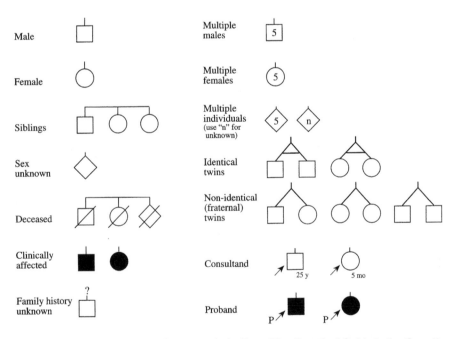

Figure 3.1. Most common pedigree symbols. From The *Practical Guide to the Genetic Family History* (p. 46), by R. L. Bennett, 1999, New York: Wiley-Liss. Copyright 1999 by Wiley-Liss, a subsidiary of John Wiley & Sons. Reprinted with permission.

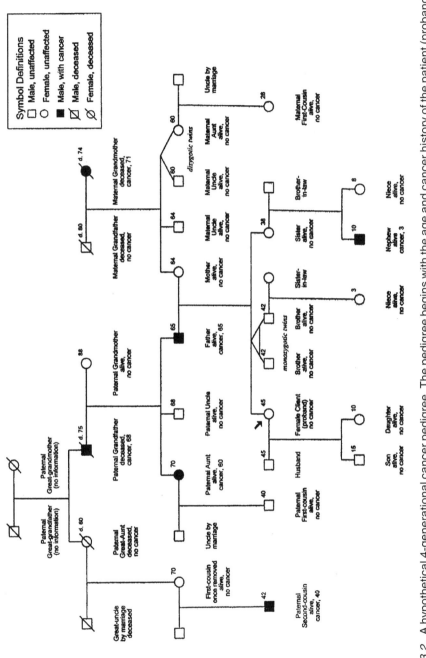

Figure 3.2. A hypothetical 4-generational cancer pedigree. The pedigree begins with the age and cancer history of the patient (proband) who is designated by an arrow. The 4-generational pedigree includes the following information on each relative: current status (alive or deceased), current age or age at death, and cancer history. From *Counseling About Cancer: Strategies for Genetic Counseling* (p. 317), by K. Schneider, 2002, New York: Wiley-Liss. Copyright 2002 by Wiley-Liss, a subsidiary of John Wiley & Sons. Reprinted with permission.

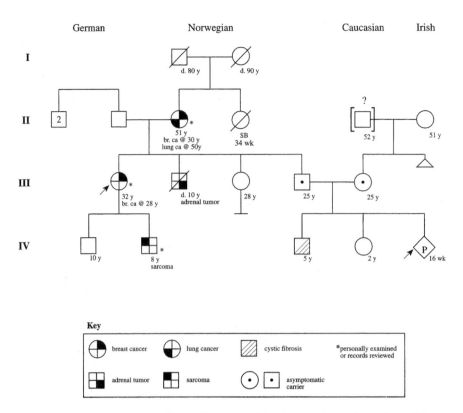

Figure 3.3. A hypothetical pedigree illustrating inheritance of a variety of conditions. From *The Practical Guide to the Genetic Family History* (p. 51), by R. L. Bennett, 1999, New York: Wiley-Liss. Copyright 1999 by Wiley-Liss, a subsidiary of John Wiley & Sons. Reprinted with permission.

Connotation of Relationships on a Pedigree

Pedigrees reflect the social relationships between family members with use of standard links. Marriage, divorce, remarriage, adoption, twinship, out-of-wedlock relationships bearing children, and so on can all be shown in the lines drawn between the symbols. Cancer diagnoses on a pedigree may be written out or may be denoted with the following initials (Bennett, 1999): BR for breast cancer, OV for ovarian cancer, CRC for colorectal cancer, BT for brain tumor, and LK for leukemia.

Creating Pedigrees

Several computer software programs are designed to draw and label pedigrees. The most commonly used are Cyrillic (Cherwell Scientific Publishing, 744 Antonio Road, Suite 27A, Palo Alto, CA 94303) and Progeny

(Progeny Software, LLC, 1025 Widener Lane, South Bend, IN 46614). The cost for the software is between $500 and $900. Patients may also make use of genealogy software available on the Internet to create their own pedigrees in anticipation of a genetic counseling visit.

Genograms

Daly et al. (1999) suggested that genograms designed for use in family therapy (McGoldrick & Gerson, 1985) can be usefully combined with the family history pedigree as an adjunct to genetic counseling. The genogram uses standardized lines drawn between individuals on the pedigree to describe the nature of the interaction between them (see Figure 3.4 for an explanation of the genogram symbols and an example of their use). Family relationships may have important implications for dissemination of genetic information within the family and for the impact of test results; therefore, combining the medical and emotional information into one drawing has clear benefits (see chap. 7, "A Family Matter," for elaboration of the ways in which familial relationships affect genetic testing). Genograms, however, are not appropriate to use with all patients. Some will resent any attempt to condense the complexity of their family interaction into a single representative drawing.

Risk Assessment

Did I Inherit a Cancer Gene?

The first part of the risk estimate involves the risk that the individual inherited a deleterious mutation in a gene that predisposes him or her to one or more types of cancer. The genetic counselor's review of the pedigree will establish the likelihood that a gene is responsible for the pattern of cancers in the family and which gene that is. The next question is to determine, on the basis of the pattern of cancers, the likelihood that the person being counseled inherited the mutated gene. Because most cancer predisposition genes are autosomal dominant, the estimate of the person's risk for having inherited a deleterious mutation will depend on how distant the individual is from a relative with the identified cancer or cancers where there is a known mutation. If the individual's parent had cancer attributable to hereditary effects, the individual seeking counseling has a 50–50 chance of having inherited the mutated gene. Similarly, if it is a sibling who has had a cancer of hereditary origin, there is also a 50% chance that he or she inherited the same mutation from their parents (assuming it is a full sibling).

Siblings, parents, and children are all considered first-degree relatives of the individual. If it is a grandmother, grandfather, aunt, or uncle (all

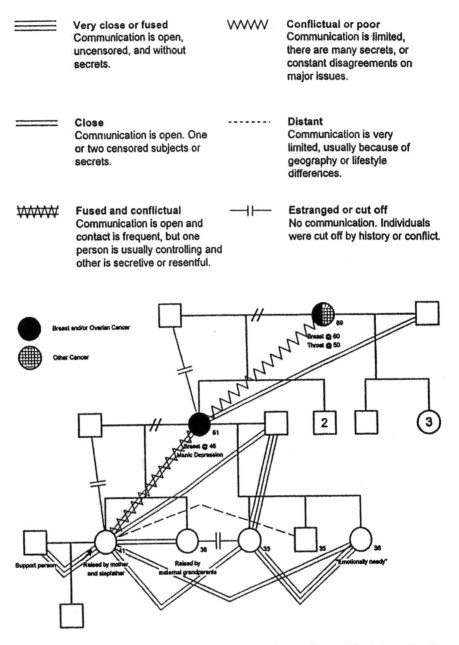

Very close or fused
Communication is open, uncensored, and without secrets.

Conflictual or poor
Communication is limited, there are many secrets, or constant disagreements on major issues.

Close
Communication is open. One or two censored subjects or secrets.

Distant
Communication is very limited, usually because of geography or lifestyle differences.

Fused and conflictual
Communication is open and contact is frequent, but one person is usually controlling and other is secretive or resentful.

Estranged or cut off
No communication. Individuals were cut off by history or conflict.

Breast and/or Ovarian Cancer

Other Cancer

Figure 3.4. A genogram and genogram symbols. From "Exploring Family Relationships in Cancer Risk Counseling Using the Genogram," by M. Daly et al., 1999, *Cancer Epidemiology, Biomarkers, and Prevention, 8,* p. 396. Copyright 1999 by American Association of Cancer Research. Reprinted with permission.

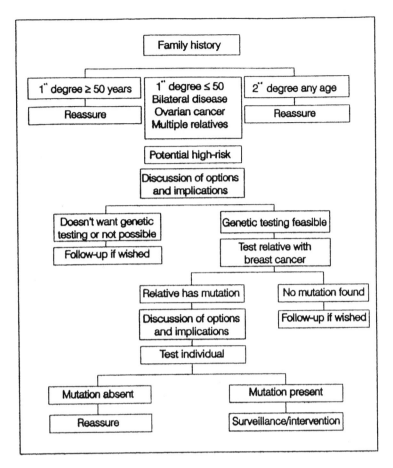

Figure 3.5. Steps in genetic investigation of women with a family history of breast/ ovarian cancer. From "Management of Women With a Family History of Breast Cancer," by P. Curry and I. S. Fentiman, 1999, *International Journal of Clinical Practice, 53,* p. 194. Copyright 1999 by Blackwell Synergy, a subsidiary of Blackwell Publishing, Inc. Reprinted with permission.

second-degree relatives) who had cancer of known hereditary origin, the risk estimate will be a 25% risk of having inherited the dominant, deleterious mutation. Other factors may play into the calculation as well. Figure 3.5 illustrates the steps in evaluation of hereditary risk for breast and ovarian cancer.

Several statistical models have been developed to calculate the risk that an individual will develop breast cancer. Each model takes into consideration some factors related to family history and other, nonhereditary factors, such as age. No model is ideal. The most commonly used are those by Gail and Benichou (1992) and Claus, Risch, and Thompson (1991). Because some models are better for estimating hereditary cancer risk than others

(Cummings, 2000; Rubinstein, O'Neill, Peters, Rittmeyer, & Stadler, 2002), the decision about which model to use will be made by the genetics professional on the basis of the nature of the family history data presented and on the individual's medical history. In addition, a computer program known as BRCAPRO (http://astor.som.jhmi.edu/brcapro/) calculates the likelihood that an individual carries a BRCA1/2 mutation and, from that, calculates age-specific breast cancer risk. From the pattern of cancers in the family history, it uses a Bayesian analysis to estimate the "conditioned" probability that a BRCA1/2 mutation is present. This method of risk estimation depends heavily on the penetrance estimate used and on knowledge of the frequency of mutated BRCA1/2 genes in the ethnic population to which the individual belongs. An extensive consideration of the pros and cons of each breast cancer risk estimation model can be found on the Internet in the National Cancer Institute PDQ Cancer Genetics Summary (http://www.cancer.gov/cancerinfo/pdq/genetics/breast-and-ovarian) in the section on Breast and Ovarian Cancer. It is not advisable for individuals without genetics training to use these models to estimate their own breast cancer risk. They should seek help from a genetics professional who understands the limitations of all risk estimation models.

Will I Get Cancer (or Get Cancer Again)?

This question is at the core of most genetic counseling sessions. If a cancer risk model or simple Mendelian estimates has been used, these form the basis of the scientific discussion. The discussion is typically even more complex than the discussion of the patient's risk of having inherited a deleterious mutation.

One important clarification is the period of time that the risk estimate covers. Cancer risk data can be broken down into the risk of developing cancer in the next 5 or 10 years, or it can be described as "lifetime risk." The lifetime risk of breast cancer is the risk that an individual will develop breast cancer at some point in his or her life, sometimes further defined as the risk to age 70 or the risk to age 85. Especially in forms of hereditary cancer in which the cancers occur at earlier than usual ages, this distinction is important and can be somewhat confusing. The risk in the general population for forms of cancer, such as breast cancer, goes up with age, especially after age 60. The risk of *hereditary* breast cancer, however, actually *declines* after age 50 because a hallmark of hereditary breast cancer is young age at diagnosis. Although the lifetime risk for a BRCA1/2 mutation carrier can be extremely high, if the person reaches age 60 without developing breast or ovarian cancer, her risk of getting breast cancer caused by genetic factors diminishes. Her population risk, however, increases like anyone else's in the population. (See chap. 1, "Genes and Cancer: The Basics," for further discussion of the implications of penetrance and chap. 2, "Cancer Genes and Cancer Risk," for discussion of age-related cancer risks.)

Further complicating the discussion of cancer risk is the fact that inherited mutations in cancer genes frequently predispose individuals to several kinds of cancer. Thus, there is not one but multiple cancer risk estimates that the genetic counselor and patient must discuss. Because these cancers tend to occur at different ages and have different levels of risk and because there may be many cancers involved in a hereditary cancer syndrome, the patient may be confused about his or her cancer risk or overwhelmed by the complexity of the information provided. This is why genetic counselors often make themselves available to answer patients' questions by phone and may arrange to schedule a follow-up visit.

Helping people at increased genetic risk to understand that they continue to be at risk for sporadic (nonhereditary) cancers is also part of the mission of genetic counselors. Counselors must be sure that their patients understand that their nonhereditary risks of developing cancer during their lives will remain, even if they are not carriers of cancer genes. A review of appropriate screening procedures for noncarriers may be included in the initial counseling session or may occur once a negative genetic test result is known.

Explaining Testing and Screening and Surveillance Options

Usually within the first genetic counseling visit, the counselor will discuss whether genetic tests are available that would offer further clarification of whether the patient is a mutation carrier. One outcome of genetic counseling is that the counselor may find no indication that the cancers in the patient's family are genetic, perhaps because of the advanced age at which the cancers have occurred, the fact that the types of cancer are unrelated in light of the currently known hereditary cancer syndromes, or the finding that the number of cancers is within typical population norms. Sometimes clarification of the medical family history can considerably alter the likelihood that the family has a hereditary cancer predisposition syndrome. This might include clarifying that the cancer status of an aunt who is married to the patient's uncle has no bearing on the patient's risk or determining through a medical records search that a relative's cancer was not the type it was originally thought to be. If what was thought to be colon cancer in a grandfather was really stomach cancer, or if a tumor in the breast of another relative was actually a metastasis of a primary lung cancer, the likelihood the family has a hereditary colon or breast cancer syndrome is significantly reduced. Genetic counseling does help many women to recognize that one or two cases of breast cancer, especially if they have occurred in older female relatives, are not by themselves evidence of markedly increased breast cancer risk or even of a likely genetic link. Individuals at intermediate risk, defined as less than a 20% risk for breast cancer, may benefit from a specialized counseling program that addresses their concerns (Burke et al., 2000). The goals of such counseling are to help individuals at intermediate risk understand how their families differ from high-risk families and to make their own risk estimation more realistic. The counselor would also remind the patient that he or she does have at least population or slightly elevated risks of developing cancer and would review currently recommended screenings, as appropriate, for Pap smear, mammogram, clinical breast exam, prostate screening, rectal exam, or colonoscopy.

If the counselor determines from the pedigree a reasonable likelihood that a mutation in a cancer predisposition gene exists in the patient's family, he or she will discuss whether genetic testing is a reasonable option. Even in some families in which a mutation is suspected, there may be little likelihood that genetic testing of a particular individual (someone who has not had cancer) would reveal clinically useful information. If there are no living family members who have had cancer, there is no known mutation site, and the patient is not a member of an ethnic group with identified high rates of a particular mutation, finding a mutation in his or her DNA would not be of much value because it would still be unclear whether it was related to cancer predisposition. Also, estimates suggest that from 16% to 66% of high-risk breast and ovarian cancer families do not carry detectable mutations (Ford et al., 1998; Frank et al., 1998; Hakansson et al., 1997). It may be difficult for patients to hear that, despite significant family history, they may not be able to determine whether they carry a deleterious mutation. In these cases, the same options would be discussed as if the person had been found to be a mutation carrier because that possibility cannot be excluded. Screening recommendations and options for risk-reducing surgical and chemoprevention, as appropriate, would be discussed. The counselor and patient would also discuss the possibility that in the future, as additional cancer-causing mutations are identified or additional cancers occur in other family members, a mutation might be found that could make possible more informative genetic testing for healthy relatives. (Chap. 2, "Cancer Genes and Cancer Risk," discusses these issues in greater detail.)

If there are genetic tests that might offer useful clarification about cancer risk, the counselor initiates another layer of discussion focusing on the mechanics of the test (drawing of a blood sample), access to the test and its cost, the test's accuracy and limitations, and the social and psychological risks of being tested. The counselor will typically ask the patient to consider his or her likely reaction to testing positive and to testing negative. The counselor will also ask the patient to imagine how other relatives would react to positive or negative test results. This usually leads to a discussion of if, how, and when the patient thinks he or she would share information about the testing with family members. If the patient appears reluctant to consider sharing genetic information with at-risk relatives, the genetic counselor is likely to pursue discussion of the reasons for the hesitancy. Genetic counselors, in addition to being well informed, must have the skills of a good listener to assess what counselees understand, to recognize whether their minds are prematurely closed to reasonable options, to hear the depth of concerns about family impact, and to be able to identify when patients have come to a decision that is ego-syntonic, or right for them.

Screening and Surveillance Recommendation and Prophylaxis Options

Yet another focus of the first genetic counseling session is a discussion of the options for *screening* (looking for symptoms of cancer in a healthy individual), *surveillance* (looking for symptoms of recurrent or second malignancies in someone who has had cancer), or *prophylaxis* (measures to reduce the risk of developing cancer through surgery or medication). This session usually involves discussion of a complex series of risk-reduction estimates for a variety of options. All of the information introduced in the first session may increase the patient's sense of being cognitively and emotionally overwhelmed, which must be taken into consideration in deciding whether additional time is needed for decision making. For this reason, many genetic counselors ask that a patient go home and consider all of the topics covered in the first meeting rather than make a decision on the spot about whether to pursue genetic testing. The counselor is also likely to encourage the patient to discuss his or her plans and concerns with family members. Programmatic, cost, and geographic considerations often make the option of a second pretesting counseling session more difficult. Sometimes it is possible to have blood taken for testing at the first visit and held until the patient is certain he or she wants testing. Alternatively, it may be possible for the patient's own primary care physician to draw and send blood if the patient decides to be tested. Other patients may feel that they were already sure when they arrived for counseling that they wanted genetic testing. If a patient is sure that he or she wants blood drawn for testing and if the counselor sees no major contraindications (discussed later in the chapter), the next step is taken. The genetic counselor will review and administer an informed consent form about the risks and benefits of the testing and will have the patient's blood drawn. Instructions will be given about how long the analysis takes and how the follow-up visit will be scheduled. In most centers, genetic test results are given in person. Patients must understand that no result, including a negative result, is delivered on the telephone so that they do not assume they have a positive result when called to schedule a disclosure session to discuss the outcome of testing.

Informed Consent

Some genetic counseling occurs under research protocols and some is done in a clinical setting. What difference does it make? In many cases, the differences are subtle, but they may be important to some patients.

Research Protocols

If patients are participants in a genetic testing research project, they should expect the following.

1. Patients will be required to sign an informed consent form expressing willingness to participate in the research.
2. Patients likely will have to provide additional information or complete additional measures to provide data related to researchers' questions. Questions could involve, for example, a comparison of the effectiveness of various forms of genetic counseling or an assessment of the emotional outcomes of genetic testing.
3. Patients may have some greater protection for the confidentiality of research results. Results would not necessarily have to go into patient medical records but could remain in separate research files. The researchers might have been able to get a Certificate of Confidentiality from the National Institutes of Health that would make it more difficult, but not impossible, for records to be subpoenaed. There is no guarantee, at least in the United States, that records can be kept completely confidential if a court requests them.
4. Patients might be able to be tested at a reduced rate or free of charge. If cost is a major impediment to testing, enrollment in a research project related to genetic testing may enable a patient to be tested.

Clinical Testing Programs

A clinical testing program may also require review and signature of an informed consent form focused on the risks and benefits of the genetic test. Demographic, medical, and lifestyle information may be requested, and there may be a brief screen of psychological symptoms as part of the clinical visit. Confidentiality of results may differ somewhat from what is available in some research programs. Clients should ask the following about the privacy protections offered in the clinical setting:

- "Who will know my result?"
- "Will the result appear in my medical chart?"
- "Under what conditions will my result or my having been tested be available to my insurer?"
- "Who can request and get copies of my result?"

In some clinics, especially when terminally ill patients undergo testing, there are forms that can be completed giving other relatives permission to learn the genetic test result of the ill person after his or her death. Knowing that a son, daughter, sister, or spouse can legally have access to the genetic test result when desired can offer comfort to some people who worry that they could die before the result is available or before their relative is ready to receive the information.

Cost

Costs for breast and ovarian cancer gene testing can vary from $300–$400 to nearly $3,000, depending on whether there is a known mutation in the family. Testing for the genes that may cause hereditary nonpolyposis colon cancer or familial adenomatous polyposis costs between $1,600 and $2,000 (Myriad Genetic Laboratories, Inc., Salt Lake City, UT). Patients who have had cancer are more likely to request that their insurance company pay for genetic testing because it is unlikely that the result would further impair their ability to get or keep health insurance. Unaffected people may not want their insurer to have a right to learn their test result, as would be the case if the insurer paid the bill for testing. In these cases, patients may prefer to pay for testing themselves, but this can be a hardship for some people. As more laws are enacted to protect the privacy of genetic information and to prohibit discrimination on the basis of genetic status, there may be less reason to avoid insurer knowledge of one's genetic test result. Because there is much flux in current legislation about genetics, it is important for the genetic counselor to discuss the extent of current legal protections as one of the considerations in the decision to be tested.

DISCLOSURE VISIT

For those who do get tested, the disclosure visit is typically held 4–6 weeks after the blood is drawn and sent to the laboratory for testing. The scheduling of a disclosure visit with a patient occurs when the laboratory returns a test result. The call or reminder card to call for an appointment that initiates the appointment arouses considerable anxiety in a majority of those tested. Many say that in the period after giving blood, their worry about their genetic cancer risk is put "on the back burner," but a reminder call or card triggers concern. Others state that the entire period of waiting for the result was marked by anxiety and preoccupation far greater than that experienced prior to having their blood drawn. In either case, a call to schedule the disclosure visit heightens emotional focus on the results. Patients may negatively interpret the caller's tone of voice, whom they assume knows their result unless they are told otherwise by the program in advance. High anxiety is the norm when patients arrive for disclosure of their test result.

The disclosure visit provides the opportunity to accomplish the following:

1. Clarify that the patient wants to receive his or her genetic test result.
2. Identify any major family or personal health issues or other events of relevance to the patient's genetic concerns (e.g., new diagnoses of family members, death of a relative, patient's marital separation, etc.) that have occurred since the testing process began.
3. Identify any major psychological distress that might be made worse by disclosure.
4. Provide the test result.
5. Interpret the meaning of the test result for the patient's cancer risk.
6. Discuss the implications of the result for the cancer risk of close relatives (children, siblings, etc.) and plans for communicating results to family members.
7. Review with new relevance the surveillance or screening recommendations.
8. Discuss whether any further genetic testing, either now or in the future, may be appropriate.
9. Discuss whether visits to other medical specialists should be considered.
10. Assess the patient's state of mind and suggest, if needed, referral for further psychological evaluation or treatment.
11. Establish a follow-up plan or reassert the counselor's availability to help with later questions, patient and family members' concerns, and referrals.

Despite this long list of agenda items for the disclosure visit, the result must be delivered as quickly as possible, given the anxiety that patients experience. A well-organized counselor will have a plan for quickly establishing the patient's wish to receive the results; determining whether there are any new, major, relevant developments in the patient's life; and briefly assessing the patient's state of mind to determine whether there is any unusual or extreme symptomatology beyond the expected level of anxiety. Most patients say that the wait within the disclosure session seems interminable, no matter how rapidly the result is delivered. This is not a time for extensive reviewing of materials because patients' rising anxiety will make it impossible for them to remember what has been said. Calm, clear delivery of the results is ideal.

Patients usually receive one of the following results.

When there is a known mutation in the family, patients receive either a

- positive result or a
- true negative result.

When there is not a known mutation in the family but patients appear to come from a high-risk family and have been tested for mutations that are unusually common in their ethnic group, they receive either a

- positive result or an
- uninformative negative result.

When patients who have had one of the component cancers in the suspected cancer predisposition syndrome are tested to see whether they have a significant mutation, they receive a

- positive result, a
- result called a variant of unknown significance, or a
- negative result.

(See chap. 5, "Opening Pandora's Box," for further explanation of the meaning of each of these results and of typical psychological reactions to receipt of the results.)

A fourth circumstance is that, often against advice, unaffected patients without a known familial mutation or increased risk because of membership in an ethnic group with increased frequency of particular deleterious mutations may decide they want their full gene sequenced to see if they have a deleterious mutation. Their results may not be informative because, at least in some cases, it will not be clear whether alterations in the gene are related to cancer predisposition or whether they are normal changes without medical implications. The latter are called "polymorphisms of unknown or uncertain significance." Also, if no genetic alterations or mutations are found, it will not be known whether this is a true finding of a lack of a cancer predisposing mutation or whether it is a function of not having known where to look for a mutation. Such uncertain outcomes are not reassuring, and the individual would be advised to continue to follow recommended cancer screening guidelines for a mutation-positive individual.

After allowing time to absorb the result, the genetic counselor usually talks briefly about what the test means, attempting to hear back enough from patients about their understanding of the result and its implications to be sure they have the correct general information. The counselor takes a reading of the patient's emotional state, and together they discuss what the patient is likely to do with the information, who he or she will tell, what he or she plans to do with the information in the short run. The counselor may help the patient think about how to tell particular family members or medical providers. In some cases, this may lead the counselor to suggest that the patient take additional time to adjust to the result before telling others. The counselor and patient will talk briefly about what the next steps might be in terms of medical visits or whether there is reason to suggest psychological referral. Although distress is usually greatest among patients receiving positive results, patients receiving indeterminate results or, occasionally, even patients receiving negative results may be upset. The range of patients' emotional reactions to disclosure of cancer genetic testing results is discussed in chapter 5, "Opening Pandora's Box."

Follow-Up by the Genetic Counselor

Because many patients say they do not take in much of the rest of the information provided in the disclosure session after they hear their test result, genetic counselors will often follow up with patients by telephone, whether the result was positive or negative. Some patients return for a third session of counseling to concentrate on information about risks to self or offspring and options for screening or prophylaxis that they did not completely absorb during the first visit when carrier status was hypothetical or during the disclosure visit when emotions were heightened.

PSYCHOLOGICAL ISSUES

Non-Directiveness

A classic theoretical argument running through much of the genetic counseling literature is whether counselors should remain neutral in their discussions of decisions their patients are considering. Unlike physicians who are often directive about what they think patients need, genetic counselors of some schools believe that their role is to inform and to discuss, not to offer advice about what clients should do with the genetic information they have received (Fine, 1993). This attitude has its beginnings in a period when genetic counselors were largely working with pregnant mothers who had to make decisions about whether to abort a fetus found to carry a genetic abnormality (Anderson, 1999). With the advent of cancer genetic counseling, clients are most often seeking counseling about their own genetic makeup, not that of an unborn child.

Kessler (2000) offered enlightened distinctions between the nondirectiveness of Rogerian psychotherapy versus non-directiveness in genetic counseling, by which he means genetic counselors' fervent support and promotion of autonomous actions on the part of their patients. He stresses the importance of counseling skills that give patients new cognitive and emotional sets to approach problems and helps them to usefully reframe issues in ways that are consonant with their own ways of thinking. Kessler's work stresses the critical importance of interactive, rather than informational, aspects of genetic counseling, stating that, without the dialogue of the genetic counseling process, counselors could be replaced by videos or written materials. He emphasizes the genetic counselor's role in maximizing the "fit" between the patient's attitudes and emotions and the decisions they make about genetic issues.

Hazards of Gathering Family History Information

Gathering medical information by reviewing hospital and physician records can be an unexpectedly emotional endeavor. Reading medical records, especially those of a deceased parent, may reveal little-known details of the treatment or the reactions to it that can be highly affecting. A mother's stated desire to "keep fighting" for the sake of her then-young children can be painful to read in light of the failure of that effort. Some patients feel closer to their deceased relatives by reading about day-to-day changes in their condition, but usually with some added measure of sadness and fear about their own future health. Such efforts may also uncover new information about the types or extent of the cancer that the relative endured. Counselees may also find errors in information provided either to an ill relative or to them. Also, information now known to have potential genetic connections to the same mutated gene, such as hereditary breast and ovarian cancer, may have wrongly been considered unrelated diseases at the time, inciting anger about lost time and lost hope. Patients long for certainty and would like to be able to trust all that medical providers tell them. It angers some family members to recognize the extent to which scientific "facts" at one point in time may be altered by new knowledge within just a few years. Genetic counselors can assist patients in processing information that may become known during the gathering of medical information.

Comprehension

A major question in genetic counseling is how much information patients can retain of the large amount they receive, often for the first time, during cancer genetic counseling sessions. Implicit in this question is the assumption that some information is more important and relevant to the patient's concerns than others. Research has verified that patients assign greater value to issues about family communication and that genetic counselors give more importance to information about genetic tests, diagnosis, and prognosis (Michie, French, Allanson, Bobrow, & Marteau, 1997). Another factor that adds to the complexity of the communication during counseling sessions is the uncertainty resulting from our incomplete knowledge of cancer genetics and cancer risk (van Zuuren, Van Schie, & van Baaren, 1997). Conveying the complexity of what is and is not known is a formidable task for genetic counselors. To help patients retain or have access to more of the information contained in cancer genetic counseling centers, some groups have developed interactive CD-ROMs to be used in connection with counseling sessions and to have available for home review or sharing with relatives (Green, Biesecker, McInerney, & Fost, 2001).

Patients seek certainty and are often disappointed to find out how many gaps exist in knowledge that is of great importance to them. They also do not always understand that much of what is conveyed about genetic risk is subject to change when future research studies look at different populations or are able to take advantage of more advanced techniques.

Assessment of Emotional Well-Being and Patient Safety

The genetic counselor, either formally or informally, makes an ongoing assessment of patients' mental competence to provide informed consent, their emotional capacity to withstand the uncertainty and waiting involved in genetic testing, and their resilience to cope with the potential disappointment of an undesired test result. If problems are noted in any of these areas, further assessment is required. Causes for psychological evaluation of patients prior to deciding to undergo testing or disclose results include the following:

1. The patient is not capable of giving consent, for example, because of psychosis or significant mental retardation.
2. The patient's acute distress makes rational decision making impossible. A genetic test result is not something that can be undone once it is delivered. It is important that the patient be capable of making a well-reasoned decision about receiving the result. Severe depression or anxiety should be carefully evaluated for its relationship to testing and disclosure. If there is an expectation that the uncertainty of not knowing the result is adding to the distress and if there is some expectation that the individual will be able to understand and accept whatever the test result is found to be, then disclosure, with

support provided, may be indicated. Marked ambivalence about receiving the result should be treated by erring on the side of not disclosing the result until the individual can be clearer about his or her wishes.

3. The patient is experiencing other major life events. Situational variables, imminent job change of the insurance holder, pending divorce proceedings, or a recent loss may indicate that testing should be postponed. Not infrequently, genetic testing occurs in the context of terminal illness of a family member. In some of these cases, discussion of testing leads to recognition that completing testing at a time when the concurrent stressor is diminished is preferable, and testing or disclosure is postponed. A woman whose sister is dying may feel torn between her own emotions regarding her test result and her desire to focus on her sister. In other cases, dying individuals feel strongly that they want testing for the benefit of their relatives. This may be a parting gift of sorts. Alternative approaches, including having the patient give permission for the relatives to receive the results after his or her death, may be explored if it seems that focus on the test result is either physically or emotionally interfering with caretaking or grieving.

Depression and anxiety are commonly seen in individuals seeking cancer genetic testing. Given the extensive loss histories and cancer experiences of those who come for counseling, this is not surprising. Some of these patients have strong systems of support from a psychotherapist or psychopharmacologist or from relatives or friends who can help provide assistance during the period of counseling, waiting, and test result disclosure. Others may find that their usually strong support network is compromised by opposition to testing from those closest to them. Some may not want to share the testing experience with others close to them or may not want to decide what to tell others until after the result is known. This may increase the burden on the testing team to evaluate the person's vulnerability effectively.

Although it is rare for a counseling patient to be in a state of acute, severe deterioration or distress when they present for counseling, it is not unknown. Genetic counselors take seriously suicidal or homicidal implications or threats or the suggestion that the individual might not be able to live with knowledge of an undesirable test result. Part of the assessment of the potential danger of undergoing genetic testing is the degree to which the patient's ongoing depression or distress is related to genetic issues or cancer fear. The worry is that the patient's psychological equilibrium might be tipped by receiving an undesirable test result. Some patients have lived with significant cancer fear for many years but nonetheless expect to be devastated if they learn with certainty that they are mutation carriers and may realize that they have passed on a cancer gene to their children. Others may not have realized until they came for counseling that, if found to be a mutation carrier, they are at increased risk for recurrence or for second primary cancers, and this information can be very threatening. Some cancer patients think that, having had cancer, the receipt of a positive genetic test result will not have much emotional impact. Research suggests, however, that this group is much more emotionally affected than they anticipate (Dorval et al., 2000).

Some genetic counseling programs have a psychologist who is available to help evaluate the patient or consult with the genetic counselor about the need for further evaluation. The psychologist's help may be needed to make a differential diagnosis of the extent to which current symptoms and distress are due to the stresses of being tested or to long-standing depression, anxiety, or other conditions related to the patient's cancer experience or family history of loss. The program psychologist can also serve as a liaison with the patient's therapist, if permission is granted. If the patient is in ongoing treatment, his or her therapist may be best able to determine the depth and causes of a patient's depression or emotional ability or to assess cognitive abilities. The therapist can also make a judgment about the potential impact that receiving an adverse genetic test result will have on the patient. Communication between the therapist and the genetic counselor or testing program psychologist can be a valuable two-way information trade. It can provide clarification of what genetic testing may reveal and can provide the genetics professional with insight into the patient's strengths and vulnerabilities. In some cases, postponement of further counseling or of a decision about testing may be recommended until the patient can discuss the emotions experienced during the initial counseling session with his or her therapist. In other cases, the patient may require help in finding a therapist with whom to work on current sources of distress.

Some programs, especially research genetic testing programs, include administration of several measures of psychological symptoms or coping strategies in their pretest battery. These may include the Brief Symptom Inventory (BSI; Derogatis & Spencer, 1982), the Ways of Coping (Folkman & Lazarus, 1980) or COPE (Carver, Scheier, & Weintraub, 1989) measures, the Medical Outcome Study (MOS) short-form health survey (Ware & Sherbourne, 1992), one of several depression scales, the State–Trait Anxiety scale (Spielberger, Gorsuch, Lushene, Vagg, & Jacobs, 1983), or a self-esteem measure such as the Rosenberg Self-Esteem Scale (Rosenberg, 1965). Inclusion of standard psychological measures can provide useful assessment, but several caveats should be considered before reacting to the scores alone. First, these measures were not developed for individuals in this situation.

It is normal to be anxious when receiving potentially life-threatening news. Because review of a family history marked by illness and loss is a part of genetic counseling, it may stir up sad or depressed feelings. Communication with family members about genetic concerns may prove to be less than ideal, deepening feelings of isolation, sadness, or anger.

Genetic testing may actually threaten feelings of solidarity that members of an at-risk family have shared because of their common disease risk. Also, counseling and testing may occur soon after a cancer diagnosis in the counselee or a close relative, which may be the focus of the anxiety or depression reflected in test scores. Despite these caveats, standard measures can provide some useful assessment of the extent of the symptoms expressed by or observed in patients. The issue to be decided is whether the patient has sufficient coping abilities to undertake the increased vulnerability of undergoing testing without serious risk of major adverse psychological outcomes (i.e., suicide, major depression, psychosis, or homicide, or violence against others). The genetic counselor will likely also inquire about emotional support available to the patient (e.g., a caring spouse; a close relationship with a sibling, child, or other relative; a therapist) as part of the assessment of the patient's ability to find sufficient support to endure the wait for results and to cope with a possibly distressing test result. The genetic counselor with such concerns should first discuss them with the patient and, if concern persists, should discuss them with a mental health professional familiar with genetic issues.

Patients usually want to get on with testing rapidly once they have decided that this is the path they wish to pursue. Also, once a DNA analysis is begun, charges are incurred. It is far preferable that any significant ambivalence about testing be resolved before the patient's blood is sent to the laboratory for analysis. This means that when the patient's blood is drawn at the first counseling session there may be a short window of time for a consultation between the genetic counselor and the mental health professional and, possibly, a meeting between the patient and the psychologist to occur, after the session and before the DNA analysis begins. Therefore, it is crucial that any genetic counselor making such assessments have an established consultation relationship with a psychologist, social worker, or psychiatrist who is aware of the issues with which the counselor is working. This allows for rapid consultation and, possibly, further assessment of the patient by a mental health professional.

If a counselor and the mental health consultant continue to feel uncomfortable about a patient's level of emotional or behavioral risk in the event of an adverse test result, they should share their concern with the patient and determine which steps to take. In some cases, psychotherapy or assessment for psychotropic medication may be indicated. Testing can and should be postponed or refused if the counselor, with input from a mental health professional, feels the patient is at risk for harming him- or herself or others. Acute deterioration in the counselor's office is highly unlikely. Nevertheless, the situation combines considerable uncertainty, vulnerability because of the high emotional content of the information being revealed, and potential for anger and misunderstanding, and thus the potential exists for severe emotional distress. It is wise to work out a plan for patient and professional safety in the unlikely event of an acute emergency, including plans to call the police and request transport of the patient to a local emergency unit for psychiatric evaluation.

Companions

Patients may come alone, or they may bring a significant other to the session for support and to be available later to discuss the complex information presented. One caution about the choice of a companion is that it is usually preferable to bring a relative or friend who is not at risk for the same hereditary disease because it may be difficult for an at-risk individual to be supportive if he or she is worried about the implications of the information for themselves as well. Some siblings, parent–child dyads, or other blood relatives, however, feel strongly about coming to the educational sessions together. Some counseling groups also prefer to have large family meetings to discuss the factual genetic information together.

Patients who are contemplating bringing a companion should consider the roles they would like that person to have and their own preferences for how the person will be involved. When patients are grateful to a friend, relative, or spouse for coming to the session, they may feel that the companion's wishes should guide their decisions. Sometimes recognition of a desire to be alone at the time of disclosure or to have a not-at-risk relative such as a spouse, but not a sister, present when the result is revealed is important to reducing the stress on the person receiving results. If siblings or other pairs in which both members are at risk are given results on the same day, it is strongly advised that the results be disclosed separately, but in close succession, to allow each to feel, at least for a few minutes, the impact of one's own result before having to be with and show concern for the balance between their relative.

Consideration should also be given to the potential burdens of being a companion to someone receiving genetic counseling or testing. Although most relatives and friends accept this role without hesitation, the counselor and patient should try to think about the particular position of the person being asked. Parents sometimes feel guilty when they learn a child has inherited a deleterious mutation. Therefore, thought should be given to whether the counseling session is the best place for parents to receive news of a positive result, particularly if they are ill or elderly. Friends may feel a special closeness after sharing the intimate experience of receiving a genetic test result, but, depending on the nature and stability of the relationship, this can later be experienced as a burden. One girlfriend who served as a companion reported that she felt somewhat uneasy a few months later when the relationship ended. She felt that because she had been his companion during this complex time, she had taken on a lifelong responsibility to provide support to her ex-boyfriend and would try to do so, despite the end of their romantic relationship.

PSYCHOLOGISTS AND GENETIC COUNSELING

Psychologists will have many new opportunities as a result of recent advances in genetics, particularly cancer genetics (Patenaude, Guttmacher, & Collins, 2002). Some will work directly or in consultation with genetic counselors. Other psychologists will encounter genetic concerns in the clinical practice of psychotherapy with patients who have cancer family histories suggestive of or proven to be of hereditary origin.

The task of the psychologist is not to attempt to deliver genetic counseling or indicate to patients whether their family appears to have inherited risk for cancer. Rather, the psychologist's role is to recognize when patients might benefit from assessment by a genetics specialist. The ability to describe for patients what a visit to a genetic counselor entails is within the scope of psychologists' practice in the 21st century. Their job is to understand the potential benefits that a visit with a genetic counselor is likely to confer to the concerned patient in terms of providing answers to important questions and, it is hoped, reducing the patient's anxiety. The psychologist should also be able to discuss the potential risks of such a visit, including the risk that the patient might learn more than he or she wants to know about familial cancer risk.

The psychologist with an extensive sense of a patient's coping skills, information style, and vulnerabilities is in a good position to help weigh the pros and cons of genetic assessment and counseling. His or her role is to support the patient in the back and forth of decision making and in the pursuit of self-actualizing, appropriate actions in this realm, as in all others. The psychologist may, in addition, be a source of referral information about the location of an appropriate genetic counselor or geneticist who can respond to personal genetic questions. If the counselor or geneticist is not known to the psychologist, he or she can suggest criteria to evaluate the capability of the counselor to be able to answer the specific questions about which the patient is most concerned.

If the patient wishes, the psychotherapist could consult directly with the geneticist or genetics counselor after the genetic counseling session to learn what the patient has been told and to be better prepared to help the patient make decisions based on that information. Consulting with the genetic counselor will also allow the psychotherapist to provide information about the patient's coping style and psychological status. The psychologist may also help the counselor differentiate the patient's current level of anxiety in approaching genetic testing and his or her typical functioning. The genetic counselor and the therapist may both work with the patient to compare various options (testing, prophylactic surgery, etc.) in light of the personality characteristics of the patient. The psychologist may also help the patient prepare to talk with family members to gather an accurate family history and to communicate information about the relatives' possible vulnerability to inherited genetic susceptibilities. Finally, the therapist may help the patient integrate and cope with the genetic test result and provide ongoing support and a neutral location in which to discuss the personal and family ramifications of genetic awareness.

*   *   *

Case Example.   A woman who described herself as being in the terminal phase of advanced breast cancer requested BRCA1/2 testing to provide information of potential use to her daughter, who was in her late 20s. The woman said her condition was precarious enough to lead her to inquire about how to ensure that her result could be given to her daughter in the event that she died before it became available. She was currently feeling well enough to come in for counseling but feared a rapid demise if her condition worsened. During the initial genetic counseling session, it came to light that she was hoarding a stash of pain medication in sufficient quantity to end her life. This alarmed the genetic counselor, who recommended that the patient speak with the program psychologist. The counselor's main question was whether the psychologist judged the patient to be a suicide risk in the event that she were to be found to carry a genetic mutation. Would she feel so guilty with regard to possibly having passed this vulnerability on to her daughter that she would consider taking the pills she was putting aside? In the extended discussion between the psychologist and the patient, it became clear that procuring and saving the pain pills was the result of an incident that had occurred a few months earlier. The patient had been in excruciating pain and felt she had been unable to obtain adequate medication. She had wished for death but also for control over her own destiny. To gain mastery over her fear that such an experience might recur as she neared death, she was saving a supply of pain pills that she knew would ease her pain, even if death resulted. She hoped never to need them and to die under her doctor's care, but she was, she said, prepared to use them if the doctor's attempts at pain control failed. As for the anticipated genetic test result, she thought it likely that she would be positive. Her saving the pills appeared to have nothing to do with the anticipation of a positive result. She wanted her daughter to have access to this information and thought of testing as doing something valuable for her daughter before she died, regardless of the result. She hoped that her being tested might one day prevent a similar outcome for her daughter. She had no intention of using the pills if she were found to be a mutation carrier. The psychologist encouraged her to talk with her physician about her desires for a pain-free terminal phase and death. The psychologist also reported to the genetic counselor that there were no psychological contraindications to proceeding with the genetic testing.

* * *

SUMMARY

In summary, cancer genetic counseling is an interactive process in which patients not only gain useful, personalized information about their genetic risk and that of their close relatives but also begin to consider the impact of this information on their well-being and health behaviors. This process generates considerable emotion, especially in families marked by extensive cancer histories and premature loss. Psychologists can work closely with genetic counselors, genetic nurses, oncologists, geneticists, epidemiologists, and primary care physicians who provide genetic counseling to support patients as they go through genetic counseling and as they consider actions based on what they learn from counseling.

The next chapter considers what patients bring to genetic counseling out of their personal experience with cancer or their membership in a family with a significant cancer history. Their loss of close relatives from cancer and their awareness of their own risk color what patients do to try to prevent or detect cancer and how they view the counseling process and the possibility of genetic testing. To understand patients who come for counseling, one needs to consider the emotional factors and family experience that have formed their views about cancer.

REFERENCES

Anderson, G. (1999). Nondirectiveness in prenatal genetics: Patients read between the lines. *Nursing Ethics*, 6, 126–136.

Bennett, R. L. (1999). *The practical guide to genetic family history*. New York: Wiley-Liss.

Bennett, R. L., Steinhaus, K. A., Uhrich, S. B., O'Sullivan, C. K., Resta, R. G., Lochner-Doyle, D., et al. (1995). Recommendations for standardized pedigree nomenclature. *American Journal of Human Genetics, 56*, 745–752.

Brandeis University Genetic Counseling Program. (1998). *Master's degree program in genetic counseling* [Catalogue]. Waltham, MA: Author.

Burke, W., Culver, J. O., Bowen, D., Lowry, D., Durfy, S., McTiernan, A., et al. (2000). Genetic counseling for women with an intermediate family history of breast cancer. *American Journal of Medical Genetics, 90*, 361–368.

Carver, C. S., Scheier, M. F., & Weintraub, J. K. (1989). Assessing coping strategies: A theoretically based approach. *Journal of Personality and Social Psychology, 56*, 267–283.

Claus, E. B., Risch, N. J., & Thompson, W. D. (1991). Genetic analysis of breast cancer in the cancer and steroid hormone study. *American Journal of Human Genetics, 48*, 2322–2342.

Cummings, S. (2000). The genetic testing process: How much counseling is needed? *Journal of Clinical Oncology, 18*(Suppl. 21), 60–64s.

Daly, M., Farmer, J., Harrop-Stein, C., Montgomery, S., Itzen, M., Costalas, J. W., et al. (1999). Exploring family relationships in cancer risk counseling using the genogram. *Cancer Epidemiology, Biomarkers, & Prevention, 8*, 393–398.

Derogatis, L. R., & Spencer, P. M. (1982). *Brief Symptom Inventory (BSI): Administration, scoring, and procedures manual.* Baltimore: Clinical Psychometric Research.

Dimond, E., Calzone, K., Davis, J., & Jenkins, J. (1998). The role of the nurse in cancer genetics. *Cancer Nursing, 2*, 57–75.

Dorval, M., Patenaude, A. F., Schneider, K., Kieffer, S. A., DiGianni, L., Kalkbrenner, K., et al. (2000). Anticipated versus actual emotional reactions to disclosure of results of genetic testes for cancer susceptibility: Findings from p53 and BRCA1 testing programs. *Journal of Clinical Oncology, 18*, 2135–2142.

Fine, B. A. (1993). The evolution of nondirectiveness in genetic counseling and implications of the human genome project. In D. Bartels, B. S. LeRoy, & A. Kaplan (Eds.), *Prescribing our future: Ethical challenges in genetic counseling* (pp. 101–117). New York: Aldine de Gruyter.

Folkman, S., & Lazarus, R. S. (1980). An analysis of coping in a middle-aged community sample. *Journal of Health and Social Behavior, 21*, 219–239.

Ford, D., Easton, D. F., Stratton, M., Narod, S., Goldgar, D., Devilee, P., et al. (1998). Genetic heterogeneity and penetrance analysis of the BRCA1 and BRCA2 genes in breast cancer families. *American Journal of Human Genetics, 62*, 676–689.

Frank, T. S., Manley, S. A., Olopade, O. I., Cummings, S., Garber, J. E., Bernhardt, B., et al. (1998). Correlation of mutations with family history and ovarian cancer risk. *Journal of Clinical Oncology, 16*, 2417–2425.

Gail, M. H., & Benichou, J. (1992). Assessing the risk of breast cancer in individuals. In V. T. DeVita, S. Hellman, & S. A. Rosenberg (Eds.), *Cancer prevention* (pp. 12–15). Philadelphia: Lippincott.

Garber, J. E., Goldstein, A. M., Kantor, A. F., Dreyfus, M. G., Fraumeni, J. F., Jr., & Li, F. P. (1991). Follow-up study of twenty-four families with Li–Fraumeni syndrome. *Cancer Research, 51,* 6094–6097.

Green, M. J., Biesecker, B. B., McInerney, A. M., & Fost, N. (2001). An interactive computer program can effectively educate patients about genetic testing for breast cancer susceptibility. *American Journal of Medical Genetics, 103,* 16–23.

Hakansson, S., Johannsson, O., Johannsson, U., Sellberg, G., Loman, N., Gerdes, A. M., et al. (1997). Moderate frequency of BRCA1 and BRCA2 germ-line mutations in Scandinavian familial breast cancer. *American Journal of Human Genetics, 60,* 1068–1078.

Hopper, J. L., & Jenkins, M. A. (1999). Modeling the probability that Ashkenazi Jewish women carry a founder mutation in BRCA1 or BRCA2. *American Journal of Human Genetics, 65,* 1771–1775.

Kessler, S. (2000). *Psyche and helix: Psychological aspects of genetic counseling.* New York: Wiley-Liss.

Kieffer, S. A., & Vockely, C. W. (1997). Expertise of genetic counselors clarified. [Letter]. *Oncology (Huntington), 12,* 1015.

National Society of Genetic Counselors. (n.d.). Retrieved June 22, 2001, from http://www.nsgc.org/TrainingProgram.asp? What=ShowAll

McGoldrick, M., & Gerson, R. (1985). *Genograms in family assessment* (pp. 1–38). New York: Norton.

Michie, S., French, D., Allanson, A., Bobrow, M., & Marteau, T. M. (1997) Information recall in genetic counseling: A pilot study of its assessment. *Patient Education and Counseling, 32,* 93–100.

Patenaude, A. F., Guttmacher, A. E., & Collins, F. S. (2002). Genetic testing and psychology: New roles, new responsibilities. *American Psychologist, 57,* 271–282.

Peters, J. A., & Stopfer, J. E. (1996). Role of the genetic counselor in familial cancer. *Oncology, 10,* 159–166.

Richards, M. P. M., Hallowell, N., Green, J. M., Murton, F., & Stratham, H. (1995). Counseling families with hereditary breast and ovarian cancer: A psychosocial perspective. *Journal of Genetic Counseling, 4,* 219–233.

Rosenberg, M. (1965). *Society and the adolescent self-image* Princeton, NJ: Princeton University Press.

Rubinstein, W. S., O'Neill, S. M., Peters, J. A., Rittmeyer, L. J., & Stadler, M. P. (2002). Mathematical modeling for breast cancer risk assessment. *Oncology, 16,* 1082–1094.

Schneider, K. A., & Marnane, D. (1997). Cancer risk counseling: How is it different? *Journal of Genetic Counseling, 6,* 97–110.

Spielberger, C., Gorsuch, R., Lushene, R., Vagg, P., & Jacobs, G. (1983). *The handbook of the State-Trait Anxiety Inventory.* Palo Alto, CA: Consulting Psychologists Press.

Van Zuuren, F. J., van Schie, E. C., & van Baaren, N. K. (1997). Uncertainty in the information provided during genetic counseling. *Patient Education and Counseling, 32,* 129–139.

Ware, J. E., Jr., & Sherbourne, C. D. (1992). The MOS 36-item short-form health survey (SF-36). I. Conceptual framework and item selection. *Medical Care, 30,* 473–483.

Watson, E. K., Shickle, D., Qureshi, N., Emery, J., & Austoker, J. (1999). The "new genetics" and primary care: GP's views on their roles and educational needs. *Family Practice, 16,* 420–425.

4

EMOTIONAL BAGGAGE: UNRESOLVED GRIEF, EMOTIONAL DISTRESS, RISK PERCEPTION, AND HEALTH BELIEFS AND BEHAVIORS

Cancer families are not all alike. A family history of cancer that suggests an inherited mutation implies a history of illness or premature deaths that has many ramifications. Implicit in eligibility for cancer genetic testing are some factors that are useful to consider when thinking about the emotional state of individuals who seek cancer genetic counseling or testing.

As this chapter emphasizes, the role of the therapist can be central in helping many patients who receive genetic information understand and act effectively on what they learn. To be helpful, the therapist must recognize the layers of personality variables and cognitive barriers through which genetic information passes. Genetic information is particularly subject to personal filtering because it is complex, involves many areas of uncertainty, and is not static but changes frequently as new discoveries are made. Wide media coverage of genetic advances—some of it well researched and informative and some of it misleading—affects patients' understanding of genetic issues. Therapists may help patients find deeper psychological acceptance of the realities and issues involved in genetic testing and may improve the likelihood that effective action will be taken and anxiety reduced. In this role, the mental health professional may find it useful to ask the patient for permission to speak with their genetics professionals to ensure that all concerned are uniform in their understanding of the patient's genetic risk status.

MRS. P.: A CASE AND ANALYSIS ILLUSTRATING THE CHALLENGES OF LIFE IN A HIGH-RISK CANCER FAMILY

Mrs. P. was 56 years old when her gynecological oncologist first referred her for symptoms of agoraphobia. She had been largely unwilling to leave her house since having a double mastectomy six months earlier. Mrs. P. had been diagnosed with cancer in one breast but had both breasts removed because of her extensive family history of cancer. This was not her first prophylactic surgery for cancer. Six years earlier, she had her ovaries removed, hoping to avoid the ovarian cancer that had led to the deaths of two of her sisters in their early 40s and of their mother at a similar age. Mrs. P. hoped that having an oophorectomy (removal of her ovaries) would make her feel "safe." Unexpectedly, routine biopsy of the removed ovaries revealed the presence of ovarian cancer. Mrs. P.'s response was to be glad that she had had them removed rather than wait for the cancer to be detected at a much later time. For a while after the oophorectomy, life had progressed normally. She took good care of herself, swam nearly daily, and enjoyed her family. By the time her breast cancer was diagnosed, however, her 31-year-old daughter had been diagnosed twice with breast cancer. When Mrs. P. presented for psychological treatment, she was refusing to leave her house, except with her husband after much coaxing, and then only occasionally. She was anhedonic (felt nothing was pleasurable), ate little, was depressed, had difficulty getting out of bed in the morning, and had persistent sleep difficulties. She admitted to having passive thoughts about suicide, thinking about how to have an "accident" while driving, but never taking active steps in that direction. Despite support from her husband, she felt despair and unworthiness about her perceived lack of femininity.

This case illustrates components of the stress that arises from living in a family in which a genetic predisposition to cancer has resulted in multiple, early cases of cancer.

Unresolved Grief

The literature on grief discusses successful grieving as a continuum, with painful memories most prominent nearer the time of the loss, and gradual distancing from the loss with increasing time (Bowlby, 1980; Parkes & Weiss, 1983; Rando, 1984). In "cancer families," many of the griefs and losses appear never to reach resolution, possibly because of the rapidity with which new diagnoses and deaths overtake those coping with earlier losses. Diagnosis of a serious disease, like cancer, necessitates a psychological adjustment not only for the patient, but also for spouses, children, siblings, and parents of the patient. Recurrence of cancer, hospitalizations, and, finally, death constitute multiple traumas. When multiple cases of the same cancer have been seen in the same family, and especially when death has been the outcome of earlier illness episodes, a new diagnosis of the same disease in another family member arouses great fear. Mrs. P. had incurred many stresses by the time she reached psychological services. Her mother and two sisters had suffered through ovarian cancer, only to lose their battles in their 40s. Mrs. P. felt lucky that knowledge of the family susceptibility to ovarian cancer had led to her prophylactic surgery, which she felt was the reason she had been spared the family curse. Just surviving to age 50 was a triumph of sorts, but it was not without more family cancer experiences (i.e., first the diagnosis of breast cancer in her daughter and then her own breast cancer diagnosis). If one imagines all of the anxieties and decisions and arrangements that this cascade of illness must have initiated, it is easy to imagine that there might not have been much emotional energy to resolve earlier losses. Energies had to be directed to surviving.

One part of the resolution of grief is a differentiation of oneself from the person who has died, here made much more difficult by the repeated linking of one relative's cancer with another's. Mrs. P.'s sister had taken offense when, at the time of the second sister's cancer diagnosis, Mrs. P. had blurted out, "Oh, I must be next." Although this was a normal reaction and may have reflected some guilt at having been spared to that point, the sister apparently resented that the focus of Mrs. P.'s comments was herself, not her sister. It is easy to see how families under such strains quarrel and how the "lucky" and the "unlucky" find it difficult to communicate. Especially when families are close and when family members assume considerable physical care for each other, it is difficult for the well members not to envision themselves in the beds of their already-diagnosed relatives. It is also easy to see why some might become numb and others quite distressed. Mrs. P., who felt lucky compared to her two sisters, had devoted herself to their care, ignoring her own feelings and needs. When she became ill herself, she applied the same emotional forces she had marshaled to care for her sister, distancing herself from her own emotions, with the resulting development of serious psychological symptoms.

Multi-Generational Cancer Experience

Mrs. P.'s worry about breast cancer included concern not only about herself, but also for her daughter, who appeared to be coping well after her mastectomy and reconstruction, and concern for her granddaughters who remained healthy. Her tendency to focus on others led to considerable focus on informing the granddaughters and worrying that they might not take seriously the need for very early breast surveillance, given the very early age at which their aunt (Mrs. P.'s daughter) had been diagnosed.

Family Communication Problems

Mrs. P.'s son refused to talk about the family cancer history. They were estranged to the point where she had not heard from him after her own breast cancer diagnosis. Mrs. P. felt it important that his daughter, her 19-year-old granddaughter, know about all of the diagnoses in the family so that she could see a breast-ovarian cancer specialist and work out a surveillance plan. Although Mrs. P. worried about whether informing her granddaughter about her illness and her daughter's would lead to further estrangement from her son, she resolved that it was more important to warn her granddaughter of the extent of the family cancer burden. She thought she could not trust this role to her son, since she feared he would not tell his daughter. She contemplated when and how to contact the granddaughter so that the message could be heard without distortion or misunderstanding of her motives.

Importance of a Supportive Spouse:
Dominance of Self-Perception of Body Image

Mrs. P.' s spouse was never seen in the treatment, but she consistently reported that he was supportive of her decision regarding the mastectomies and seemed not to have lost any of his sexual interest in her as a result of her surgery. He sought ways to make her feel better, and was genuinely worried about her. Nonetheless, Mrs. P.'s image of her physical self when she entered treatment was of an "ugly" creature, without any feminine characteristics or traits. Although she was grateful for her husband's emotional support and understood his frustration at not being able to make her feel feminine, her own views carried more weight and were the determinants of her feeling that she was, in the absence of ovaries and, especially, breasts, an unattractive, gender-less being.

Value of Psychotherapy in Resolution of Grief and Mobilization of Resilience

The three months of therapy that Mrs. P. undertook were successful in reducing her depression, increasing her mobility and socialization, and allowing for sufficient alteration in her self-perception to enable her to feel good about her appearance again. Her resumption of swimming classes and her enjoyment of the physical mobility and socialization that the classes provided was a triumph and a tribute to her willingness to re-visit some of the difficult periods of her past and to consider more deeply the concept of "femininity." Mrs. P. remained adamant that having had both breasts removed at once had been the best decision, since she would not have wanted to undergo multiple surgeries. It did seem that more time and attention pre-surgery to the potential emotional and physical outcomes of surgery might have helped to better prepare her for the loss of both of her breasts.

Enormous Destructive Power of Cancer Genes

The diagnosis of a recurrence of her cancer shortly after Mrs. P.'s hard-won psychological achievement was a reminder that within these families feeling healthy, even briefly, seems like hubris. Family members feel punished for any optimism or future orientation they experience when yet another cancer is diagnosed or a negative turn occurs in a relative's illness course. The difficulty in maintaining hope in such an environment in the face of multiple diagnoses, relapses, and deaths in very young and relatively young people is very apparent. It is all too easy to see how family communication is made more difficult as some prepare for dying, others try desperately to distance themselves from cancer, and all wonder who will be the next to fall under the family "curse." In these families it is difficult to enjoy good health, as it is always experienced as a temporary phenomenon, without the blissful denial of mortality which most of us exist in (Becker, 1973).

DISTRESS

A major question that researchers have attempted to answer early in research on cancer genetic testing is whether individuals who seek testing have higher than average levels of psychological problems. A number of researchers have found what the clinical example just described would lead us to expect: Levels of distress are greater among members of "cancer families" reporting for genetic testing than in the general population. Kash, Holland, Halper, and Miller (1992) found 27% of at-risk women to have distress scores (Global Symptom Index; GSI) above the 90th percentile on the Symptom Checklist—90 (SCL–90; Derogatis, 1983). Whereas 10% of the women in the general population score at a level consistent with clinical symptomatology, nearly three times that many at-risk women score in the clinical range. Audrain, Schwartz, Lerman, Hughes, and Peshkin (1997) found moderate levels of both general and cancer-specific distress among women self-referred for genetic counseling and possible *BRCA1* testing. Means for this group were just half a standard deviation below the cut-off for clinical levels of distress on the Hopkins Symptom Checklist—25 (Derogatis, Lipman, Rickels, Uhlenhuth, & Covi, 1974). Higher distress was associated with higher perceptions of breast cancer risk and lower perceptions of control over developing breast cancer.

Anxiety was noted to be high among the women reporting for counseling in the Watson et al. study (1998), with 33.6% scoring at or above the clinically significant level of psychological morbidity on the General Health Questionnaire (Goldberg & Williams, 1988), a well-known British measure of psychological symptomatology. These authors suggest that "a substantial minority of clinic attenders are very anxious women for whom psychological counseling might be helpful" (p. 738) and went on to question the availability of sufficient mental heath staff to meet the needs of these patients.

In the Netherlands, a study compared individuals presenting for genetic testing for a number of genetic conditions, including members of families with high incidence of breast and ovarian cancer and familial adenomatous polyposis (DudokdeWit et al., 1997a). They found that those at-risk for neurodegenerative disease were more distressed, as evidenced by higher avoidance and intrusion scores on the Impact of Event Scale (Horowitz, Wilner, & Alvarez, 1979) than individuals at risk for a cancer syndrome. Individuals who reported high levels of intrusion tended to be those with painful memories of how the illness had affected parents and other close family members in the past. The authors questioned whether low distress scores for some might indicate denial. They believed that at-risk individuals might "try to convince themselves that there is no reason to worry and report low distress scores, while in fact they are emotionally affected by the predictive test" (p. 387). They also hypothesized that worrying was a means of rehearsing or preparing for the test result, so that those who were avoidant might be most at risk for later distress. Among 85 women who were either first- or second-degree relatives of known *BRCA1/2* carriers, 26% had increased scores on measures of general distress on the Hospital Anxiety and Depression Scale (Zigmond & Snaith, 1983). In another report, the same group describes the need for "a multidisciplinary team including a psychologist" (DudokdeWit et al., 1997b, p. 70) to offer counselors help and supervision concerning intertwining individual and family motives and reactions. The availability of psychological referral to those undergoing testing was also suggested.

In a study of 430 women attending the High-Risk Clinic at the UCLA Revlon Breast Center, Lindberg and Wellisch (2001) found that 40% to 45% of the women scored above the clinical cutoff for both state and trait anxiety. The also found a significant association between state and trait anxiety and anxiety related to undergoing mammograms and breast self-examination. Higher levels of distress and anxiety were found among women versus men who had donated blood for hereditary nonpolyposis colon cancer (HNPCC) testing. Other factors correlated with distress were younger age, non-White race, lower level of formal education, and less satisfaction with social support (Vernon et al., 1997).

Coping style, particularly style of processing medical information, has been shown to be associated with the emotions and perceptions of high-risk women. Genetic counseling requires substantial ability on the part of the patient to seek out and take in large quantities of medical information. The information is complex and must be integrated personally with the particular family and individual medical histories of the person seeking counseling. This requires a willingness to attend to and cope with a large body of abstract, personally threatening information. This is no doubt a significant factor in why the majority of individuals who come forth for cancer genetic testing are highly educated. Yet among this population there is nonetheless some variation in the cognitive processing and interpretation of the information provided. Miller, Roussi, Caputo, and Kruus (1995) described as "monitors" those who tend to focus on the threatening aspects of the information provided, perseverate on negative outcomes, and continue somewhat compulsively to search for new information that they hope will allay their fear. Their style is contrasted to "blunters," individuals who intuitively shield themselves from the threat component of information provided to them. Women at increased risk for ovarian cancer who are high monitors have more elevated cancer risk perceptions and more intrusive cancer ideation and general distress (Schwartz, Lerman, Miller, Daly, & Masny, 1995). More recently, it has been shown that anxiety during the period of waiting for *BRCA1/2* results is greater for women who are high monitors (Tercyak et al., 2001). These authors recommended that tailored "psychological management" be made available to women who are high monitors to reduce distress during the period of waiting for results.

LOSS, UNRESOLVED GRIEF, CAREGIVING, AND DISTRESS

The experience of being part of a cancer family affects the lives of individuals within the family in many ways. It is not only the diagnoses of cancer or the deaths of young parents that affect healthy family members. The omnipresence of cancer changes day-to-day life, often resulting in strained finances, restricted social interaction, and heightened tensions among family members. These individuals are cast into caretaking roles for ill relatives, sometimes, as in Mrs. P.'s case, many times over. The repetition of these experiences within the family translates grief into trauma, as devastating experiences occur in close proximity to each other, with little time for resolution and relief before the next tragedy. Although not everyone who comes for cancer genetic testing has had the extent of loss that Mrs. P. has experienced, they are, by definition, individuals who have had more frequent than normal family experiences of cancer. Many have watched a parent die at an early age because one of the cruel aspects of at least some hereditary cancer syndromes is the early age at which the cancers occur. It is hoped that the focus on high-risk cancer families resulting from the availability of genetic testing will lead to more opportunities for psychological intervention, especially with bereaved children, to help reduce the long-term distress that many experience.

Early experiences with cancer and the death of close relatives, especially mothers, from cancer contribute to the overestimation of cancer risk that occurs in members of high-risk families (see Risk Perception later in the chapter). This in turn deepens worry about cancer and adds to the intensity of desires for genetic testing and risk-reducing activities, including prophylactic surgeries. Many of the women who undergo prophylactic mastectomy report that their major motivation is to be alive to help their children grow up, unlike their own experience of having their own mother die when they were young.

The connection between maternal loss and psychological distress among high-risk women has been demonstrated in a number of studies. Zakowski et al. (1997) found that women with positive family histories of breast cancer whose mother had died of breast cancer had elevated levels of psychological distress. DudokdeWit et al. (1997a) similarly reported that individuals at-risk for several genetic conditions, including breast–ovarian and colon cancers, with "disease specific key experience" related to illness in a close relative had high levels of intrusive thought. Erblich, Bovbjerg, and Valdimarsdottir (2000) compared women with positive family histories (FH+) of cancer (one or more first-degree relatives with breast cancer) and women from the same community without such family histories (FH−) on general distress (Brief Symptom Inventory scores) and breast-cancer-related distress on the Impact of Event Scale. They found higher cancer-related distress in women whose mothers had died of breast cancer; even higher levels of distress were found among women who had cared for their mothers with breast cancer and whose mothers later died from the disease. This latter group had depressive symptoms that were significantly greater than women whose mothers had died but who had not cared for the mothers or those who did not have a family history of cancer. What is particularly striking is that the mothers of women in this study had died an average of 14 years earlier, suggesting the long-lasting impact of these traumatic family experiences.

Some dissenters believe that levels of distress among at-risk individuals seeking testing are exaggerated and that screening for distress among individuals seeking genetic testing is costly and unjustified. Coyne, Benazon, Gaba,

Calzone, and Weber (2000) studied 464 at-risk women who were members of a hereditary breast and ovarian cancer registry. They were studied during a period when the women were anticipating being offered genetic testing. Of the women in this sample, 23% scored in the clinically distressed range on the Hopkins Symptom Checklist—25, a standard psychological distress measure (Derogatis et al., 1974), but only 1% met the criteria for major depressive disorder using the Structured Clinical Interview for DSM–IV (First, Spitzer, Williams, & Gibbon, 1995). These authors dismissed the scores on the Hopkins Symptom Checklist as representing transient distress at levels below some primary medical care, community, and other medical samples (including wives of myocardial infarction patients, female congestive heart failure patients, and a group of divorced women who did not have custody of their children). The authors posited that "the experience of living with familial risk of cancer may well have organized psychological resources and fostered resiliency that more than compensates for any vulnerability associated with it" (p. 871). Although this study raises a number of interesting questions about the importance of acquiring empirical data in this area, there are problems in the methodology (Paterson et al., 2001), including a lack of equivalence of the comparison samples, the dismissal of self-reported distress measured by standard instruments, and the underlying assumption of the study that only distress that interferes with comprehension or adherence is significant in the lives of those undergoing genetic testing.

RISK PERCEPTION

A major question for individuals seeking genetic counseling and testing concerns their beliefs about their level of vulnerability to disease as a result of the hereditary predisposition in their family. Although objective risk can be estimated by genetic counselors using pedigrees and the statistical models discussed in chapter 3, self-perception of risk may be an even more potent force in determining how stressful individuals find life in a high-risk cancer family. Risk perception is an important factor in the use of screening and surveillance behaviors and interacts strongly with psychological distress. One of the central aims of genetic counseling is to ensure that individuals have accurate understanding of their current estimated risk and of the implications of the risks revealed through testing. I address here questions about how to present risk information to improve understanding and then address the question of how much difference the presentation of objective risk information makes to the risk perception of individuals whose family experience has been so heavily affected by cancer.

Which Risk Are We Talking About?

Risk can be expressed in a number of ways, and various risk estimates can be calculated for any one person. A person might be asked to estimate his or her risk for a particular disease by choosing a number from 1 to 100 to represent the percentage risk. An alternate approach would be to describe a comparative risk, that is, risk relative to the general population for the disease. This would likely be in the form of a 1- to 5-point Likert-type scale, with items such as *much lower risk, slightly lower risk, same risk, slightly higher risk, much higher risk*. When scientists and doctors talk about risk as a ratio or comparison with other groups, they speak of "relative risk" and describe it numerically. An example might be the relative risk of developing ovarian cancer for a woman who has a mother or sister who had ovarian cancer before age 30. In a relative risk comparison, this risk would be compared with the risk for women in the general population. This relative risk (RR) would be expressed as RR = 4.8 (Stratton et al., 1999), meaning that the woman from an ovarian cancer family with a FDR who had ovarian cancer would have 4.8 as many chances of developing ovarian cancer as a woman in the general population. To know just how likely she would be to develop ovarian cancer, it would be necessary to know the absolute lifetime risk of developing ovarian cancer. Absolute risk is usually expressed as a percentage. Absolute risks can be lifetime risks, risks by current age, or risks within a given time period, say the next 5–10 years. The absolute lifetime risk of ovarian cancer for women in the general population is about 1%, which means that first-degree relatives of the woman with ovarian cancer under age 30 would have about a 5% chance of developing ovarian cancer before age 85.

Overestimation of Cancer Risk

Weinstein (1982, 1984) posited that "unrealistic optimism" guides people's comparison of their risk for getting a disease compared with the risk of others similar to themselves. He believes that despite what people may give as their objective risk estimate, when asked how much they are at risk compared, say, with others their age, they are likely to consider themselves at a lower risk. This theory may help to explain why women without a family history in the McCaul and O'Donnell (1998) study described themselves as at less risk than other people their age, despite giving personal breast cancer risk estimates that were three times the actual population risk. Risk estimates increase with perceived lack of control of the disease and with personal knowledge of someone who has had the disease, both prominent features of the experience of living in a family with increased cancer rates. In these families, experience generates the opposite conclusions—that is, unrealistic pessimism. When several close relatives have all developed the same or related cancers, it feels as if cancer is the norm rather than the exception. Many people with extensive family histories of cancer say they feel it is not a question of *if* they will develop cancer but *when*. Research discussed below illustrates how personality factors and life events influence risk perceptions and also demonstrate that perceived risk is difficult to influence through provision of objective risk information.

A number of studies have shown that, in general, women overestimate their risk for breast cancer. This is especially true for women who have first-degree relatives with breast cancer. Perhaps because of the vast public information campaign about breast cancer and growing public knowledge about the genetics of hereditary breast/ovarian syndromes, women who are first-degree relatives of someone with the disease tend to think their lifetime risk of breast cancer is four times or more that of women in the general population (McCaul & O'Donnell, 1998). Because of the media attention to breast cancer genetics and to holistic ways to try to decrease one's risk of breast cancer through diet, exercise, and other factors, these tend to be in the forefront of women's minds when asked to estimate their own risk for breast cancer. In the McCaul and O'Donnell study, 76% of the women used "genetics" as a factor in determining their personal breast cancer risk estimate; 61% cited "lifestyle choices" (i.e., diet, exercise, breast-feeding) as factors they had considered in estimating their risk. Only 7% used the widely publicized "1 in 9" population lifetime risk figure (Offit, 1998) in their estimation of personal risk, despite the fact that 53% of the sample had no family breast cancer risk and thus should be at or below the population risk for breast cancer. The 1 in 9 risk denotes the approximately 11% risk that a woman will develop breast cancer if she lives to age 85 (Offit, 1998). Women's estimates of genetic risk did not seem to take into consideration the fact that only 5% to 10% of breast cancer is thought to be hereditary in etiology.

Zakowski et al. (1997) showed that the death of a parent from cancer led women who were undergoing mammography screening but had no abnormal findings to have significantly higher estimates of their lifetime risk of breast cancer (mean estimated lifetime risk = 70%) than similar women who did not have a parent die of cancer (mean estimated lifetime risk = 53%) or women in the general population of similar age who had no family history of cancer and were recruited through advertisement (mean estimated lifetime risk = 32%; p < .05). The authors conjectured that the death of a parent from cancer raises the threat of a cancer diagnosis to an extreme and challenges normal feelings of invulnerability. Of interest is that these women had been asked to rate their risk of *developing*, not dying from, breast cancer, yet they perceived themselves at increased likelihood to develop the disease, presumably because the threat of cancer loomed larger in their experience than in the experience of women who had not lost a parent to the disease. In the Zakowski et al. study, death of a parent from cancer was also correlated with more intrusive thoughts about breast cancer and scores indicating greater avoidance of cancer. Recency of parental death was not correlated with increased distress, reflecting again how long-lasting the psychological effects of losing a parent to cancer can be on an individual's sense of his or her own vulnerability to the disease. This point is especially important to remember when treating older patients whose parent died from cancer many years earlier. As a case in point, an interviewer elicited tears from a 70-year-old man during a telephone interview about breast cancer genetic testing as he recalled his inability to attend his mother's funeral, 50 years earlier, after she died from breast cancer while he was serving as a soldier in World War II.

If an individual has a first-degree relative who had breast cancer, that individual's overall risk estimate is increased, but not nearly so much as women appear to think (Cannon-Albright, Bishop, Goldgar, & Skolnick, 1991). In the McCaul and O'Donnell (1998) study, women with a first-degree relative with breast cancer thought, on average, that they had a 55% lifetime risk of the disease, and women with no family history thought, on average, that they had a 35% risk of breast cancer. Given the 11% population breast cancer risk, it is striking that so many women significantly overestimated their risk. In a report of 192 healthy, asymptomatic women at high risk for breast cancer, 67% of the women overestimated their breast cancer risk (Kash, Holland, Miller, & Osborne, 1999). This overestimation suggests that the level of anxiety about breast cancer in U.S. women far exceeds what is realistic.

An English study (Evans, Burnel, Hopwood, & Howell, 1993) of risk estimates given by women attending a cancer genetics clinic also showed distortion of the women's understanding of both population risks and of their personal risk of breast cancer. Errors included both overestimation and underestimation, however. Only 11% of the women correctly estimated the population lifetime risk for breast cancer; 30% of the women thought the population lifetime risk of breast cancer was 1 in 50 or lower. Forty-four percent correctly estimated their own risk (as calculated according to the Claus model [Claus, Risch, & Thompson, 1990] by the clinic geneticist or oncologist). Of those who incorrectly estimated their personal risk, 29% underestimated by more than 50% and 23% overestimated their risk by 50% or more. Given such discrepancies, one can imagine that the women at the ends of the continuum of estimates would have very different reactions to hearing actual population and personal risk estimates during genetic counseling.

Ovarian cancer risks are even less well understood than breast cancer risk. In the Hallowell study (1998), 43% of the women stated that their level of risk as determined through genetic counseling was actually lower than what they had previously believed. After counseling, however, 23% still inaccurately described their risk in absolute terms, that is, either as certainty that they would develop cancer (15%) or certainty that they would not develop cancer (8%). The authors believe their data illustrate the extent to which women reframe the information they have been given to allow themselves to continue to maintain their preexisting, emotional sense of cancer risk. So if neither population statistics nor personalized risk estimates inform women's ideas of their own genetic risk, what do they use as the basis for their thinking? It appears that they use their own life experience. All of the women who thought it inevitable that they would get cancer referred to their family cancer experience as the basis for their belief that cancer would eventually be their fate as well.

How Women Think About Risk

Some question whether women naturally think of risk in numerical ways at all and whether studies of the success of genetic counseling that employ changes in women's numerical estimates of their own risk of breast cancer are measuring the wrong variable. A British study interviewed unaffected women referred to a cancer family history clinic for genetic counseling for hereditary breast and ovarian cancer about how they thought about their risk for breast and ovarian cancer (Hallowell et al., 1998). Interestingly, upon entry to the program, 83% of the women said they did not think of their risk numerically and 70% could not cite the population risk for breast or ovarian cancer, yet 76% of the women perceived themselves to be at greater risk compared with women in the general population. What this highlights is that, at least prior to genetic counseling, women are guided by a general, psychological sense of being at increased risk, not by numbers that they attach either to their own risk or to that of women in general. It may be difficult for these women to evaluate the various numerical risks they may read or be told about because they lack a good understanding of the baseline risk of breast or ovarian cancer for a woman in the general population.

How Women With Cancer Think About Risk

One might wonder whether women who have had cancer have more realistic ideas about the likelihood of their carrying a genetic mutation responsible for their cancer. A study (Iglehart et al., 1998) of 200 women with family histories suggestive of genetic risk who were diagnosed with breast cancer (91%), ovarian cancer (7%), or both (3%) at age 56 or earlier showed no correlation between the women's baseline (i.e., precounseling) estimates of their likelihood of carrying a mutation in their *BRCA1/2* genes and the risk estimates of an expert panel or of the much-utilized carrier probability model, BRCAPRO (Berry, Parmigiani, Sanchez, Schildkraut, & Winer, 1997; Parmigiani, Berry, & Aguilar, 1998). When estimates were arranged by quartile (risk from 0%–25%, 26%–50%, 51–75%, and 76%–100%), 55% of the women differed in their personal risk estimate by more than two quartiles from the risks estimated by professionals. When 100 of the women were given genetic mutation screening tests (an abbreviated search for certain known mutations) and the results were compared, there was again no correlation between the findings and the risk estimates of the women. In other words, women's estimates and the estimates of professionals diverged markedly, with women vastly overestimating their risk for carrying a BRCA1/2 mutation.

Perceived Risk for Colon Cancer

Perceived risk for colon cancer and perceptions of risk relative to the general population were higher among first-degree relatives of colorectal cancer patients who accepted genetic testing for HNPCC versus those who declined (Codori et al., 1999). One third of those who declined testing said that they thought their risk was lower than the risk for the general population. Decliners also tended to be nonadherent to colonoscopy recommendations. Decliners were more likely to think it would be difficult to cope with knowing one was a mutation carrier compared with those who accepted testing. In that study, the uptake of testing among individuals who lived within 50 miles of the test center was 58%.

An Australian study (Collins, Halliday, Warren, & Williamson, 2000) found a positive correlation between risk perception for colorectal cancer and cancer worry. All but the highest perceived risk group found that they worried less following a genetic testing session, suggesting that they had significantly overestimated their risk. Over half of the attendees at the familial colorectal cancer clinic in Melbourne were very worried about colorectal cancer. That study found a positive relationship between cancer worry and adherence to screening behavior recommendations.

Petersen et al. (1999) studied 1,373 individuals who had at least one first-degree relative with colon cancer. They found that 78% believed they had a higher colon cancer risk than the general population, and most thought that they would want genetic testing. Concern about developing colon cancer increased, not surprisingly, with the number of relatives with colon cancer, and these individuals were willing to pay more for genetic testing (up to $1,000) than others in the sample. Women expressed more worry than men.

In general, although individuals at risk for HNPCC have expressed high rates of interest in genetic testing (Glanz, Grove, Lerman, Gotay, & Le Marchand, 1999; Petersen et al., 1999), the acceptance rates have been only slightly higher than rates of uptake for *BRCA1/2*. Lerman et al. (1999) found that 43% of HNPCC family members accepted genetic testing and 57% declined. Depression was associated with the decision not to be tested, especially among women; depressed women were 4 times less likely to be tested than women who were not depressed. Acceptance rates for familial adenomatous polyposis testing have been higher; 82% of asymptomatic adults enrolled in a colorectal cancer registry and 95% of minors underwent genetic testing (Petersen & Boyd, 1995). An English study showed nearly 100% of those at risk had undergone genetic testing (Whitelaw, Northover, & Hodgson, 1996).

Prostate Cancer Risk Perception

Prostate cancer accounts for 29% of cancer cases (Greenlee, Murray, Bolden, & Wingo, 2000); about 5% to 10% of prostate cancer cases are likely to represent inherited mutations. It appears somewhat more difficult to find and define these hereditary families because age of onset is somewhat, but often not strikingly, younger then in sporadic cases. Only about 10% of prostate cancers occur under 60 years of age. In addition, the range of expression and the rate of progression of the disease in a single family varies significantly, making it more difficult to predict the type of disease experience that the presence of an inherited mutation conveys (Ostrander & Stanford, 2000).

Although there is not yet clinical testing for prostate cancer genes, some research has been conducted on how men perceive their risk, how interested they say they are in genetic testing, and how these factors relate to screening practices (Bratt et al., 2000). Unaffected male relatives (50–72 years of age) of men from 118 Swedish families with three or more connected cases of prostate cancer were studied via mail questionnaire. The estimated lifetime risk of prostate cancer in this sample was 35% to 45%. Risk overestimation was common; the median estimate of personal risk was 50%; 40% of the men perceived their risk to be greater than 67%. Risk perception was significantly positively correlated with the number of relatives who had died from prostate cancer. A quarter of the men worried fairly or very much, but only 3% said that prostate cancer worry affected their daily life very much. Worry was associated with higher depression and anxiety scores. Depression was correlated with risk overestimation. These findings are similar to many about risk perception in women from high-risk breast and ovarian cancer families.

A study that conducted focus groups for Caucasian, African American, and Asian men in a community sample found those with a family history of prostate cancer saw themselves at increased risk for the disease, as did those who had experienced non-cancer-related prostate problems (Doukas, Fetters, Coyne, & McCullough, 2000). A high level of interest in and support for prostate genetic testing was found among the Caucasian and Asian men, but more concern was noted among the African American men about possible misuse of genetic information.

Does Genetic Counseling Change Risk Perception?

It is often difficult to change people's deeply held health beliefs and usual health behaviors through provision of objective risk information alone. One indication of the strength of underlying attitudes and health beliefs is data on the limited extent to which genetic counseling changes beliefs, attitudes, and plans. In the Burke et al. (1997) study of women at intermediate risk of breast cancer who received highly individualized counseling, estimates of personal risk and population risk were lowered from the original overestimates. Among the women at intermediate risk (means of 12%–13% breast cancer risk by the Gail [Gail et al., 1989] and Claus models [Claus, Risch, & Thompson, 1994]) who received genetic counseling, personal risk estimates greater than 50% dropped from 48% to 17% 6 months after counseling. A control group of intermediate risk women who did not receive counseling maintained their high levels of overestimation, with only a 4% reduction from 54% to 50% 6 months later. More important, however, the majority of the women who received counseling continued to consider themselves good candidates for BRCA1/2 genetic testing, despite counseling to the contrary. Prior to genetic counseling, 82% of counselees and 93% of control participants thought that they were definitely or probably eligible candidates for genetic testing. The percentage among control participants was unchanged but dropped only to 60% among those who received the counseling. The women's interest in genetic testing was similar, dropping from 91% before counseling to 58% for those who received counseling and only to 88% among control participants. The authors suggest that, although the women in this program derived benefits from counseling and, on average, reduced the inaccuracy of their risk estimation, even further refinement is needed in the design of counseling protocols to achieve more realistic risk appraisal and to better guide behavior.

Another study reviewed women's reactions to being informed by letter of their ineligibility for genetic testing for hereditary breast cancer after completing a screening questionnaire (Bottorff et al., 2000). The letter stated clearly that the reason for the ineligibility was that the women did not appear to be at high risk of developing breast cancer. Nonetheless, the women responded with anger, frustration, fear, and disappointment, refusing for the most part to accept that they were not at high risk. Fewer than half, however, contacted their physician to discuss the ineligibility letter, as recommended.

Others have found similar disjunctive results in the counseling of high-risk women. A study in Wales compared the impact of standard consultation with breast surgeons with specialized, multidisciplinary genetics assessment of women with a family history of breast cancer. They concluded that specialized genetics services did not result in cost-effective improvements in anxiety, breast cancer worry, or perceived risk. The slight improvement in knowledge about breast cancer did not justify the extra cost, the authors believe, because the level of knowledge achieved was not considered optimal, even among the counseled group (Brain et al., 2000).

Watson et al. (1998) found that among 115 consecutive women with a family history of breast cancer who received genetic consultation at one of two London hospitals, only 41% accurately reported the risk estimate for breast cancer that they had received during counseling a month after having had the counseling; 25% overestimated their risk, 11% underestimated their risk, and another 25% could not remember or did not know their risk. Those who received an audiotape of the consultation were no more likely than those without a tape to remember their risk accurately. Interestingly, increased cancer worry was associated with increased risk perception, regardless of actual risk. In other words, women's personal beliefs about their risk appeared to guide how much they worried about getting cancer, not the objective risk information they received during counseling.

Lindberg and Wellisch (2001) found that 77% of the 430 at-risk women in their study overestimated their risk by more than 10%, but they found overestimation of risk unrelated to women's general anxiety. They concluded that

> overestimation of risk is not a function of women's immediate worries or general anxious states. Rather, we believe that overestimation of risk appears clinically to be a function of an ongoing internalized self-perception of vulnerability to breast cancer. This self-perception, we hypothesize, is developmental in nature and is related to identification, introjection, and internalization of the ill family member, especially the mother. (p. 303)

This interesting hypothesis attempts to integrate the history of loss with the risk perception and distress of high-risk women. It supports the heavy impact of emotional overlay in what is sometimes conceived of as a cognitive task. It also speaks to the need to provide cancer risk education that addresses the underlying psychological issues and processes as well as providing factual risk information.

HEALTH BELIEFS

Preexisting, deep-seated health beliefs, then, can be obstacles to realistic assessment of one's risk for disease. Misconceptions about the inheritance of breast cancer were common among a group of 200 well-educated (55% had some college or college degrees or some graduate education), high-risk women who had breast cancer (Iglehart et al., 1998). Among these women, 86% believed that 1 in 10 women carry a *BRCA1/2* mutation, and 62% believed that half of all breast cancer cases are caused by *BRCA1/2*. (In reality, 1 in 8 or 1 in 9 women get breast cancer, and only 5% to 10% of breast cancer is thought to be due to inheritance of cancer susceptibility genes.) Furthermore, 56% of these women did not believe that fathers can pass along mutations in *BRCA1/2* as easily as mothers.

Oppenheim, Brugieres, Chompret, and Hartmann (2001) report on the diverse etiologies that members of Li–Fraumeni syndrome families ascribed to the relentless occurrences of cancer within their families. Some believed it was a "curse," others that it stemmed from blood donations. When the results of genetic testing showed the cause to be genetic, one man was described as "relieved. There was a logic to it, a beginning, a middle, and an end" (p. 174). The authors went on to say, however, that he believed the mutation had its origins with Original Sin and reported that he had become a Jehovah's Witness to ensure he would not be given blood transfusions. Such vignettes are not unique as illustrations of the desire to find meaning amid the helplessness of feeling one's family has been singled out, generation after generation, for misfortune. The authors suggest that medical professionals inquire about the patients' beliefs about the origin of their familial misfortune when caring for members of high-risk cancer families, recognizing that self-perceived beliefs about etiology are often much more powerful and immutable than those that come as facts from outside medical sources.

Cultural Differences

Cultural background heavily influences attitudes toward medical information and medical providers. To date, genetic testing for cancer genes has tended to involve a relatively homogeneous group of highly educated, high-income, Caucasian people. This is likely to change as more genes are found and genetic counseling and testing for a wider variety of disorders becomes the standard of care. This change will demand attention to the forms of counseling we use and the cultural appropriateness of measures used to assess patient distress and outcomes and to indicate satisfaction.

Causal attribution for illness is influenced by the sense of perceived control or helplessness experienced by members of various cultures (Die-Trill, 2000). Other factors, including religious beliefs, level of education, and ideas about self-responsibility affect views on why illness occurs in one's family with high frequency. Illness attribution can occur at more than one level, with individuals able to repeat what doctors have told them is the cause for their own or their child's illness, but, if asked, also revealing their highly cathected, personal views of the illness etiology. In a study of mothers of children with cancer, most said that medical providers had told them there was no known cause for their child's illness (which is generally true for pediatric cancers). Nevertheless, 83% described their personal views about factors they believed were responsible for the child's cancer (Patenaude, Basili, Fairclough, & Li, 1996). These factors ranged from environmental toxins, genetics, parental behavior during pregnancy, parental sexual behavior, drug use, smoking, stress, and earlier childhood illness. Mothers' attributions controlled much of the way families coped with the illness, leading one family, for example, to move from a house the mother believed had electromagnetic environmental hazards she held responsible for her child's cancer and another to dispose of its microwave oven, which the mother blamed for her child's illness.

Different cultures perceive cancer differently. In some, such as the Japanese, it is associated with shame, fostering a climate of noncommunication within families and frequent nondisclosure of diagnosis to the patient (Fukui et al., 2000). Breast cancer patients in Israel varied in their ideas about the cause of their cancer depending on whether they had a Western orientation, attributing the breast cancer to science-oriented factors over which some control was possible, or whether they had an Eastern orientation, which associated cancer with fatalism and helplessness (Baider & Sarell, 1983). In one study, African American women were found to associate breast cancer with bumping or bruising of the breast, smoking, and use of oral contraceptives (Royak-Schaler, Cheuvront, Wilson, & Williams, 1996).

Hughes et al. (1997) compared knowledge about *BRCA1* testing between 407 African American and Caucasian women who had at least one first-degree relative with breast and/or ovarian cancer. They found significant differences by ethnic group in knowledge and perception of benefits. African American women had significantly less knowledge about breast and ovarian cancer genetics and genetic testing, but they were also more positive about the potential benefits of testing. The authors concluded that African American women might base their decisions about testing on different information and beliefs than Caucasian women.

Recommendations given to those at high risk for hereditary breast and ovarian cancer include surveillance and screening options such as mammography and risk reduction options such as chemoprevention and prophylactic surgery. It has been shown that in addition to individual differences in the acceptability of various forms of prophylactic surgery, there are also cultural differences in the acceptability of these three forms of early detection and risk reduction (Julian-Reynier et al., 2001). A comparison of English, French, and French Canadian women showed that the French women were least accepting of prophylactic mastectomy, the French and French Canadian were least accepting of prophylactic oophorectomy, and the English women were more in favor of chemoprevention. Cultural biases may reflect professional attitudes and recommendations within each country but may also reflect more basic cultural attitudes and values about illness, about control over nature, and about the factors that make life worthwhile.

The participation of African Americans in clinical genetics studies has been even lower than their participation in biomedical research in general (Royal et al., 2000). It is believed that this is a function both of the paucity of African American genetics professionals to encourage participation and of the historically negative experiences of African Americans in research on sickle cell disease, another genetic disease. In 1998, the American Society of Human Genetics reported that only 1.1% of their membership (composed of medical geneticists, genetic counselors, and cytogeneticists) was African American (Mittman, 1998). A group of African American biomedical and social scientists formulated a "Manifesto on Genomic Studies," which stated that acceptable studies would include African American community representatives. The manifesto encouraged the involvement of African American professionals in all aspects of research, not simply as suppliers of research participants (Jackson, 1998). It encouraged recognition of the heterogeneity of diverse African American subcultures and the tailoring of research invitations and materials to the characteristics of these groups. It also encouraged flexibility in the recruiting of participants, including evening hours and home visits. It linked the success of projects with African American participants to the degree of attention paid to the diverse needs of participant populations.

The familial focus of cancer genetics magnifies the cultural lens through which patient–provider communication occurs. Professionals are often blind to how cultural assumptions can color the ways in which information about families is gathered. We take for granted, for example, the notion of bilateral kinship systems with maternal and paternal lines of inheritance and ask family history questions to complete a pedigree accordingly. Meiser et al. (2001b) describe incompatibility between some cultural views of kinship and assumptions underlying Mendelian genetics. Many Asian and Middle Eastern families, for example, define a kindred through male lines of descent, making it difficult to overlay questions that seek to uncover patterns of inherited disease coming from both maternal or paternal lines. They point out that there is cultural variation in how people of various cultures view assistance (such as genetic counseling) from outside the family and the revelation of detailed health information to strangers. In addition, they cite language and literacy barriers, lack of awareness of genetic services and related risk-reducing treatments or preventive measures, lack of access to medical records for diagnostic confirmation, and lack of referral for genetic services as factors limiting the access of minority patients to genetic counseling and testing. In addition, the scarcity of minority genetic counselors is, in itself, not conducive to encouraging minority patients to seek genetic counseling (Royal et al., 2000).

Health Behaviors of At-Risk Individuals

Perceptions of control over disease, risk perception, and psychological distress all affect an individual's attitudes regarding the importance of carrying out health practices recommended to minimize increased hereditary risk for disease. If people do not believe much can be done to affect whether a disease develops or at what stage it is discovered, then they are not highly motivated to carry out the recommended testing or examination. If people perceive themselves to be at low risk, then their motivation to adhere to recommendations is again likely to be low. If people believe they are at extremely high risk, they may find it difficult to undergo screening or surveillance activities because the anxiety the testing process generates is likely to be unpleasant, perhaps even paralyzing. If distress is very high, even people who believe they can take some control by following recommended surveillance guidelines may be too anxious or depressed to overcome the normal barriers to making and keeping appointments. The fact that many women, including high-risk women, do not adhere to recommendations, that many men from hereditary prostate cancer families do not have regular exams and prostate specific antigen tests, and that both average and high-risk men and women avoid screening colonoscopies leads to serious questions about whether campaigns to raise awareness about cancer risk have failed to adequately address the significant emotional and cultural barriers that prevent optimal early detection.

Many researchers suggest that there is an optimal range of anxiety for individuals at potentially increased risk. A certain amount of anxiety motivates an individual to overcome the hassle of finding appropriate services and making and meeting appointment times. If anxiety is too low, these barriers impede such action. Fear of discrimination, lack of insurance coverage for such services, and hesitancy to use existing coverage create additional barriers. If the patient perceives there is a high likelihood that "bad" information may be forthcoming from such a consultation, appointments may be repeatedly cancelled. Similarly, once personalized risk information is received, there may be an optimal level of anxiety to keep individuals going for regular screening or surveillance checks. If, after counseling, the information received heightens a woman's anxiety, making her believe that it is likely a lump she has found in her breast is cancer, it could have the undesired effect of having her put off going to a doctor for an evaluation of the lump for a longer period of time than she would have without the personal risk information.

What do we know, then, about the health behaviors of individuals who come for cancer genetic counseling or testing? Screening of at-risk individuals varies considerably depending on the nature of the cancer risk and type of testing or examination recommended. Valdimarsdottir et al. (1995) found that high-risk women had higher levels of generalized distress than did women in the general population, both at the time of getting a mammogram and even one month following receipt of a normal result. Women at high risk of breast and ovarian cancer tend, in general, to be relatively faithful to the recommendations for mammograms at earlier-than-usual ages and more frequent clinical breast exams. Yet although most women at high-risk for breast and ovarian cancer report that they get regular mammograms, many do not do breast self-examination (BSE) monthly as general population recommendations propose (Kash et al., 1992). Breast self-examination is difficult to do for many women at high risk for breast cancer, who report that they are too frightened of finding a lump to do regular self-examinations. Lindberg and Wellisch (2001) reported a negative correlation between anxiety about BSE and compliance. They hypothesized that it is difficult for women to perform BSE because it is the one early detection procedure performed when the woman is alone. Their recommendation is for highly supportive, targeted training for BSE.

A Canadian study of women from families with likely inherited ovarian cancer, most of whom had relatives with ovarian or breast cancer (or both), illustrated an inverse relationship between adherence to surveillance recommendations for ovarian cancer and perceived risk. Risk perception was assessed following a genetic counseling session. Individuals who perceived themselves to be at high risk were five times less likely to adhere to the recommended surveillance practices than those who perceived themselves to be at moderate or low risk (Ritvo et al., 2002).

Surveillance for colon cancer among the general population is at much lower levels than mammography (Vernon, 1997). In a recent study of individuals who had had colorectal cancer or who had a first-degree relative with colon cancer, the majority had no knowledge of genetic testing for colon cancer genes, although they were aware of breast cancer genetic testing (Kinney, DeVellis, Skrzynia, & Millikan, 2001). When informed about the options for testing, those surveyed thought that testing positive would result in greater adherence to recommendations for colonoscopy, although they found that expectation distasteful. Another study found total lack of awareness about genetic testing options among first-degree relatives of colon cancer patients in St. Louis and Indianapolis. When those participants were informed, considerable distrust about potential outcomes of testing were elicited (Todora et al., 2001). Even among individuals who have undergone HNPCC cancer genetic counseling and genetic testing, the level of colon cancer surveillance is sub-optimal.

Because of the range of cancers present in Li–Fraumeni syndrome, at-risk individuals should have regular checkups. It is also essential that they have a physician who is knowledgeable about their family history and about Li–Fraumeni syndrome so that they can rapidly and appropriately evaluate any symptom that might indicate a malignancy. Among a sample of individuals from Li–Fraumeni syndrome families at 90% lifetime risk for a variety of cancers, many did not follow even general population recommendations for cancer screening. It is ironic that some individuals who come for *p53* genetic testing did not even have a personal physician (Patenaude, 1997).

Factors beyond cancer family history, such as socioeconomic status, geographic distribution, media attention, and physician recommendation, also affect screening and surveillance adherence for at-risk individuals. As such, it is extremely difficult to compare screening rates across hereditary cancers. It is also true that, in most cases, we have data largely on that part of the at-risk population who are willing to participate in research studies or be seen in high-risk clinics. It could be hypothesized that this group may be the most motivated and thus may also be more adherent than those unwilling to be research participants or to come to high-risk clinics. This hypothesis is among several issues in need of further research within the population of at-risk individuals who do not undergo genetic counseling or testing.

Although the men and women who have been tested for breast cancer genes to date have tended to be from better educated levels of society, even among these groups significant misunderstandings exist about the meaning of negative or indeterminate results. In some cases, this appears to result from the complexity of the information delivered; in others cases, it is due to the persistence of preexisting personal beliefs about cancer. In the future, as more individuals with lower levels of education and literacy, people who do not speak English or are nonnative English speakers, and people who come from more diverse cultural backgrounds are tested, greater confusion can be expected. This anticipated confusion speaks to the need for research on the cultural meanings of genetic information and on effective means of delivering this information. It also speaks to the need for culturally sensitive psychologists who can help patients from diverse backgrounds integrate genetic information into their views of themselves, their families, and the larger society.

Physician education and physician recommendations are also important factors in screening behaviors of at-risk populations. In a sample of gastrointestinal specialists, only 16% were recommending appropriate surveillance for HNPCC patients (Batra, Valdimarsdottir, McGovern, Itzkowitz, & Brown, 2002). In an earlier study, 30% of the physicians giving HNPCC genetic test results to patients misinterpreted the meaning of a negative result (Giardello et al., 1997).

A number of studies have pointed out that there are both psychological and medical implications of participating in any kind of disease screening. Marteau, van Duijn, and Ellis (1992) showed that individuals found to carry the gene for Tay–Sachs disease, a degenerative neurological disease, reported less optimism about their future than noncarriers, even though their being a carrier had no effect on their own health or expected life span. Perceived health at present was not significantly different between carriers and non-carriers. The authors concluded that when people learn they carry a mutation for a serious disease, it has subtle but significant and long-lasting effects on their perception of themselves and their health. A study in Israel by Gilbar (1998) showed that women who know they are at increased risk for breast cancer who come for evaluation of a possible breast cancer symptom have similar lag times to the lag time of women without a family history; about 50% of both groups wait more than six months to go to the doctor. However, women with a family history are much more distressed at the time of the doctor's visit. A recent Australian study has suggested that after women are informed that they are carriers of BRCA1/2 mutations, they adhere less strictly to recommendations about mammograms and other surveillance behaviors than before undergoing testing (Meiser et al., 2001a). There is a great need for more follow-up studies in this area. The fruits of new genetic knowledge and effective counseling programs can only be realized if at-risk individuals are not left so anxious about the cancers for which they are at high risk that they adopt patterns of denial and avoidance, decreasing the likelihood of early detection through screening. Here again, mental health professionals have a major role to play. Advanced molecular biology cannot help people who are paralyzed by cancer fears to get regular checkups or make medical appointments to evaluate suspicious symptoms.

In addition to worries about reduced ability to diagnose cancer early, we should also be concerned with the development of cancer phobia symptoms in people without actual symptoms. Jimmie Holland, a respected psycho-oncologist, has noted that family experience with cancer is prominent in the histories of healthy individuals experiencing extreme cancer phobia (Holland, 1989). Ryle (1948) reported that 39% of patients with cancer phobia had experienced a death in the family from cancer. Bianchi (1971) noted that media focus on a particular disease or medical concern is often accompanied by increased reports of phobias related to that condition. Media focus on genetic testing for breast cancer has certainly been intense over the last 5–10 years. Holland (1989) also noted that although it is difficult to diagnose, cancer phobia in individuals at increased risk of cancer can sometimes lead to dysfunction. Some women for whom such fear is overwhelming seek prophylactic surgical solutions rather than cope with the anxiety through other means. Kerr et al. (1998) noted that that some patients falsely report histories of hereditary cancer because of excessive concern about the disease and a desire to undergo testing. Careful follow-up of medical records in suspicious cases and referral for psychological assessment and treatment are recommended, preferably before surgery or other irreparable actions are taken.

One of the stronger motivations for seeking genetic testing that people cite is the belief that knowing their genetic risk status will help them improve their health behaviors (Esplen et al., 2001; Julian-Reynier et al., 1996). It is interesting that this motivation is described as an expected outcome of testing positive, but sometimes also as an expectation of what will change if the test result is negative. Many at-risk individuals consider failure to fully comply with diet and exercise recommendations as a personal weakness that they think they would be motivated to correct if they knew with certainty that they were at high risk for cancer. Many also believe that a negative test would increase their personal investment in their future health and well-being and would decrease their worry about cancer, which would lead to improvement in their motivation to take care of themselves. They hope that knowing their gene-negative status would improve the likelihood that surveillance procedures would provide repeated evidence of the absence of cancer, rather than a positive diagnosis.

The ultimate medical goals of genetic counseling and testing for cancer genes are to reduce the number of at-risk individuals who develop cancer and the number who die from the cancers that do develop. The creation of targeted risk-reduction measures for mutation carriers is in its infancy. Over the decades to come, through pharmacogenomic improvements and increasing knowledge about which procedures and risk-reduction activities are truly preventative, we will be able to clarify prevention and screening recommendations. It is hoped, for example, that risk-reduction measures less disagreeable than colonoscopies and with fewer sequelae than prophylactic mastectomy will be developed and that these measures will have equal or superior efficacy. In the meanwhile, many individuals will have difficult decisions to make. Mental health professionals have much to offer these people and their family members at each step in the progression from genetic counseling to testing and, if needed, to planning for risk-reducing surgeries and screening or surveillance activities. Individualized planning that takes into consideration the psychological style, cultural health beliefs, and strengths of the individual is most likely to yield optimal rewards in terms of adherence to recommendations and diminished distress, two of the ultimate goals of the Human Genome Project.

SUMMARY

I have briefly described some of the complex issues present in families heavily burdened by hereditary cancer. Much remains to be learned about the interaction of these factors in determining who makes use of genetic technologies, who experiences emotional distress related to testing, and who will develop cancer.

Cancer genetic counseling offers at-risk individuals knowledge about the likelihood of an inherited risk factor in their family, an estimate of their individual risk, and a recommendation about the likely utility of genetic testing. For some, cancer genetic testing provides more definitive information about personal risk. Whether knowledge of personal cancer risk is more of an asset than a liability depends on the balance between the individual's coping style, psychological vulnerability, objective and perceived risk, and the impact such knowledge has on his or her health behaviors and outcomes.

The role of separating the effects of unresolved grief reactions, possible posttraumatic stress disorder, and a family experience heavily linked to illness on the emotions of individuals contemplating or reacting to cancer genetic testing will fall, with increasing frequency, to mental health professionals, both within cancer centers and in the community. Psychotherapy may be seen in some cases as a prerequisite to the genetic testing of distressed individuals, a follow-up adjunct to testing, or, in some cases, even an alternative to testing. Some people seeking testing want to resolve issues that are actually psychological in nature and will not be relieved by provision of more accurate risk information alone. Some seek testing in the hope of finding better ways to cope with feelings of guilt or doom that are more properly the work of therapists than genetic counselors. Others are referred for longer term psychotherapy to resolve deeper conflicts or emotions aroused by the prospect or impact of genetic counseling and testing. Sometimes both genetics counselors and mental health professionals are needed to answer the patient's questions. The collaboration between genetic counselors and psychologists is a natural one; the two professions share similar goals and support the ultimate aims of genetic advances. The goal of genetic counseling is not to improve individuals' accuracy in repeating statistics about cancer risk, but rather to reduce worry and clarify the appropriateness of genetic testing and preventive, risk-reduction, or early detection strategies. The optimal end point of genetic testing is improvement in the quality, and whenever possible, the quantity of life for individuals at increased risk of cancer through clarification of individual risk.

REFERENCES

Audrain, J., Schwartz, M. D., Lerman, C., Hughes, C., & Peshkin, B. N. (1997). Psychological distress in women seeking genetic counseling for breast-ovarian cancer risk: The contributions of personality and appraisal. *Annals of Behavioral Medicine, 19*, 370–377.

Baider, L., & Sarell, M. (1983). Perceptions and causal attributions of Israeli women with breast cancer concerning their illness: The effects of ethnicity and religiosity. *Psychotherapy and Psychosomatics, 39*, 136–143.

Batra, S., Valdimarsdottir, H., McGovern, M., Itzkowitz, S., & Brown, K. (2002). Awareness of genetic testing for colorectal cancer predisposition among specialists in gastroenterology. *American Journal of Gastroenterology, 97*, 729–733.

Becker, E. (1973). *The denial of death.* New York: The Free Press.

Berry, D. A., Parmigiani, G., Sanchez, J., Schildkraut, J., & Winer, E. (1997). Probability of carrying a mutation of breast-ovarian cancer gene BRCA1 based on family history. *Journal of the National Cancer Institute, 89*, 227–238.

Bianchi, G. N. (1971). Origins of disease phobia. *Australia-New Zealand Journal of Psychiatry, 5*, 241–257.

Bottorff, J. L., Balneaves, L. G., Buxton, J., Ratner, P. A., McCullum, M., Chalmers, K., Hack, T., et al. (2000). Falling through the cracks: Women's experience of ineligibility for risk of breast cancer. *Canadian Family Physician, 46*, 1449–1456.

Bowlby, J. (1980). Loss, sadness & depression. In *Attachment and loss* (Vol. 3). London: Hogarth Press.

Brain, K., Gray, J., Norman, P., France, E., Anglim, C., Barton, G., et al. (2000). Randomized trial of a specialist genetic assessment service for familial breast cancer. *Journal of the National Cancer Institute, 92*, 1345–1351.

Bratt, O., Damber, J.-E., Emanuelsson, M., Kristoffersson, U., Lundgren, R., Olsson, H., & Gronberg, H. (2000). Risk perception, screening practice and interest in genetic testing among unaffected men in families with hereditary prostate cancer. *European Journal of Cancer, 36*, 235–241.

Burke, W., Peterson, G., Lynch, P., Botkin, J., Daly, M., Garber, J. E., et al. (1997). Recommendations for follow-up care of individuals with an inherited predisposition to cancer 1: Hereditary nonpolyposis colon cancer. *Journal of the American Medical Association, 277*, 915–919.

Cannon-Albright, L. A., Bishop, D. T., Goldgar, D., & Skolnick, M. H. (1991). Genetic predisposition to cancer. In V. T. De Vita, S. Hellman, & S. A. Rosenberg (Eds.), *Important advances in oncology* (pp. 39–55). Philadelphia: Lippincott.

Claus, E. B., Risch, N. J., & Thompson, W. D. (1990). Age at onset as an indicator of familial risk of breast cancer. *American Journal of Epidemiology, 131*, 961–972.

Claus, E. B., Risch, N., & Thompson, W. D. (1994). Autosomal dominant inheritance of early-onset breast cancer: Implications for risk prediction. *Cancer, 73*, 643–651.

Codori, A.- M., Petersen, G. M., Miglioretti, D. L., Larkin, E. K., Bushey, M. T., Young, C., et al. (1999). Attitudes toward colon cancer gene testing: Factors predicting test uptake. *Cancer Epidemiology, Biomarkers, & Prevention, 8,* 345–351.

Collins, V., Halliday, J., Warren, R., & Williamson, R. (2000). Cancer worries, risk perceptions and associations with interest in DNA testing and clinic satisfaction in a familial colorectal cancer clinic. *Clinical Genetics, 58,* 460–468.

Coyne, J. C., Benazon, N. R., Gaba, C. G., Calzone, B., & Weber, B. L. (2000). Distress and psychiatric morbidity among women from high-risk breast and ovarian cancer families. *Journal of Consulting and Clinical Psychology, 68,* 864–874.

Derogatis, L. R. (1983). *SCL–90 Administration, scoring, and procedures manual.* Baltimore: Clinical Psychometric Research.

Derogatis, L. R., Lipman, R. S., Rickels, K., Uhlenhuth, E. H., & Covi, L. (1974). The Hopkins Symptom Checklist (HSCL): A self-report symptom inventory. *Behavioral Sciences, 19,* 1–15.

Die-Trill, M. (2000). Beliefs about cancer causation and their influence on family function. In L. Baider, C. L. Cooper, & A. K. De-Nour (Eds.), *Cancer and the family* (2nd ed., pp. 119–130). Chichester, England: Wiley.

Doukas, D. J., Fetters, M. D., Coyne, J. C., & McCullough, L. B. (2000). How men view genetic testing for prostate cancer risk: Findings from focus groups. *Clinical Genetics, 58,* 169–176.

DudokdeWit, A. C., Tibben, A., Duivenvoorden, H. J., Frets, P. G., Zoeteweij, M. W., Losekoot, M., et al. (1997a). Psychological distress in applicants for predictive DNA testing of autosomal dominant, heritable, late onset disorders. *Journal of Medical Genetics, 34,* 382–390.

DudokdeWit, A. C., Tibben, A., Frets, P. G., Meijers-Heijboer, E. J., Devilee, P. L., Klijn, J. G. M., et al. (1997b). *BRCA1* in the family: A case description of the psychological implications. *American Journal of Medical Genetics, 71,* 63–71.

Erblich, J., Bovbjerg, D., & Valdimarsdottir, H. B. (2000). Looking forward and back: Distress among women at familial risk for breast cancer. *Annals of Behavioral Medicine, 22,* 53–59.

Esplen, M. J., Madlensky, L., Butler, K., McKinnon, W., Bapat, B., Wong, J., et al. (2001). Motivations and psychosocial impact of genetic testing for HNPCC. *American Journal of Medical Genetics, 103,* 9–15.

Evans, D. G. R., Burnel, L. D., Hopwood, P., & Howell, A. (1993). Perception of risk in women with family history of breast cancer. *British Journal of Cancer, 67,* 612–619.

First, M., Spitzer, R. L., Williams, J. B., & Gibbon, M. B. (1995). *Structured Clinical Interview for DSM–IV (IP).* New York: New York State Psychiatric Institute, Biometrics Research Department.

Fukui, S., Kamiya, M., Koike, M., Kugaya, A., Okamura, H., Nakanishi, T., et al. (2000). Applicability of a Western-developed psychosocial group intervention for Japanese patients with primary breast cancer. *Psycho-Oncology, 9,* 169–177.

Gail, M. H., Brinton, L. A., Byar, D. P., Corle, D. K., Green, S. B., et al. (1989). Projecting individualized probabilities of developing breast cancer for white females who are being examined annually. *Journal of the National Cancer Institute (Bethesda), 81*, 1879–1886.

Giardello, F. M., Brensinger, J. D., Petersen, G. M., Luce, M. C., Hylind, L. M., Bacon, J. A., et al. (1997). The use and interpretation of commercial APC gene testing for familial adenomatous polyposis. *New England Journal of Medicine, 336*, 823–827.

Gilbar, O. (1998). Coping with threat: Implications for women with a family history of breast cancer. *Psychosomatics, 39*, 320–339.

Glanz, K., Grove, J., Lerman, C., Gotay, C., & Le Marchand, L. (1999). Correlates of intentions to obtain genetic counseling and colorectal cancer gene testing among at-risk relatives from three ethnic groups. *Cancer Epidemiology, Biomarkers, & Prevention, 8*, 329–336.

Goldberg, D., & Williams, P. (1988). *A user's guide to the General Health Questionnaire*. London: NFER-Nelson.

Greenlee, R., Murray, T., Bolden, S., & Wingo, P. (2000). Cancer statistics, 2000. *CA: A Cancer Journal for Clinicians, 50*, 7–33.

Hallowell, N. (1998). "You don't want to lose your ovaries because you think, 'I might become a man.'" Women's perceptions of prophylactic surgery as a cancer risk management option. *Psycho-Oncology, 7*, 263–275.

Holland, J. C. (1989). Fears and abnormal reactions to cancer in physically healthy individuals. In J. C. Holland & J. H. Rowland (Eds.), *Handbook of psycho-oncology: Psychological care of the patient with cancer* (pp. 13–21). New York: Oxford University Press.

Horowitz, M., Wilner, N., & Alvarez, W. (1979). Impact of Event Scale: A measure of subjective stress. *Psychosomatic Medicine, 41*, 209–218.

Hughes, C. H., Comez-Caminero, A., Benkendorf, J., Kerner, J., Isaacs, C., Barter, J., & Lerman, C. (1997). Ethnic differences in knowledge and attitudes about BRCA1 in women at increased risk. *Patient Education and Counseling, 32*, 51–62.

Iglhehart, J. D., Miron, A., Rimer, B. K., Winer, E. P., Berry, D., & Shildkraut, J. M. (1998). Overestimation of hereditary breast cancer risk. *Annals of Surgery, 228*, 375–384.

Jackson, F. (1998). Scientific limitations and ethical ramifications of a non-representative human genome project: African-American responses. *Science and Engineering Ethics, 4*, 155–170.

Julian-Reynier, C. M., Bouchard, L. J., Evans, D. G., Eisinger, F. A., Foulkes, W. D., Kerr, B., et al. (2001). Women's attitudes toward preventive strategies for hereditary breast or ovarian carcinoma differ from one country to another. *Cancer, 92*, 959–968.

Julian-Reynier, C., Eisinger, F., Vennin, P., Chabal, F., Aurran, Y., Nogues, C., et al. (1996). Attitudes towards cancer predictive testing and transmission of information to the family. *Journal of Medical Genetics, 33*, 731–736.

Kash, K. M., Holland, J. C., Halper, M. S., & Miller, D. G. (1992). Psychological distress and surveillance behaviors of women with a family history of breast cancer. *Journal of the National Cancer Institute, 84*, 24–30.

Kash, K. M., Holland, J. C., Miller, D. G., & Osborne, M. P. (1999) Intervention for women at risk for breast cancer. *Psycho-Oncology, 8(Suppl. 6)*, 9.

Kerr, B., Foulkes, W. D., Cade, D., Hadfield, L., Hopwood, P., Serruya, C., et al. (1998). False family history of breast cancer in the family cancer clinic. *European Journal of Surgical Oncology, 24*, 275–279.

Kinney, A. Y., DeVellis, B. M., Skrzynia, C., & Millikan, R. (2001). Genetic testing for colorectal carcinoma susceptibility: Focus group responses of individuals with colorectal carcinoma and first-degree relatives. *Cancer, 91*, 57–65.

Lerman, C., Hughes, C., Trock, B. J., Myers, R. E., Main, D., Bonney, A., et al. (1999). Genetic testing in families with hereditary nonpolyposis colon cancer. *Journal of the American Medical Association, 281*, 1618–1622.

Lindberg, N. M., & Wellisch, D. (2001). Anxiety and compliance among women at high risk for breast cancer. *Annals of Behavioral Medicine, 23*, 298–303.

Marteau, T. M., van Duijn, M., & Ellis, I. (1992). Effects of genetic screening on perceptions of health: A pilot study. *Journal of Medical Genetics, 29*, 24–26.

McCaul, K. D., & O'Donnell, S. M. (1998). Naive beliefs about breast cancer risk. *Women's Health: Research on Gender, Behavior, and Policy, 4*, 93–101.

Meiser, B., Butow, P. N., Barratt, A. L., Schnieden, V., Gattas, M., Kirk, J., et al. (2001a). Long-term outcomes of genetic counseling in women at increased risk of developing breast cancer. *Patient Education and Counseling, 44*, 215–225.

Meiser, B., Eisbruch, M., Barlow-Stewart, K., Tucker, K., Steel, Z., & Goldstein, D. (2001b). Cultural aspects of cancer genetics: Setting a research agenda. *Journal of Medical Genetics, 38*, 425–429.

Miller, S. M., Roussi, P., Caputo, G. C., & Kruus, L. (1995). Patterns of children's coping with an aversive dental treatment. *Health Psychology, 14*, 236–246.

Mittman, I. S. (1998). Genetic education to diverse communities employing a community empowerment model. *Community Genetics, 1*, 160–165.

Offit, K. (1998). *Clinical cancer genetics: Risk counseling and management.* New York: Wiley-Liss.

Oppenheim, D., Brugieres, L., Chompret, A., & Hartmann, O. (2001). The psychological burden inflicted by multiple cancers in Li–Fraumeni families: Five case studies. *Journal of Genetic Counseling, 10*, 169–183.

Ostrander, E. A., & Stanford, J. L. (2000). Genetics of prostate cancer: Too many loci, too few genes. *American Journal of Human Genetics, 67*, 1367–1375.

Parks, C. M., & Weiss, R. S. (1983). *Recovery from bereavement.* New York: Basic Books.

Parmigiani, G., Berry, D. A., & Aguilar, O. (1998). Modeling risk of breast cancer and decisions about genetic testing. *American Journal of Human Genetics, 62*, 145–158.

Patenaude, A. F. (1997). *Li–Fraumeni Syndrome genetic testing project interviews.* Unpublished manuscript.

Patenaude, A. F., Basili, L., Fairclough, D. L., & Li, F. P. (1996). Attitudes of 47 mothers of pediatric oncology patients toward genetic testing for cancer predisposition. *Journal of Clinical Oncology, 14,* 415–421.

Paterson, A. G., Trask, P. C., Schwartz, S. M., Deaner, S. L., Riba, M., & Holland, J. C., et al. (2001). Screening and treatment of distress. *Journal of Consulting and Clinical Psychology, 69,* 339.

Petersen, G. M., & Boyd, P. (1995). Gene tests and counseling for colorectal cancer risk: Lessons from familial polyposis. *Journal of the National Cancer Institute Monographs, 17,* 67–71.

Petersen, G. M., Larkin, E., Codori, A. -M., Wang, C. -Y., Booker, S. V., Bacon, J., et al. (1999). Attitudes toward colon cancer gene testing: A survey of relatives. *Cancer Epidemiology, Biomarkers, & Prevention, 8,* 337–344.

Rando, T. (1984). *Grief, dying, and death: Clinical interventions for caregivers.* Champagne, IL: Research Press Co.

Ritvo, P., Irvine, J., Robinson, G., Brown, G., Murphy, K. J., Matthew, A., & Rosen, B. (2002). Psychological adjustment to familial-genetic risk assessment for ovarian cancer: Predictors of nonadherence to surveillance recommendations. *Gynecologic Oncology, 84,* 72–80.

Royak-Schaler, R., Cheuvront, B., Wilson, K. R., & Williams, C. M. (1996). *Journal of Clinical Psychology in Medical Settings, 3,* 185–199.

Royal, C., Baffoe-Bonnie, A., Kittles, R., Powell, I., Bennett, J., Hoke, G., et al. (2000). Recruitment experience in the first phase of the African-American hereditary prostate cancer (AAHPC) study. *Annals of Epidemiology, 10,* S68–S77.

Ryle, J. A. (1948). The Twenty-First Maudsley Lecture: Nosophobia. *Journal of Mental Science, 94,* 1–17.

Schwartz, M. D., Lerman, C., Miller, S. M., Daly, M., & Masny, A. (1995). Coping disposition, perceived risk and psychological distress among women at increased risk for ovarian cancer. *Health Psychology, 14,* 232–235.

Stratton, J. F., Thompson, D., Bobrow, L., Dalal, N., Gore, M., Bishop, D. T., et al. (1999). The genetic epidemiology of early-onset epithelial ovarian cancer: A population-based study. *American Journal of Human Genetics, 65,* 1725–1732.

Tercyak, K. P., Lerman, C., Peshkin, B. N., Hughes, C., Main, D., Isaacs, C., & Schwartz, M. D. (2001). Effects of coping style and BRCA1 and BRCA2 test results on anxiety among women participating in genetic counseling and testing for breast and ovarian cancer risk. *Health Psychology, 20,* 217–222.

Todora, H. M. S., Skinner, C. S., Gidday, L., Ivanovich, J. L., Rawl, S., & Whelan, A. J. (2001). Perceptions of genetic risk assessment and education among first-degree relatives of colorectal patients and implications for physicians. *Family Practice, 18,* 367–372.

Valdimarsdottir, H., Bovbjerg, D. H., Kash, K. M., Holland, J. C., Osborne, M. P., & Miller, D. G. (1995). Psychological distress in women with a familial risk for breast cancer. *Psycho-Oncology, 4*, 133–141.

Vernon, S. W. (1997). Participation in colorectal cancer screening: A review. *Journal of the National Cancer Institute, 89*, 1406–1422.

Vernon, S. W., Gritz, E. R., Peterson, S. K., Amos, C. I., Perz, C. A., Baile, W. F., & Lynch, P. M. (1997). Correlates of psychologic distress in colorectal cancer patients undergoing genetic testing for hereditary colon cancer. *Health Psychology, 16*, 73–86.

Watson, M., Duvivier, V., Wade Walsh, M., Ashley, A., Davidson, J., Papaikonomou, M., et al. (1998). Family history of breast cancer: What do women understand and recall about their genetic risk? *Journal of Medical Genetics, 35*, 731–738.

Weinstein, N. D. (1982). Unrealistic optimism about susceptibility to health problems. *Journal of Behavioral Medicine, 5*, 441–460.

Weinstein, N. D. (1984). Why it won't happen to me: Perceptions of risk factors and susceptibility. *Health Psychology, 3*, 431–457.

Whitelaw, S., Northover, J. M., & Hodgson, S. V. (1996). Attitudes to predictive DNA testing in familial adenomatous polyposis. *Journal of Medical Genetics, 33*, 540–543.

Zakowski, S. G., Valdimarsdottir, H. B., Bovbjerg, D., Borgen, P., Holland, J., Kash, K., et al. (1997). Predictors of intrusive thoughts and avoidance in women with family histories of breast cancer. *Annals of Behavioral Medicine, 19*, 362–369.

Zigmond, A. S., & Snaith, R. P. (1983). The Hospital Anxiety and Depression Scale. *Acta Psychiatrica Scandanavia, 67*, 361–370.

5

OPENING PANDORA'S BOX: DISCLOSURE OF THE RESULTS OF CANCER GENETIC TESTING

PREPARING TO HEAR

Some patients take months to schedule their appointment for disclosure of genetic testing results. Others count the hours until they can have the answers they seek. Some bring a spouse, parent, sibling, grown child, or friend. Others insist on going alone. Although the length of discussion before disclosure is usually kept to a minimum, for some it is still much too long. Others say later they wished health care providers had talked longer before "dropping the bomb."

Genetic testing results are usually revealed in person by a genetic counselor, geneticist, or physician. Usually the counselor who conducted the initial counseling visit either delivers the result or is present when a geneticist or medical oncologist does so. This is useful so that discussions following disclosure can focus on the implications of the results that are likely to be most salient for that individual. If a physician is present, he or she can focus on the medical implications while the counselor relates more directly to genetic issues and the patient's emotional and familial concerns.

DELIVERY OF THE TEST RESULT

Whenever it comes, delivery of the test result is a dramatic moment for everyone involved. It is an intimate moment when professionals feel privileged to be present at a turning point in the life of another person. At the same time, the professional delivering the message shoulders the burden of responsibility for the manner of the delivery, the clarity of the recommendations, and the oversight of the individual's emotional response. At times, it is difficult not to feel responsible for the content of the message as well, however irrational that may be. The results have implications not only for the individual at the disclosure visit, but also for other generations; the impact is, in some ways, more far-reaching and profound than the diagnosis of a malignancy. For carriers who are members of high-risk cancer families, the answer links them to relatives who have had cancer and separates them from those not at increased risk. For noncarriers, the result may be experienced as separation from the many experiences of illness and loss that they may have witnessed or heard of among their relatives and from those family members who are known to be at risk or whose status is unknown. Providers should be mindful that despite receiving "good" news, these individuals may still experience some, often unanticipated, sense of loss or disconnection at this juncture.

What the Patient Is Told

The information conveyed in cases with a known mutation in the family is relatively uncomplicated. In those cases, disclosure is a relatively simple message: "Yes, you do have the mutation in your family" or "No, you do not have the mutation that your relatives with cancer have." The definitive nature of the information leaves little room for interpretation.

When there is not a known mutation in the family, the disclosure may involve a more complicated explanation of the result. This circumstance occurs when someone is the first in his or her family to be tested or if there are no living or consenting relatives with cancer in whom to look for a mutation. Under these circumstances, the test is not an attempt to match a known deleterious mutation at a specific site with the presence or absence of a mutation at that site in the blood of the tested individual, but a search for any alterations from what is considered "normal." With current genetic knowledge, the result cannot always be interpreted.

A positive result in an affected individual means that a mutation was found that is known to interfere with the gene's function. This alteration is sufficient to justify the conclusion that the mutation is responsible for causing the cancer. This is the mutation that can then be looked for in the DNA of other family members who have not had cancer.

If no mutations or variants are found, the result is considered an indeterminate negative. This result

> may decrease the likelihood that the client has an inherited predisposition to cancer but does not eliminate the possibility. The family could have a mutation in the analyzed gene that cannot be detected by current technologies or could have a mutation in a gene which has not yet been identified. (Schneider, 2002, p. 262)

The third possibility in this circumstance is that of a polymorphism of unknown significance, a new change of unclear importance. The possibilities range from being significant enough to cause cancer to being minor enough not to interfere with the function of the gene at all.

Both indeterminate negative and polymorphism of unknown significance results are complex, abstract, and difficult to interpret. Recipients of such information cannot be completely reassured because the meaning of the information is unclear. In many ways, the uncertainty they face is as great as that they had before initiating testing. One hopes that they were prepared for the possibility of an uncertain outcome during the genetic counseling stage, although such uncertainty is emotionally difficult to anticipate and easy to dismiss as unlikely. Because of the "fuzzy" nature of the information received, that is, that this result may or may not be significant with regard to cancer risk, it is also open to misinterpretation or reinterpretation. Such abstract and uncertain scientific information can be difficult to comprehend, even under ideal circumstances. Patients may come away believing that they must be a mutation carrier at increased risk because something was changed in their DNA, or, at the other end of the spectrum, that this result is definitive proof that they don't have a "bad" mutation. Repetition of the complex and uncertain meaning of their test result and a chance to ask questions and discuss the person's beliefs about the information conveyed are especially important parts of the counseling process for those with indeterminate negative results or polymorphisms of unknown significance.

Another situation that can lead to an indeterminate result is when there is no known mutation in a family, but the person undergoing testing is a member of an ethnic group in which particular mutations occur with greater than usual frequency. The individual can be tested looking only for those mutations. This is currently the case with Ashkenazi Jews who are tested for the two BRCA1 and one BRCA2 mutations known to exist in increased frequency among members of this group. A positive result confirms that the individual is at increased genetic risk for breast and ovarian cancer. Just how much the risk is increased may vary depending on how much knowledge there is about the penetrance of the mutation in the patient's ethnic group. For example, in the case of Ashkenazi Jews, it is currently believed that testing positive for one of the three mutations conveys a 56%

risk for breast cancer as well as a significantly increased risk for ovarian cancer and smaller increases in risk for colon and prostate cancers (Struewing et al., 1997). (See chap. 2, "Cancer Genes and Cancer Risk," for further discussion of cancer risks and founder mutations.) A negative result in this circumstance is not a true negative because 10% of mutations in Ashkenazi Jews with hereditary breast and ovarian cancer occur at sites other than those where the three classic mutations occur. This result is referred to as an indeterminate negative.

The finding of a polymorphism of unknown significance or of an indeterminate negative can be disappointing to people receiving this complex result because it leaves them without clear information about their risk, despite the considerable expense incurred for testing and the lengthy wait for results. Further assessment of the result may reveal if the polymorphism of unknown significance has been found in other families and, if so, if it has been associated with cancer.

It is well known that anxiety interferes with learning and decision making (Janis, 1983). Certainly disclosure of a genetic test result is a moment of high anxiety and preoccupation and not the ideal environment for conveying information that can have such complex meaning and implications. Although genetic counselors and geneticists make valiant efforts, most patients report that they remember accurately little factual information from disclosure sessions. For these reasons, follow-up, in person or by telephone, after the disclosure session, especially with carriers, is useful in correcting misconceptions and discussing options for screening, surveillance, and risk reduction.

Acceptance

Some people appear well prepared to hear the results of testing. Others have a firm belief that they are or are not carriers, which may be confirmed or disproved at disclosure. There are tears of joy, tears of sorrow, and tears of relief at the end of an anxiety-filled wait. Often there are also tears of grief aroused by thoughts of ill or deceased relatives. Many are stoic in the face of a positive result, saying that they expected this result and had always known their chances of getting cancer were high. "This is nothing new. I have always thought I would get cancer. It was just a question of when. This doesn't change anything." Some take comfort in the counselor's restating that this is not a cancer diagnosis, only a clear warning of an increased, but not inevitable, likelihood of getting certain types of cancer.

* * *

Case Example. Rick was engaged to be married. He and his fiancée came together to the genetic testing research setting for the genetic counseling session and again, several months later, for the result. A *p53* mutation had been found to explain the excessive cancers in Rick's family. Rick had been contacted as part of the research program and decided he wanted to know if he was a carrier. He worked in a family business and did not have health insurance. He also did not have an ongoing relationship with a primary care physician or an internist; he only went to the doctor if he had a problem, and he had not been ill for several years. He said he didn't worry about cancer too much, but he thought that if he was positive for the mutation, he would take better care of himself. He also believed that it could influence the decision he and his fiancée made about having children. He held hands with his fiancée as the doctor delivered his result. Rick did, in fact, carry the *p53* familial mutation. His fiancée clenched his hand tighter, and then they embraced. He winced almost imperceptibly. It felt like a verdict had been delivered. His New England roots seemed to prohibit showing more emotion. He was sad and disappointed, he said, but it was better to know. He would find insurance, he would find a doctor, although he thought he wanted one who lived in a different town, so he could be more secure that his status would not become common knowledge. They would still get married, they had decided that beforehand. His fiancée would worry for him and with him about taking care of himself. She felt this was a role she wanted to take on and help him with. Maybe they wouldn't have kids. During a follow-up interview six months later, Rick described what had changed in his life since the disclosure session. The wedding had occurred. He had a health insurance policy, but still no doctor. His wife was after him about that and, more generally, about his health. His thoughts about children had changed. He had decided that they probably would have children. He thought about the fact that if his parents had known the same genetic information he now knew and they had made the decision not to have children, he wouldn't have been born. He reasoned that he was healthy and over 30 and that if he had children that might well be the case for them, too. Thirty years from now, things might be different. There might be better ways to prevent cancer, even in people with "bad genes." He and his bride were doing fine, he said. He rarely thought about cancer.

* * *

The data that are emerging suggest that most people accept the news that they carry a deleterious mutation with less than clinical levels of distress and reestablish equilibrium in their daily lives, at least outwardly. Some put it out of mind, as Rick did. For others, it is a source, at least initially, of significant distress and intrusive thought. Family members, too, react, and it changes their lives as well.

DISTRESS AND DEPRESSION

Since the advent of the availability of genetic tests for cancer susceptibility in the mid-1990s, there has been a great deal of concern in medical and ethical circles about whether learning the results of cancer genetic tests causes serious emotional and interpersonal harm. Because there are also continuing questions about the medical benefits of knowing one's genetic cancer susceptibility status, it remains challenging to determine whether the benefits merit the risk of possible emotional distress or exposure to social stigma.

The first cancer genetic testing protocols were based on those developed for research programs investigating the impact of genetic test results on individuals at increased risk for Huntington's disease (HD). Individuals who develop HD have four to eight times the suicide rate of the general population (DiMaio et al., 1993; Schoenfeld et al., 1984). The worry was that telling people from families with HD that they had tested positive for a degenerative condition with no treatment or cure would elicit self-defeating, self-injurious, or even suicidal behaviors. A worldwide review of the adverse outcomes of genetic testing for HD showed that less than 1% of tested individuals had either attempted or committed suicide following disclosure of their results. There were 5 completed suicides and 21 attempts (Almqvist, Bloch, Brinkman, Craufurd, & Hayden, 1999).

To date, few studies have considered the impact of cancer genetic testing. Most of those that do exist compare mean baseline scores from administrations of standard measures of psychological distress at entry into a counseling program with mean scores after disclosure of test results. Most of the reports show only small effects on the average participant in a cancer genetic testing program. All the authors caution in generalizing from this data, however, because these early studies were conducted in controlled research environments using extensive genetic counseling and psychological support and follow-up.

PSYCHOLOGICAL OUTCOMES OF BREAST–OVARIAN CANCER PREDISPOSITION TESTING

The first people to be offered genetic testing for common cancers were from high-risk breast and ovarian cancer families. Studies of the outcomes of genetic testing generally take at least several years, and to date only relatively short-term findings are available about the impact of testing. Lerman et al. (1996) found that depressive symptoms of men and women carriers of BRCA1 mutations were not, on average, significantly changed at one month following disclosure compared with predisclosure levels. At one month, noncarriers showed a decline on the Center for Epidemiological

Studies—Depression Scale (CES–D; Radloff, 1977) depression scores, and decliners of testing showed no appreciable change in their scores. Croyle, Smith, Botkin, Baty, and Nash (1997) found that among 60 women tested for *BRCA1*, mutation carriers had (not surprisingly) greater levels of test-related distress after disclosure than noncarriers. Baseline anxiety scores were correlated with anxiety at follow-up. General (state) anxiety was also significantly diminished for noncarriers, but mean anxiety scores were relatively unchanged for carriers. Cancer experience also moderated the effect in that women found to carry a mutation who had not had cancer or experienced cancer-related surgery (i.e., those with less prior personal cancer experience) appeared most affected by positive results. The authors concluded that because many women seeking genetic testing for breast cancer susceptibility are likely to be those who have not had either cancer or prophylactic surgery, the relatively high anxiety experienced by such women in this study should be addressed in future planning of testing programs.

Other groups have found indications that disclosure of a genetic test result is more stressful for cancer patients than originally appreciated. Dorval et al. (2000) found cancer patients less likely than noncancer patients to accurately anticipate their emotions following disclosure. Cancer patients tended to underestimate how worried and sad they would feel upon hearing definitively that they were mutation carriers. Underestimating the emotional impact of a test result was associated with a significant increase in distress at six months postdisclosure. A French study of 23 cancer patients who were mutation carriers for *BRCA1/2* or a colon cancer predisposition gene found high anxiety in a third of the cancer patients at six weeks postdisclosure. Qualitative interviews revealed that for a third of the cancer patients, learning their carrier status had evoked deep fear related to the possibility of developing a second cancer and concern about their children's cancer risk (Bonadona et al., 2002).

One issue that researchers and practitioners consider now that clinical testing for *BRCA1/2* has become relatively available outside of research programs is the extent to which the outcomes of testing are similar in the two settings. At the same institution as the Lerman study, Schwartz et al. (2002) studied women tested through a clinical program rather than a research study. They found, as did the Croyle et al. (1997) study, that unaffected participants who had positive results did show "modestly" elevated distress compared with participants who had negative results. The difference was due to decreases in distress among individuals who tested negative for *BRCA1/2* mutations that had been found in other family members. Among women with cancer who tested positive, there was no difference in cancer-specific or general distress compared with women who had had cancer and whose results did not show a mutation (and were thus uninformative). The generalizability of this study and of many other studies of outcomes of *BRCA1/2* testing may be limited, however, because of the homogeneity of the samples, especially the lack of cultural diversity, the high socioeconomic status of the participants, and the fact that these women received intensive, personalized, genetic counseling. The majority in the Schwartz study, for example, were college-educated Caucasian women with family incomes over $75,000.

Family Effects on Outcome of BRCA1/2 Testing

Some reports suggest that the method of analyzing even standard measurement data can alter the interpretation of the impact of results. Smith, West, Croyle, and Botkin (1999) found that if the result status for all family members was taken into consideration, elevations in distress were noted among several groups of tested individuals that had not been apparent when all carrier or noncarrier scores were analyzed together. Upon initial analysis, there was no significant difference in distress between male carriers and noncarriers of BRCA1 mutations. However, when analyzed further, it was found that male mutation carriers who were the first tested in their family and who had other siblings awaiting results were significantly more distressed than those who had siblings who had all tested negative. Male noncarriers with siblings who were all positive were also distressed. In the initial analysis, female carriers of BRCA1 mutations did score significantly higher on the Impact of Events Scale (Horowitz, Wilner, & Alvarez, 1979) than noncarriers at one week postdisclosure. Women who were mutation carriers and had all negative siblings (i.e., they were the only positives in their sibship), however, had very high Impact of Events Scale scores. These carriers had scores equivalent to those of women diagnosed with cancer within the past 10 weeks. Women carriers with sisters still awaiting results also had greater distress after disclosure.

The interacting effects of one's own test result and that of others in the family in determining the level of distress experienced was seen also in a study in the Netherlands of outcomes of BRCA1/2 testing. Lodder et al. (2001) found that among women who had been tested, 20% of those found to be mutation carriers had anxiety at or above borderline levels of anxiety on the Hospital Anxiety and Depression Scale (Zigmond & Snaith, 1983). Posttest anxiety was significantly correlated with pretest anxiety. Among noncarriers, 11% of tested women who did not have a mutation tested above clinical cutoffs for anxiety after learning they were negative. Half of the noncarrier women who had had high anxiety before disclosure continued to have high anxiety after receiving their normal test result. One third of the mutation carriers who had low anxiety scores before disclosure had high scores following disclosure. Depression scores were high for 12% of the mutation carriers and 4% of the noncarriers. Family experience interacted with result, such that noncarriers who had a sister who had recently tested positive had significantly higher posttest levels of depression than the other noncarriers. The results suggested the influence of both familial and individual factors, as well as the test result itself, on emotional outcomes following *BRCA1/2* testing.

Personality Factors in Breast and Ovarian Cancer Genetic Testing Outcomes

A study from the Georgetown University School of Medicine shows that coping style, particularly monitoring versus blunting of health threat information (discussed in chap. 4), influenced the level of a woman's anxiety during the period of waiting for test results but did not play a role in the heightened distress experienced by mutation carriers once the test result was known (Tercyak et al., 2001). Anxiety immediately following disclosure was significantly higher for mutation carriers versus noncarriers. Many patients mention the anxiety of waiting as a difficult aspect of the testing experience. The period between providing the blood sample for DNA analysis and receiving the test result is becoming shorter with technological improvements in genetic tests, but this interval may still be a time when individuals who focus on the anxiety-provoking aspects of medical information would find psychotherapeutic support or behavioral interventions helpful.

COLON CANCER GENETIC TESTING OUTCOMES

Remarkably little difference in anxiety scores between individuals testing positive and negative for hereditary nonpolyposis colorectal cancer mutations was found in a Finnish study that followed 271 individuals for one year after genetic testing (Aktan-Collan, Haukkala, Jukka-Pekka, Uutela, & Kaarianen, 2001). Immediately after disclosure, mutation carriers scored slightly, but significantly, higher on the State–Trait Anxiety Inventory (Spielberger & Lushene, 1970). Both at the one month and at the one year follow-up points, however, there was no longer any significant difference in anxiety scores between carriers and noncarriers. Mutation-positive individuals were consistently more afraid of cancer, as measured by the Aro adaptation of the Illness Attitude Scale (Aro, Absetz, van den Elderen, van der Ploeg, & van der Kamp, 2000) than were those who were mutation negative. It seems that the distress of cancer genetic testing is relatively specific and that it appears to peak at the time of disclosure in many cases.

Only a few studies have considered the impact of genetic testing for APC mutations in families with familial adenomatous polyposis. (Chap. 8 considers the outcomes for children in these families from the three recent studies.) In a study done in the United Kingdom and Australia, 43% of tested adults scored in the clinical range of anxiety after receiving their mutation-positive results versus 20% among those who received mutation-negative results ($p < .001$; Michie, Bobrow, Marteau, & FAP Collaborative Research Group, 2001). Mean depression scores for adults in this study were not significantly different for those who tested positive versus those who tested negative.

Parents of children who were tested for familial adenomatous polyposis in a U.S. study (Codori et al., 2003) had significantly higher depression rates at long-term follow-up (23–55 months) when their children had mixed testing outcomes (that is, one or more child was positive and one or more was negative) than parents of children who were all positive or parents of children who were all negative. Parents' mean depression scores remained in the nonclinical range, although about 5% of parents who began with nonclinical depression scores had scores in the clinical range at follow-up. Four of the five were unaffected parents, and three were parents whose children had mixed testing outcomes.

SOMATIZATION—MEN2A

It is somewhat surprising that few reports describe somatization among individuals tested for cancer genes. The literature on carriers of *RET* mutations predisposing to MEN2, however, contains several references to somatic symptoms and complaints among disease carriers. Trichotillomania (hair pulling to the point of baldness, lack of eyelashes, etc.), stomach pains, and night nausea were reported in a 13-year-old girl tested for RET (Giarelli, 1999). Grosfeld, Lips, and Beemer (1996) also reported that 41% of applicants to a MEN2 testing program in the Netherlands reported somatic complaints and 46% reported sleep disturbance 1 week after entering the research program. Anxiety (46%) and depressive (29%) symptoms were also prominent in this group. Two weeks following disclosure, these complaints remained high in both carriers and noncarriers. Somatic complaints were reported by 46% of positives and 33% of negatives and sleep complaints by 58% of positives and 46% of negatives. Carriers began to be preoccupied with symptoms of MEN2 and even reinterpreted past events as possible signs of the onset of the illness. Noncarriers were worried about the status of other family members and also found it stressful to adjust to the differentiation within the family group of some being at risk and others not. The authors reported that the MEN2 families had often been reluctant to discuss the illness with nonfamily members and thus had been dependent on support from other family members. The differentiation of at-risk status within the family changed the dynamics of that support network. A year after disclosure, somatic complaints were considerably lower (21% for positives and 14% for negatives), as were sleep complaints (7% for positives and 10% for negatives).

A SPECIAL ISSUE: LYING

There are several forms that lying can take with regard to cancer genetic testing. The first is the presentation of false family history data to mislead providers into considering the individual as someone at increased genetic risk for cancer and as eligible for genetic testing. A very small number of cases are reported in the literature, but the number will likely increase as social awareness of genetic testing increases. Kerr et al. (1998) reported on five families in their clinic (or 0.5% of their cases to date) in which family history information was intentionally falsified by the person seen in the clinic or by his or her relative. Signs indicating that the family history was false included lack of concordance in diagnoses and age at diagnosis reported to different members of the clinic, unrealistic length of survival based on clinical features reported, and lack of detailed knowledge of the illness in close relatives. Several women reporting false family history had a history of benign breast disease themselves or had at least one family member with breast cancer. This is in keeping with the general finding that women with Munchausen syndrome often have a true personal or family history of some serious illness (Masterton, 1995). Recognizing the possible presence of a Munchausen syndrome requires careful evaluation of the family history information provided. Checking of medical records is recommended when a reported family history appears inconsistent or is provided by someone who evokes suspicion. If the medical history is found to be false or significantly embellished, involvement of a mental health professional is encouraged to confront the individual and to help explain that such behavior is usually indicative of a need for psychological treatment of the underlying insecurities and anxiety.

Sometimes patients lie to family members or significant others about the results of a genetic test. This may be an attempt to gain time to come to a state of acceptance about an unexpected result: The person cannot believe that they are mutation positive, and telling someone else would confirm the reality of the result. They feel they have no option other than lying, often for the expressed reason of sparing the other person. Sometimes it is an attempt to avoid feelings of regret and responsibility for having passed (or potentially having passed) a deleterious mutation to a child. Some patients do not feel the full impact of knowing their children have a 50–50 chance of having inherited a mutation that predisposes them to cancer until the result is known. In addition, parents of older children sometimes project that the news of this "bad gene" must upset their child's romantic relationships. The parent construes that if the boyfriend or girlfriend of their adult child learns about the family's potentially high cancer risk, it might precipitate the end of the relationship. Rather than take the risk, especially in the case of a child who might not be at immediate increased medical risk, the parent might lie to the son or daughter, with plans to tell the truth later after the relationship has either resulted in marriage or ended for other reasons.

Trust is a critical dimension to family relationships. Lying about a test result is much more likely to cause permanent injury to the relationship between parent and child, among siblings, or among other relatives than is talking openly about an inherited mutation. The mutation is something one cannot control; lying is under the control of the individual and thus something for which the other person can legitimately hold the liar responsible. Good preparation for genetic testing involves thinking through who will be told and what feelings may be aroused by the disclosure. It may also involve surveying close family members about their wishes with regard to learning the test results of others in the family. Ideally, this is done before any actual test results are available, and possibly even before informing others about a definitive plan to be tested. Psychologists and other mental health professionals will increasingly be called on to help individuals discover how to talk with their family members about genetic information and how to decide whom to tell about genetic test results. Tasks for the therapist may include helping patients to distinguish personal privacy from familial responsibility, fear from guilt, and avoidance from lying. Skilled mental health providers can often help patients come to sufficient acceptance of the meaning of a positive test result to responsibly take on the burden of communicating well to other family members.

* * *

Case Example. Ted was a young, handsome man from a family riddled with cancer and identified as having a cancer syndrome. His girlfriend accompanied him to the genetic counseling visit in another state to learn more about his cancer risk. A technician took a blood sample, which would be used to determine whether he had the mutation known to be responsible for the cancer syndrome in his family. He was a firm believer in positive thinking, and he was sure he would be negative. He did not bring his girlfriend to the disclosure session but instead came with a relative who was also in the process of being tested. After getting his result, Ted called his girlfriend from the airport and told her the good news: He was not a carrier of the mutation. She was thrilled and welcomed him home warmly when he saw her in person the next night. About 10 days later, she ran into Ted's best friend. They chatted for a few minutes before he said something about how sorry he was to hear about Ted's test result. She looked at him quizzically. She realized that Ted had not told her the truth, as she saw no reason for the friend to make up such a story.

She confronted Ted that night, and he told her the truth. He had intended to tell her about the positive result, but he had not wanted to tell her on the phone. He realized that if he did not call her after the disclosure session, she would have worried. When she was so happy, he found it impossible to burst the bubble and reverse himself by telling her the truth. He had talked to his best friend and told him the truth, needing support and not wanting to make the same mistake with him. He had been too embarrassed to tell his friend that he had lied to her about the result, so he had not warned him that she didn't know. He was very sorry. In the short run, they talked a great deal about it, and the incident seemed to pass. When they broke up a few months later, however, it seemed that his lying about something so important had played a part in her growing distance from him.

* * *

These results illustrate the ways in which genetic results differ from those of other medical tests. When a family learns of a genetic predisposition in one of its members, individuals within the family evaluate their "good" or "bad" luck within the context of the results of the family as a whole. One cannot be purely happy when it is not clear how others in the family have fared in this genetic lottery. On the other hand, it is distressing to be the only one in the family who draws the short straw of increased genetic predisposition to cancer, that is, to be the only positive among a family of negatives. These reactions are even more pronounced when the cancer predisposition unevenly affects individuals of one sex or the other, as is the case with BRCA1/2 genes. When a brother is negative and his sister positive, and thus at very high risk for both breast and ovarian cancer, the guilt and distress are often intense. When hereditary predisposition genes for prostate cancer are found, it will be men who are the family members at disproportionately high risk. Both research data and clinical experience increasingly point to the importance of considering the impact of the entire testing experience on the family as a whole.

This brings up the cascade of testing effects that may occur over several generations. The period of time during which members of the adult generations of a family choose to be tested may be lengthy and spread over years or even decades. By the time all members of that generation have opted for or against testing, there are likely to be children or grandchildren reaching the age at which they can decide if they wish to be tested. Given the intertwining of impact of one person's result on others, anxiety about the potential presence of mutations in the family may be nearly perpetual in some at-risk families with closely spaced generations.

BEING SPARED: TESTING NEGATIVE

Most people, especially those who have not had cancer, approach genetic testing with the hope it will show them to be free of hereditary risk for cancer. When a true negative test result is disclosed, many express the feeling of having a great weight lifted from their shoulders, of having the future instantly become longer. The cycle is broken, one's children are not at increased risk, and the tested individual does not face a future overshadowed by the prospect of cancer.

From many, however, the message that they are not personally at increased genetic risk is quickly accompanied by feelings of guilt (discussed in the next section) with regard to those in their family who are mutation carriers. As the Smith et al. (1999) study showed, the joy of being negative is tainted for many when others in their family do not prove to be so lucky or when test results are not available for everyone and the uncertainty and worry linger.

Some negative individuals devote themselves to the physical care of affected relatives (see the case example of Mrs. P. in chap. 4). Others take on special roles with the children of ill relatives. Still others insist that the testing changes nothing. It is difficult to believe that subtle changes in the nature or editing of conversations about illness, at the very least, do not occur between siblings found to have divergent cancer genetic testing results.

Being negative for an inherited cancer predisposing mutation only provides information about the risk of cancer caused by that mutation. The individual remains at the level of population risk for sporadic cancers. Those who test negative need guidance about what those risks are and at what age they, and others in the general population, need to undertake screening activities. Genetic counselors usually address these issues in the disclosure session and any other follow-up that is provided. Like much of the rest of the cancer genetic counseling experience, however, individual psychological factors appear to govern the degree to which these recommendations are accepted. Some individuals find it difficult to give up the level of surveillance or screening they have had as a member of a high-risk family prior to being tested. This reluctance has been noted particularly in colon cancer families, in which some at-risk individuals wished to continue their annual colonoscopy screenings to experience the continuing reassurance they provided (Rhodes, Chapman, Burn, & Gunn, 1991). Women found not to carry a known *BRCA1/2* mutation in their family can be assured that they do not have increased hereditary risk for breast or ovarian cancer, but they should be reminded that they continue to be at the general population risk for breast (11% to 15% lifetime risk) or ovarian (1% to 2%) cancer. They should therefore follow the general population guidelines for screening, including breast self- and clinical examinations and mammograms (American Cancer Society, 1999). Some women who get such true negative results happily revert to population guidelines. Others find it more difficult to give up their previous anxieties about being at increased cancer risk and continue to follow screening guidelines for high-risk women.

On the other hand, some noncarriers of cancer predisposing mutations sheepishly report that after finding they did not carry a familial cancer predisposition mutation, they relaxed their concern and adopted some unhealthy habits. Using tanning machines and trading an exercise regime for life as a "couch potato" have been described as part of the process of feeling more normal and less at risk among people found to be noncarriers. These behaviors, although not usually pervasive, do raise some questions about whether "normalcy" necessarily involves less than ideal vigilance about health, especially for individuals in the 30–50 age range.

GUILT

Guilt is experienced by both mutation-negative and mutation-positive individuals. Those who test positive have guilt about perpetuating the conditions of fear and potential risk into the next and subsequent generations. They also feel guilty about the possibility of subjecting their spouse and children to the burdens of watching them become ill or die. This guilt and fear is especially marked in individuals who witnessed the cancer death of a parent from the same condition. With increases in the success of cancer treatments, more children will come to watch their parents triumph over the cancer that runs in their family, and, it is hoped, this fear will diminish. When a parent has had and survived a single bout of cancer, the children often seem particularly resilient to excess worry about cancer. These children have reason to hope that even if they have the mutation and get cancer, chances are good that they will survive. One woman from a high-risk family who had undergone a prophylactic mastectomy expressed a fear that if she did not develop cancer as a result of having had prophylactic surgery, women in the next generation of her family would worry too little about breast cancer and might not undertake adequate risk-reduction or screening measures. She hypothesized that alternate generations might act differently with regard to breast cancer prevention, depending on whether they had witnessed their mothers or aunts undergoing treatment for or dying from breast cancer.

Some who test negative in families where others are not so lucky feel guilty about their relief for themselves and their offspring to the point that it is almost palpable. Others say that it is not exactly guilt they feel, but a deep, lingering sadness that not everyone in the family can relax as they can. Although disease onset of any sort separates the lucky from the unlucky in a family, the power of the genetic dice to predict a future affected by cancer at an early age for some and not others appears to amplify those differences. Perhaps this is because fairness is a concept learned at an early age, usually in a family context. When siblings are tested in close proximity for an inherited mutation, the feelings of one having been favored in the nature of their genetic dowry elicits strong emotion. It is interesting that the suffering of the negatives for their less lucky brothers and sisters is voiced more often than is the jealousy of the mutation carriers for their negative siblings.

> When I found out I didn't have the gene [sic], I just went back to living my life. But you know, I feel guilty. My sister has had ovarian cancer and she has the gene, but she looks ok, so I just forget about it most of the time and then I feel guilty. She has had chemo a couple of times and I know that isn't good. I can't tell if she knows it isn't good. . . . We don't talk about it. I don't bring it up. She just goes on with her life and I go on with mine.

Now that genetic testing for some cancer genes has been available for a number of years, a new sort of guilt appears to be surfacing. This is guilt for not having taken some step sooner that, it is imagined, might have prevented the cancer diagnosis or death of a relative by providing information earlier about familial risk. Sometimes this guilt is about not being tested or guilt about not having pushed a hesitant, affected relative to be tested. The guilty person reasons that, had they or the relative been tested earlier, information about the mutation might have been disseminated earlier in the family, and perhaps others would have taken steps that might have led to earlier detection of the cancer.

CONFUSION

Confusion is not uncommon, given the complexity of the information, even in scientifically clear cases, about what a result does and does not mean about the risk status of others in the family. For example, although a true negative means that one's children are not at increased risk, it has no implications for the status of siblings who have an independent chance of having inherited the "bad" or "deleterious" mutation. Because people in the general population frequently have mistaken ideas about how much of their genetic makeup they share with their siblings versus their children (Richards, 1996), it is not surprising that confusion arises about the implications for relatives of an individual's genetic test result.

Confusion also exists when a mutation is not found in people with cancer who come from families with long histories of the disease. They wonder what else might have caused the recurrent cases of cancer in their family. This worry may be reduced by reviewing the fact that, even in cancers for which there is much genetic information available, other genes yet to be discovered are likely responsible for some portion of the 5% to 10% of inherited cancers. When *BRCA1* and *BRCA2* were first found, it was thought that they, in connection with *p53* and a number of other rare genetic conditions, might account for almost all cases of inherited breast cancer. Several more recent studies have suggested, however, that this is not the case (Rebbeck et al., 1996; Serova-Sinilnikova et al., 1997). It is likely that at least a *BRCA3* gene has not yet been found, and it is possible that other genes will be found in the future that are responsible for remaining cases of familial breast and ovarian cancer as well.

For a woman with breast cancer and a significant family history, the finding that she does not carry a mutation in a known breast cancer susceptibility gene opens up questions about whether another gene might have caused her cancer or whether a mistake might have been made in her testing. Patients are frustrated after a disclosure that does not provide firm answers. Self-blame may be heightened when an external cause cannot be identified. Some women conclude that they are responsible for "causing" their cancer because of a failure to exercise, watch their weight, or take care of themselves in other ways. Such women may require either further genetic counseling or, in some cases, referral for psychological counseling to help them cope with this new knowledge and work through their self-blame. For these reasons, postdisclosure discussion and follow-up about the emotions and beliefs aroused by disclosure of a genetic test are as important as clarification of the medical and scientific facts provided at the time the result is given.

Psychological processes determine much of the ways in which a person copes with an indeterminate result. Cognitive abilities, especially capacity for abstract information, may influence how well the result is understood. Anxiety, however, may interfere, leaving even those with powerful intellectual abilities confused. Optimism will lead some individuals to focus on the fact that a true mutation was not found and that they are no worse off than they were before testing. The pessimist will think of all the negative ramifications of this confusing result and may rail against the testing process itself. In truth, the individual may not be any better off for having invested time and money in testing. Genetic counseling can prepare patients for the possibility that testing might not yield any new information. They may nevertheless experience frustration in being unable to reduce their level of uncertainty, something genetic testing can do, at least in part, for those who get a positive or true negative result.

A woman who has not received a true negative test result for *BRCA1/2* but has instead received an indeterminate result or a negative without a known familial mutation cannot be "cleared" of genetic risk for breast and ovarian cancer. These women are usually told to follow recommendations for surveillance at the highest levels, that is, at the levels recommended for women known to be mutation carriers. This can add to the confusion because the result was "negative," but the recommendations for surveillance are the same as for women who received "positive" results. This mixed message is subject to whatever interpretation the patient gives it, which may vary across a full spectrum from an assumption that the result implies no need to worry about breast cancer risk to the opposite assumption that the test showed that she was truly at very high risk.

Patients are not alone in finding the explanation of an indeterminate negative result confusing. Giardello et al. (1997) found that more than 30% of primary care providers could not correctly interpret an indeterminate negative result for familial adenomatous polyposis. An indeterminate negative result may also lead the person who still wants to know if he or she has a mutation in a disease gene to be on a "waiting list" of sorts. They have the option to be tested for new genes as they are identified that may be responsible for their family disease pattern. They may also be retested if someone in the family develops cancer and tests positive, identifying the location of a familial mutation that could then be looked for in their DNA. Some of those who have found the first testing experience uninformative do not wish to be retested and to reexperience the wait and possible frustration of learning they still cannot, for whatever reason, receive a definitive result. Among those who are tested again, this time looking for mutations in a different gene, some proportion will again come up empty-handed, with no known hereditary mutation to link with the history of cancer in their family. Some will interpret this finding positively, hoping it suggests that there is not a hereditary predisposition in the family. Others will be disappointed and frustrated, feeling that their efforts have not yielded information that can help unaffected family members determine whether they are at increased hereditary risk. As the number of possible gene tests increase, people from high-risk families may have multiple opportunities to be tested. For some, the resulting frustration will limit the number of times they are willing to go through the process.

PARADOXICAL REACTIONS

One of the surprises in studies of psychological outcomes of genetic testing for Huntington's disease was that some people found not to be carriers of the gene for this disorder, as well as their spouses, expressed either immediate disappointment when given their result or gradually became depressed after disclosure (Myers, Taylor, & Sinsheimer, 1997). This seemed to occur either because of regret at a life lived in anticipation of a foreshortened life span complicated by illness or because it necessitated a change in life plan, which proved difficult. This paradoxical reaction was also found occasionally among spouses of individuals testing negative for HD. In one case, the spouse of a woman from an HD family, a high-achieving business-man, had retired early to care for his wife. When she was told she did not carry the familial mutation, he was at a loss about how to spend his time and subsequently became depressed (Huggins et al., 1992).

Paradoxical reactions such as these have also been observed in cancer genetic testing programs. For this reason, people considering testing should be encouraged to anticipate all the feelings they think they might have if they were to receive a true negative result, in addition to anticipating their reaction to a positive result.

Although most people approach genetic testing for cancer susceptibility hoping to be shown not to be mutation carriers, some rare individuals hope to be found to be carriers. In one case, this was because a woman thought carrying the familial mutation would provide a rationale for her lifelong depression. She also felt it would gain attention from a husband she perceived to be preoccupied. Her disappointment continued for a year following result disclosure and led to conflict with her husband because he could not under-stand her lack of excitement at being free of an increased cancer risk.

Paradoxical reactions can also mask suicidal wishes. Some patients have stated that finding they were mutation carriers would mean there was a foreseeable end to their emotional suffering because the odds favored their getting cancer at a relatively early age. This would allow them to anticipate an early death from a passively accepted cancer, rather than having to consider more active means of ending their lives. Such reactions are often not directly stated upon disclosure. Clinicians who think this could be a factor in their patients' seeming disappointment at their negative test result (perhaps because of previous deep depression or suicidal ideation) may have to inquire directly about whether this notion, observed in others, could possibly have any part in their patients' disappointment.

As mentioned earlier, the "separation" that occurs in some families after genetic test results become available is a phenomenon that merits further investigation. Certainly a number of patients have voiced concern about such divisions changing the dynamics of sibships or other family alliances. Results like those of Smith et al. (1999) suggest that knowledge, or lack of knowledge, of other family members' test results appears to influ-ence an individual's emotional response to his or her own result. Some have said that their family's cancer burden used to make them feel like it was "us against the world." In such cases, learning that not all family members are at increased risk for cancer may upset family cohesion based on familial difference from the general population.

REGRET

Regret is only occasionally voiced by individuals who have sought genetic testing. It is especially rare among those receiving definitive results. It is difficult to know whether this is due to the reduction in uncertainty or whether it is cognitive dissonance that makes it impossible to think that one's choice to be tested was wrong when it was so consciously rendered. Surprise, however, is not so unusual. The majority of tested individuals have a belief about what their result will be and how much the result will affect them emotionally. Regret, when seen, is often among those whose result was different from their expectations and who found it more difficult to accept than anticipated. Those who are more disturbed by what they perceive as the downside of a negative result, who regret the unlived life they might have chosen had they known earlier or who feel separated from other members of their family, may express regret. When one is positive, even if it is more upsetting than anticipated, total regret is often difficult to voice because a positive result opens up the possibility of pursuing appropriate, lifesaving medical and behavioral measures. Many individuals conclude, "Now, at least, I can do something to try to prevent cancer."

CLINICAL ASSESSMENT OF ACUTE DISTRESS FOLLOWING DISCLOSURE

Assessing the extent of distress in a person who is adversely affected by disclosure of his or her genetic test result can be a challenging task. Acute expressions of distress are certainly appropriate to the magnitude of the situation. Depending on the setting, if it is possible to let the person and his or her support person have some time to cry, talk, and regain their composure, this may be ideal. If no support person is present, the genetic counselor, a mental health professional, or other health provider may sit with the person quietly until he or she is able to listen and talk. It is not advisable to leave a distraught person alone or to allow the person to leave the testing center. Although little factual information may be retained from discussions following an upsetting disclosure, it is usually calming for the distraught person to have a medical or genetics professional repeat the facts that a positive test result is not a diagnosis of cancer, that there are ways to look for cancer and experts who can follow high-risk individuals, that children still have a 50% chance of *not* inheriting a mutation, and that not everyone with a mutation develops cancer (assuming that is the case). Having the genetics or medical professional present means that the individual can easily ask questions about the situation, about what to do next, about how others in this circumstance have coped, and about how to tell one's parent, child, or sibling. Together a plan can be forged for a return visit and for making an appointment with an oncologist or for procedures such as a colonoscopy, transvaginal ultrasound, or mammogram. A rehearsal of how the person will spread the news to others in his or her family can also be helpful. Patients are reminded that they are not obligated to tell employers and that they are not required to volunteer the information to insurers.

The vast majority of patients experience a reduction in their acute distress over the course of the disclosure session. Ongoing inquiry over the course of the meeting about the level of the person's sense of panic or anguish is helpful to gain a more accurate sense of whether the person may harbor self-destructive thoughts or be too depressed to maneuver the trip home. (This is only rarely the case.) If at the end of an hour or so there is no improvement in the person's distraught state of mind, it may be necessary for the genetic counselor to consider additional supports. This might include, if possible, immediate assessment by a mental health provider with whom the genetic counselor has a prior consultative relationship or, at least, a discussion between the genetic counselor or mental health provider about what additional steps should be taken. In rare instances, there may be a need for the genetic counselor or even a hospital security officer to accompany the patient to an emergency outpatient unit where he or she can see a psychologist or psychiatrist for further assessment. If a friend or family member accompanied the patient, he or she will likely be involved for support. Devising a plan for what the patient should do if he or she becomes acutely distressed at a later point usually provides sufficient structure to bring the session safely to a close. This can include informing the patient about the availability of professional backup or about where to seek emergency psychiatric services, making a referral to a mental health provider or recommending that the individual sees his or her ongoing therapist as soon as possible. Although the skills of a well-trained clinician are valuable here, in the vast majority of cases, the individual, despite grief and sadness, can come to a point where he or she regains the cognitive and emotional stability to leave the clinic. The follow-up of a patient who was distressed during a genetic counseling session should include a telephone call the next day to reevaluate his or her emotional stability and comfort and the need for further mental health referral or, in very rare cases, emergency evaluation. Scheduling another genetic counseling appointment is recommended because a distressed patient will likely remember little of what the counselor said.

DECLINERS

Do the people who seek genetic testing differ in marked psychological ways from those who do not? It seems likely that there are differences between "first-adapters" (i.e., those who quickly take advantage of new opportunities, such as genetic testing), those who wait for a while before considering counseling or testing, and those who dismiss counseling and testing completely. It is not easy to systematically study people who are not interested in genetic services, especially now that genetic testing is moving into clinical testing setting where people are largely self-referred. Lerman et al. (1998) studied individuals invited to a research program including genetic testing for *BRCA1/2*. Of the 396 individuals invited to participate, 43% declined to be tested, with almost everyone in that group also declining genetic counseling. At baseline (entry into the program), there was no difference in CES–D scores of individuals who eventually comprised the carrier, noncarrier, and decliner groups. The percentage of people who met the criteria for clinically significant depression was under 15% in each group. At 1 month after those tested had received their results, however, the CES–D depression scores of decliners were "dramatically" and significantly above those of the other two groups: 19% of decliners, 14% of mutation carriers, and 8% of noncarriers were depressed (CES–D scores > 16). Increases over the 1-month follow-up period were especially marked among those who scored high on depression at baseline and did not receive results; depression rates rose from 26% to 47% for decliners, stayed essentially the same for carriers (20% to 23%), and declined for noncarriers from 41% to 11%. The odds of becoming depressed over this period were reported to be 8 times greater for those who declined versus those who received negative results and 6 times greater for carriers than for noncarriers. Differences continued at 6 months, with 41% of decliners scoring in the depressed range versus 32% of carriers and 18% of noncarriers.

At risk individuals who decline testing at one point may decide to be tested in the future. The term "decliners" is often used in the literature in ways that mix together people who are categorically opposed to testing and will never be tested, those slow to warm to the idea, and those frightened but attracted to the idea of knowing their genetic status. The latter two groups may need more time to decide to be tested than is typically acceptable in a research project. The question of whether individuals who hesitate to be tested are more or less psychologically prepared to cope with the eventual result will only become clear over time.

HEALTH BEHAVIOR CHANGE FOLLOWING DISCLOSURE
OF MUTATION STATUS

The ultimate medical goal of cancer genetic testing is to improve the health of those at increased genetic risk. Most of those who come for counseling and testing believe that being tested will improve their adherence to recommended levels of surveillance or screening behaviors. But does knowing one's result actually lead to more appropriate health behaviors?

In a Canadian study (Metcalfe et al., 2000) of 79 women who tested positive for a *BRCA1* or *BRCA2* mutation, 57% said that they had changed their screening practices when assessed an average of 18 months following disclosure. It was especially women under age 50 and those with no previous cancer history who had upgraded their cancer screening behaviors. Two thirds said they had considered prophylactic mastectomy, and 21% had had prophylactic mastectomy following disclosure. About 40% of the women had had their ovaries prophylactically removed following disclosure that they were carriers. These percentages were significantly higher than those reported in several studies by Lerman and colleagues with shorter follow-up periods. The Lerman et al. (1997) study highlighted the difference between intentions stated immediately after disclosure and actual behavior. In that study, 1 week after disclosure, 31% of mutation carriers stated that they were considering prophylactic mastectomy and 48% considered prophylactic oophorectomy. At 6 months postdisclosure, however, only 1% had undergone prophylactic mastectomy and 2% prophylactic oophorectomy. By one year postdisclosure (Lerman et al., 2000), 3% of unaffected mutation carriers had undergone prophylactic mastectomy, and 13% of carriers had had a prophylactic oophorectomy. Only 21% of female carriers had had a CA-125 test, and 15% had had a vaginal ultrasound, as recommended. The adherence rate for mammography was 68% in carriers, unchanged from pretest levels. One might wonder whether some part of this discrepancy in uptake of prophylactic surgery between the U.S. and Canadian studies is a reflection of differences in the health insurance policies of the two countries.

Although some people embark on testing with clear intentions of having prophylactic surgery if found to be a mutation carrier, others react much more ambivalently and may take months or years to determine whether such an intervention is something they can live with. Genetic counselors often feel their role includes encouraging those who intend to leap from the disclosure session to the operating room to take time to think through their decision and to speak to a mental health counselor or others who have undergone surgery to be sure they are making the right decision. In other cases, the reverse may be true. Individuals strongly advised to have their colon prophylactically removed for familial adenomatous polyposis or hereditary nonpolyposis colorectal cancer may hesitate to the point that professionals fear the colorectal cancer will not be found until it has metastasized and is life-threatening. Psychotherapists can help uncover the emotional conflicts underlying refusal to accept recommendations for potentially life-saving treatment and can help patients rethink their decision. Not everyone is willing to accept drastic surgeries, even when they offer significantly improved odds of survival. Sometimes the barriers to acceptance are amenable to psychotherapeutic intervention focused on unresolved grief, feelings of unworthiness, shame, or anger, but this is not always the case. Some people prefer to avoid surgery, even though they recognize there is a possibility their gamble will not succeed. The challenge for the mental health provider is to help people explore the options in light of their own experience, beliefs, and vulnerabilities and to be sure that they have considered the alternatives to the extent possible. To live with the risk of dying is something we all do. Talking through the special issues involved for mutation carriers allows for the triumph of human dignity in the face of markedly increased threats to survival.

The Lerman et al. (2000) study also points out what may be serious problems regarding the uptake of screening or surveillance recommendations by those found to be at increased cancer risk. The fact that only two thirds of the female mutation carriers in that study had had a mammogram in the year since disclosure of their carrier state and that that rate was unchanged from the mammogram rate before genetic testing suggests a need for further exploration of the motivators and inhibitors of health protective behaviors among those who seek testing. It seems ironic that a woman would opt for high-technology genetic testing to discover her risk for breast and ovarian cancer but would then ignore the recommendation to be screened for breast cancer with mammography. When health providers' messages about the need for regular screening to detect cancer at the earliest possible time is not reaching one third of those at increased risk, further research is necessary to determine how to improve adherence. The sample in the Lerman et al. (2000) study was highly educated, suggesting that neither comprehension nor retention of the message nor cost was the problem, but that anxiety, lack of trust in medical procedures, and other more psychological factors were operating to prevent full adherence to medical advice obtained through genetic counseling and testing.

In the future, it is hoped that there will be effective, less drastic options than those currently available for individuals at increased hereditary cancer risk, making adherence to recommendations less onerous. It is still likely, however, that psychological treatment of the anxiety, grief, depression, guilt, and other symptoms that occur in the context of disclosure of the results of genetic testing will be important to maximize the positive outcomes of cancer genetic testing. Treatment of emotional symptoms such as post-disclosure anxiety in mutation carriers may facilitate the adoption of screening and risk-reduction behaviors that, in turn, may improve the odds of early detection and even, ultimately, prevention of hereditary cancers.

SUMMARY

Receiving a genetic test result is a life-altering experience. Like many of life's transition points, in a moment everything and nothing is changed. It is not surprising that the reaction to this experience varies widely from individual to individual, from family to family. We are also learning that the reaction to testing reflects concern about the test results of other family members. This is a point at which assessment of psychological well-being and support for patient and family members is especially needed. For some, this may become a focus of therapeutic discussion for years to come. Others may pay fleeting attention to feelings about the disclosure and minimize its impact.

Patients who are found to be mutation carriers are encouraged to use the genetic information they receive to tailor their health behaviors to try to detect or prevent cancer. What patients make of the information and whether they take up the call for screening or risk-reducing surgical options depends in large measure on psychological factors. In the next chapter, I consider the psychological issues involved for patients who consider and opt for prophylactic mastectomy, oophorectomy (removal of the ovaries), or colectomy. Taking a step to remove a currently healthy body part involves a great deal of faith in the predictive information that suggests that this is a beneficial action. The next chapter discusses how psychologists can help patients evaluate the impact of such a choice on their future quality of life. These dilemmas raise profound but fascinating questions that are well suited to the introspection and enlightenment that psychologists and other seasoned and knowledgeable mental health professionals can offer to those facing such challenges.

REFERENCES

Aktan-Collan, K., Haukkala, A., Jukka-Pekka, M., Uutela, A., & Kaarianen, H. (2001). Psychological consequences of predictive genetic testing for hereditary non-polyposis colorectal cancer (HNPCC): A prospective follow-up study. *International Journal of Cancer, 93,* 608–611.

Almqvist, E. W., Bloch, M., Brinkman, R., Craufurd, D., & Hayden, M. R. (1999). A worldwide assessment of the frequency of suicide, suicide attempts, or psychiatric hospitalization after predictive testing for Huntington disease. *American Journal of Human Genetics, 64*, 1293–1304.

American Cancer Society. (1999). *Cancer facts & figures—1999*. Atlanta, GA: Author.

Aro, A. R., Absetz, S. P., van den Elderen, T. M., van der Ploeg, E., & van der Kamp, L. J. (2000). False-positive findings in mammography screening induces short-term distress—Breast cancer specific concerns prevails longer. *European Journal of Cancer, 36*, 1089–1097.

Bonadona, V., Saltel, P., Desseigne, F., Mignotte, H., Saurin, J.-C., Wang, Q., et al. (2002). Cancer patients who experienced diagnostic genetic testing for cancer susceptibility: Reactions and behavior after the disclosure of a positive test result. *Cancer Epidemiology, Biomarkers, & Prevention, 11*, 97–104.

Codori, A.- M., Zawacki, K. L., Petersen, G. M., Miglioretti, D. L., Bacon, J. A., Trimbath, et al. (2003). Genetic testing for hereditary colorectal cancer in children: Long-term psychological effects. *American Journal of Medical Genetics, 116A*, 117–128.

Croyle, R. T., Smith, K. R., Botkin, J. R., Baty, B., & Nash, J. (1997). Psychological responses to BRCA1 mutation testing: Preliminary findings. *Health Psychology, 16*, 63–72.

DiMaio, L., Squitieri, F., Napolitano, G., Campanella, G., Trofatter, J. A., & Conneally, P. M. (1993). Suicide risk in Huntington's disease. *Journal of Medical Genetics, 30*, 293–295.

Dorval, M., Patenaude, A. F., Schneider, K. A., Kieffer, S. A., DiGianni, L., Kalkbrenner, K., et al. (2000). Anticipated versus actual emotional reactions to disclosure of results of genetic tests for cancer susceptibility: Findings from p53 and BRCA1 testing programs. *Journal of Clinical Oncology, 18*, 2135–2142.

Giardello, F. M., Brensinger, J. D., Petersen, G. M., Luce, M .C., Hylind, L. M., Bacon, J. A., et al. (1997). The use and interpretation of commercial APC gene testing for familial adenoma atous polyposis. *New England Journal of Medicine, 336*, 823–827.

Giarelli, E. (1999). Spiraling out of control: One case of pathologic anxiety as a response to a genetic risk of cancer. *Cancer Nursing, 22*, 327–339.

Grosfeld, F. J. M., Lips, C. J. M., & Beemer, F. A. (1996). Psychosocial consequences of DNA analysis for MEN Type 2. *Oncology, 10*, 141–157.

Horowitz, M., Wilner, N., & Alvarez, W. (1979) Impact of Events Scale: A measure of subjective stress. *Psychosomatic Medicine, 41*, 209–218.

Huggins, M., Bloch, M., Wiggins S., Adam S., Suchowersky O., Trew M., et al. (1992). Predictive testing for Huntington disease in Canada: Adverse effects and unexpected results in those receiving a decreased risk. *American Journal of Medical Genetics, 42*, 508–515.

Janis, I. L. (1984). The patient as decision-maker. In D. Gentry (Ed.), *Handbook of behavioral medicine* (pp. 326–368). New York: Guilford Press.

Kerr, B., Foulkes, W. D., Cade, D., Hadfield, L., Hopwood, P., Serruya, C., et al. (1998). False family history of breast cancer in the family cancer clinic. *European Journal of Surgical Oncology, 24,* 275–279.

Lerman, C., Biesecker, B., Benkendorf, J. L., Kerner, J., Gomez-Caminero, A., Hughes, C., et al. (1997). Controlled trial of pretest education approaches to enhance informed decision-making for *BRCA1* gene testing. *Journal of the National Cancer Institute, 89,* 148–157.

Lerman, C., Hughes, C., Croyle, R. T., Main, D., Durham, C., Snyder, C., et al. (2000). Prophylactic surgery decisions and surveillance practices one year following *BRCA1/2* testing. *Preventive Medicine, 31,* 75–80.

Lerman, C., Hughes, C., Lemon, S. J., Main, D., Snyder, C., & Durham, C. (1998). What you don't know can hurt you: Adverse psychologic effects in members of *BRCA1*-linked and *BRCA2*-linked families who decline testing. *Journal of Clinical Oncology, 16,* 1650–1654.

Lerman, C., Narod, S., Schulman, K., Hughes, C., Gomez-Caminero, A., & Bonney, G. (1996). *BRCA1* testing in families with hereditary breast-ovarian cancer: A prospective study of patient decision making and outcomes. *Journal of the American Medical Association, 275,* 1885–1892.

Lodder, L., Frets, P. G., Trijsburg, R. W., Meijers-Heijboer, E. J., Klijn, J. G. M., Duivenvoorden, H. J., et al. (2001). Psychological impact of receiving a *BRCA1/BRCA2* test result. *American Journal of Medical Genetics, 98,* 15–24.

Masterton, G. (1995). Factitious disorders and the surgeon. *British Journal of Surgery, 82,* 1588–1589.

Metcalfe, K. A., Liede, A., Hoodfar, E., Scott, A., Foulkes, W. D., & Narod. S. A. (2000). An evaluation of needs of female *BRCA1* and *BRCA2* carriers undergoing counselling. *Journal of Medical Genetics, 37,* 866–874.

Michie, S. M., Bobrow, M., Marteau, T .M., on behalf of the FAP Collaborative Research Group. (2001) Predictive genetic testing in children and adults: A study of emotional impact. *Journal of Medical Genetics, 38,* 519–526.

Myers, R. H., Taylor, C. A., & Sinsheimer, J. A. (1997). Genetic testing for neuropsychiatric disease: Experiences from 8 years of genetic testing for Huntington's disease. In L. L. Heston (Ed.), *Progress in Alzheimer's disease and similar conditions* (pp. 137–160). Washington, DC: American Psychiatric Press.

Radloff, L. S. (1977). The CES–D Scale: A self-report depression scale for research in the general population. *Applied Psychological Measures, 1,* 385–401.

Rebbeck, T. R., Couch, F. J., Kant, J., Calzone, K., DeShano, M., Peng, Y., et al. (1996). Genetic heterogeneity in hereditary breast cancer: Role of *BRCA1* and *BRCA2. American Journal of Human Genetics, 59,* 547–553.

Rhodes, M., Chapman, P. D., Burn, J., & Gunn, A. (1991). Role of a regional register for familial adenomatous polyposis: Experience in the northern region. *British Journal of Surgery, 78,* 451–452.

Richards, M. (1996). Families, kinship, and genetics. In T. Marteau & M. Richards (Eds.), *The troubled helix: Social and psychological implications of the new human genetics* (pp. 249–274). Cambridge, England: Cambridge University Press.

Schoenfeld, M., Myers, R. H., Cupples, L. A., Berkman, B., Sax, D. S., & Clark, E. (1984). Increased rate of suicide among patients with Huntington's disease. *Journal of Neurology, Neurosurgery, & Psychiatry, 47*, 1283–1287.

Schneider, K. (2002). *Counseling about cancer: Strategies for genetic testing* (2nd ed.). New York: Wiley.

Schwartz, M. D., Peshkin, B. N., Hughes, C., Main, D., Isaacs, C., & Lerman, C. (2002). Impact of BRCA1/BRCA2 mutation testing on psychologic distress in a clinic-based sample. *Journal of Clinical Oncology, 20*, 514–520.

Serova-Sinilnikova, O. M., Boutrand, L., Stoppa-Lyonnet, D., Bressac-de-Paillerets, B., Dubois, V., Lasset, C., et al. (1997). BRCA2 mutations in breast cancer families: Are there more breast cancer susceptibility genes? *American Journal of Human Genetics, 60*, 486–495.

Smith, K. R., West, J. A., Croyle, R. T., & Botkin, J. R. (1999). Familial context of genetic testing for cancer susceptibility: Moderating effect of siblings' test results on psychological distress one to two weeks after BRCA1 mutation testing. *Cancer Epidemiology, Biomarkers, & Prevention, 8*, 385–392.

Spielberger, C. G., & Lushene, R. (1970). *State–Trait Anxiety manual.* Palo Alto, CA: Consulting Psychologists Press.

Struewing, J. P., Hartge, P., Wacholder, S., Baker, S. M., Berlin, M., McAdams, et al. (1997). The risk of cancer associated with specific mutations of BRCA1 and BRCA2 among Ashkenazi Jews. *New England Journal of Medicine, 336*, 1401–1408.

Tercyak, K. P., Lerman, C., Peshkin, B., Hughes, C., Main, D., Isaacs, C., & Schwartz, M. D. (2001). *Health Psychology, 20*, 217–222.

Zigmond, A. S., & Snaith, R. P. (1983). The Hospital Anxiety and Depression Scale. *Acta Psychiatrica Scandanavia, 67*, 361–370.

6

PROPHYLACTIC SURGERY

The ultimate medical goals of cancer genetic counseling and testing are to reduce disease occurrence (morbidity) and cancer deaths (mortality) among those at immediate hereditary risk for cancer. One of the most effective risk-reducing options offered to mutation carriers is prophylactic surgery. Difficult decision making about irreversible surgical options is often carried out under stressful conditions, such as recent cancer diagnosis of oneself or a loved one. Prophylactic surgery necessitates evaluation of one's identity, body image, family history, current roles, and cancer fear. This is an area in which psychological consultation can be usefully applied. For some, decisions about prophylactic surgery take place slowly over a number of years. Some people may have vowed when a parent died of cancer that they would do anything, including prophylactic surgery, to prevent that outcome for themselves and have only questioned when was the proper time to have surgery. For others, especially those recently diagnosed with cancer, the decision making may be condensed into days or weeks. In either case, it can involve agonizing choices, painful memories, and feeling stuck between a rock and a hard place. Those who feel that it is a clear choice may proceed with abandon to find willing surgeons and to inform one's family about the decision and timing of the surgery. Others may struggle with great ambivalence with the powerful psychological conflicts that prophylactic surgery brings to the fore. In either case, it is useful to help patients gather all the necessary information about immediate and long-term physical outcomes and to help them to try to anticipate or rehearse the emotional changes that surgery will initiate.

PROPHYLACTIC MASTECTOMY

"Drastic," "disfiguring," "mutilating"—these are words used to describe prophylactic mastectomy (PM), the removal of healthy breasts to prevent the development of cancer, which is one of the options offered to women who are thought to be at very high risk for developing breast cancer. This includes women who have been found to be *BRCA1/2* carriers and are thus at 56%–85% risk of developing breast cancer during their lives and women whose family histories are strongly suggestive of a hereditary factor, but who may not have the option of genetic testing. Physicians or genetic counselors typically inform at-risk women that bilateral PM is an option that can greatly, but not completely, reduce their risk of developing breast cancer. Some women who are considered to be "cancer phobic" in ways that significantly interfere with their daily lives also often either initiate discussion of PM with their physicians or have it suggested to them. The mention of PM in all of these circumstances is typically accompanied by a caveat that this is a highly personal decision and one that a woman should not make without careful consideration and research. Depending on the personal beliefs of the professional, a physician may give the impression that PM is an extreme option that goes beyond current, typical recommendations for many women who actually have breast cancer or that PM is the recommendation of choice for those at hereditary risk who want to do everything they can to ensure their survival.

Although the importance of patient psychological factors in uptake of PM is well recognized, there has been relatively little published data on the emotional and interpersonal ramifications of PM to guide either the patient considering the procedure or the professional presenting the option. Many at-risk women report initially being appalled by the thought that anyone would ever willingly remove her healthy breasts. For many, this feeling persists, and PM is never something they seriously consider. Among women who do consider PM, many might find consultation with psychologists or other mental health counselors useful as part of the process of weighing the personal pros and cons of the procedure.

Some women diagnosed with cancer in one breast who have either strong personal histories of breast cancer or other factors that increase the likelihood of contralateral (other side) breast cancer may also consider PM. Some of these women chose to have their healthy breast removed, usually (but not always) at the same time as they undergo a mastectomy on their cancerous breast, which is referred to as a unilateral prophylactic mastectomy. In this circumstance, the decision about prophylactic surgery may be approached more as a medical issue than it is for bilateral prophylactic mastectomy in a healthy woman. Nevertheless, consideration of the psychological ramifications is equally important for women with cancer as it is for healthy women considering bilateral prophylactic mastectomy.

What Is Prophylactic Mastectomy?

Although there is theoretically a choice of either a total or a subcutaneous mastectomy for those undergoing PM, the greater residual breast tissue left in a subcutaneous mastectomy, resulting in greater risk of cancer, leads most surgeons doing prophylactic mastectomies to encourage a woman to have a total mastectomy (Eisen, Rebbeck, Wood, & Weber, 2000). In a total mastectomy, "as much breast tissue as possible is removed by excising an ellipse of skin, including the nipple and areola, and underlying breast tissue down to the fascial plane overlying the chest wall" (Eisen et al., 2000, p. 1982). In a subcutaneous mastectomy, much of the breast tissue is removed, but some, which is associated with blood supply to the nipple and areola, is left intact. Although nipple and areola remain in a subcutaneous mastectomy, they lack sensation because of scarring of the underlying nerves, and thus their role in sexual foreplay and stimulation for the woman is greatly diminished, if not absent. The slight advantage of retaining some aspects of normal shape with a subcutaneous mastectomy is outweighed by the greater cancer risk. When a total mastectomy is performed, additional surgery can create reconstruction of nipples with tattooing of the areolar area. The trade-off is that this can require multiple surgical steps and willingness to endure some period of time with a reconstructed breast that lacks a nipple.

Reconstruction

"Electing to undergo breast reconstruction carries with it the potential for significant physical and psychological benefits but also the chance for profound physical and psychological distress" (Schain, 1991, p. 1170). Women who undergo mastectomies have several options following surgery. Some women believe that a desire to reconstruct new breasts is a sign of "self-indulgent vanity" (Harcourt & Rumsey, 2001). Although older women opt not to have reconstruction more often than younger women, it should not be assumed that a woman does not want reconstruction just because she is older. The rationale that some women offer for not having reconstruction after prophylactic mastectomy is that if they wish to go to the extreme of removing their breast, they do not want to put anything into their bodies that could possibly obstruct detection of a tumor in the residual tissue. Some of these women wear external breast prostheses, but some do not. Breast prostheses can be uncomfortable and become misaligned and are, to some, a reminder of feeling changed or "abnormal" after surgery.

About 30% of U.S. women opt to have some form of breast reconstruction following mastectomy (Rowland, Diosso, Holland, Chaglassian, & Kinne, 1995). Although the form of a breast can be created, because of nerve cutting and other factors, there is usually little or no sensation in the newly formed breast.

> It should be borne in mind that a reconstructed breast has neither the function nor the physiological attributes of a natural breast. It is not therefore a true replacement. The best any surgeon can hope to achieve is "a visually satisfying breast mound of a size, shape, situation, color and skin texture that as a whole matches as nearly as possible the original." (Ward, 1981, p. 125)

Several types of breast reconstruction are commonly done. A woman decides in connection with her surgeon whether she wants implants or whether she wants the surgeon to reconstruct her breast from her own skin and fat, taken from another area of her body. Factors to evaluate include the woman's physical health because the length of the surgery varies by procedure; longer surgical time involves risks that may not be advisable for women with significant health problems or older age. A woman who wants to use her own tissue will have to be evaluated to see if her body type is appropriate, the ideal body type for this surgery being women with large breasts and minimal abdominal fat (Moran, Herceg, Kurtelawicz, & Serletti, 2000). If all biological indicators are equivalent with regard to the decision between implants and autogenous tissue reconstruction, the preference of the woman can be paramount. Some women feel strongly that they do not want anything "foreign" in their bodies and that they would worry a great deal about having implants, even those made of saline, which are the most commonly used today. On the other hand, some women do not like the idea of having surgery on multiple parts of their body and prefer implants. Considerations about the possible size of the breasts to be constructed may also play a role in a woman's decision.

A major consideration in deciding to have implants is the fact that the most commonly used implant procedure requires multiple surgeries. In staged expander-implant reconstruction, a temporary tissue expander is placed into a "pocket" under the muscles of the chest during the initial mastectomy surgery (Hughes, Papa, Whitney, & McLellan, 1999). The patient then visits the doctor's office over a number of weeks to have saline injected into the "balloons" of the imbedded tissue expander. This allows the skin to stretch gradually over the area of the new breast, which reduces the likelihood of complications. Once the desired size is reached, a permanent breast prosthesis is placed in a second, short surgery. A final step, if desired, is tattooing of skin in the "nipple" or areolar areas to darken the skin color.

There is an option for immediate placement of a permanent implant at the time of the mastectomy surgery. This can usually only be done with small-breasted women to avoid complications associated with stretching the skin. Also, the size of the breasts that are formed with this surgery is usually smaller than the woman's original breast size, which can be a concern for some women.

Implants need to be replaced every 5–15 years, which means that a young woman undergoing PM and opting for implants should be prepared to undergo surgery to replace the implants between four and eight times during her lifetime (Bostwick, 1995). Masses that develop can usually be felt on physical examination, but, in some cases, biopsy under general anesthesia may be needed to evaluate a breast lump.

The most common breast reconstruction method used today is the so-called TRAM flap (TRAM stands for transverse rectus abdominis myocutaneous, referring to the muscle flap removed from the abdomen to form the new breast). The muscle, skin, and fat of the lower abdomen are removed just as they would be if the patient were having a "tummy tuck" operation and are tunneled under the skin up to the site where the breast was removed. Patients often find the prospect of a flatter abdomen a "plus" in their consideration of this type of surgery. A connection to the blood supply is maintained via the epigastric artery and is sometimes augmented, if needed, by microsurgery from smaller blood vessels (Hughes et al., 1999). Sufficient blood supply is critical to success in maintaining the skin and the tissues that have been moved to form the breast. In some cases, a combination of TRAM surgery and expanders are used (Moran et al., 2000). TRAM flap surgery is long, requires a longer hospitalization (4–7 days), and requires 4–6 weeks of postoperative recovery time. Complications occur in about 30% of the cases, especially in women who are obese and who smoke (Watterson, Bostwick, Hester, Bried, & Taylor, 1995). The surgical result, however, often feels quite natural, which many women value highly.

One other possibility is called latissimus flap reconstruction. In this surgery, muscle and soft tissue from the back are transposed to the breast wound site to recreate a breast mound. This surgery is more difficult to do when both breasts are being reconstructed. and expanders are often needed, adding to the possible sources of complication.

It is clear that all forms of reconstruction carry significant risks of complication and offer varied advantages. The key to psychological success is for a woman considering the options to be well informed by a sensitive plastic surgeon, to have adequate time to consider how the strengths and drawbacks of each option fit her particular goals for the surgery, to have the possibility of considering the options with a psychotherapist, and, often, to have the opportunity to talk to a woman who has undergone PM surgery. Women differ a good deal in whether speed of accomplishing the surgery, suppleness, external appearance, breast size, or shape are the qualities that are most important to them. Many women have thought a great deal about having their breasts removed and much less about what kind of new breast they wish to have fashioned for them. A psychotherapist with some knowledge of the types of surgery available and with the ability to help a woman considering PM to decide whether surgery is right for her may help the woman determine which aspects of a surgical outcome are most important to her and what degree of medical involvement over what period of time is tolerable to her. If prophylactic mastectomy seems abhorrent or for other reasons is not appropriate for the individual, a psychotherapist can help the woman to feel comfortable with a screening or surveillance plan that better fits her lifestyle and coping mechanisms.

One of the issues about which patients who opt for surgery must make a decision is whether they will have reconstruction right away, at the same time they have the mastectomy, or whether they will wait. It used to be recommended that women wait, for both physical healing and psychological mourning of the lost breast to occur. The pendulum has swung, however, to the opposite view, that if a woman is going to have reconstruction, it is preferable for it to be initiated at least at the same time as the mastectomy surgery (Harcourt & Rumsey, 2001). Studies suggest that a woman's request for immediate reconstruction is predictive of good adjustment to the loss of a breast (Rowland et al., 1995) and that it is also less burdensome in reducing the number of surgeries. There is a need for more research in this area because the actual data in some studies supported earlier reconstruction (Al-Ghazal, Sully, Fallowfield, & Blamey, 2000) and in others found equal satisfaction among women having either immediate or delayed reconstruction (Schain, Wellisch, Pasnau, & Landsverk, 1985).

All patients undergoing mastectomy and reconstruction, especially women who undergo sequential surgical procedures, should be cautioned that a considerable period of time, at least a year according to Mock (1993), is likely needed to make the psychological adjustment to accept their changed body as their own. This can be a time for heightened vulnerability, especially when the patient feels that she did not have sufficient time to prepare for these changes. Intimate relationships may also undergo some readjustment during this period. Even strong partner support may not fully assuage feelings of a lack of femininity and sexual attractiveness following prophylactic mastectomy. Several researchers have described defensive coping strategies as being associated with poorer outcomes (e.g., Anderson & Kaczmarek, 1996; Rowland et al., 1993). Psychotherapeutic support may be welcomed to help women examine their underlying notions of what constitutes sexuality and attractiveness.

Cost

One concern some unaffected women voice is whether they will have to pay for PM. Insurance companies have usually paid for prophylactic mastectomy when a woman has a significant family history of breast cancer. Although the majority of women opting for PM who have a strong family history or who are BRCA1/2 mutation carriers ultimately do have their surgery paid for by their insurance carriers, problems are not unknown. Physician justification of the reasons for the surgery and the potential savings that the prevention of cancer would occasion is needed, and, in some rare cases, more drastic legal action has been required, some of which has provided legal precedents for coverage (Lynch, Severin, Mooney, & Lynch, 1995). Coverage for breast reconstruction is more variable.

A dilemma for some unaffected patients (i.e., patients who have not had cancer) who are mutation carriers is that they wish not to reveal their BRCA1/2 status to their insurer, for fear of losing all health insurance coverage, but feel that they may be forced to do so to have their surgery covered. In general, it has not been necessary to justify the need for this procedure by undergoing genetic testing or by revealing one's genetic status if testing has been done. Discussion of one's family history and estimation of objective risk for developing breast cancer by a genetic counselor or medical oncologist are usually sufficient. A recent study of insurance carriers, however, showed that the majority of reporting health insurers had no specific policy about coverage for prophylactic mastectomy. Of those responding who did, 29% had a policy of refusing to cover PM for strong family history and 24% had a policy of refusing PM to BRCA1/2 mutation carriers (Kuerer et al., 2000). Government carriers (Medicare and state Medicaid programs) were twice as likely to have noncoverage policies for PM, and a much smaller percentage had plans that specifically covered PM. This suggests that there may be significant discrepancies in the coverage for PM afforded to women of higher and lower socioeconomic status and that more advance planning may be needed to protest noncoverage for women whose health insurance is through a government plan.

The Kuerer et al. (2000) study also showed that although 32% of participating insurance companies had a specific policy allowing coverage for women with cancer who are seeking removal of their noncancerous breast at the same time they undergo mastectomy of their cancerous breast, 26% had a policy of refusing to cover unilateral prophylactic mastectomy; 42% had no policy about whether to cover this kind of prophylactic surgery.

This suggests that even women with cancer in one breast who have a significant family history that leads them to consider removing both breasts, one for cancer and one prophylactically, should seek early guidance about their insurer's willingness to cover such surgery. Because many women may be making this decision shortly after a diagnosis of breast cancer and under considerable pressure of time, it may be even more important that the insurer be approached quickly to determine whether any extra efforts will be needed to convince them to cover the prophylactic surgery. Considerations about cost are likely to contribute significantly to the anxiety of the woman making a decision or anticipating having PM, even though most women ultimately receive the desired coverage.

To What Extent Does Prophylactic Mastectomy Reduce Cancer Risk?

Although prophylactic mastectomies have been performed for several decades, data on the efficacy of the procedure are relatively recent. A retrospective 1999 study from the Mayo Clinic was the first to demonstrate a 90% risk reduction in a group of moderate- and high-risk women who had undergone PM (Hartmann et al., 1999). This study followed 639 women for a median of 14 years who had had surgery at a median age of 42 years. Breast cancers in the 214 women who were considered high risk were compared with breast cancer in their 403 sisters who had not undergone PM. Women in the moderate risk group were assigned Gail model (Gail et al., 1989) risk predictions, and actual and predicted rates of breast cancer were compared. Among moderate-risk women who had undergone PM, there were only four actual breast cancers compared with Gail model predictions of 37.4 expected breast cancers. Among the high-risk women, 3 (1.4%) of the 214 PM patients developed breast cancer, compared with 38 of their sisters without PM who were diagnosed with breast cancer after their sisters' PM. All of the seven breast cancers that occurred in women who had undergone prophylactic surgery followed subcutaneous, not total, mastectomies.

A recent Dutch study of 139 women who were BRCA1/2 mutation carriers, 76 of whom had had PM, showed similarly positive outcomes (Meijers-Heijboer et al., 2001). Although the follow-up period was only three years, none of the women in the PM group had developed breast cancer, whereas 8 breast cancers had developed in the surveillance group. A third statistical study, however, showed that to prevent one case of breast cancer among high-risk women, 6.2 women would have to undergo PM. Twenty-five women would have to undergo PM to prevent one death from breast cancer (Rhodes, Hartmann, & Perez, 2000).

It nonetheless remains crucial that women understand that PM does not guarantee they will never develop breast cancer. It seems ironic, albeit true, that women can have their breasts removed to a point where they feel that they have no breasts made of their own tissue, but there nonetheless remains enough underlying tissue to cause breast cancer. Most women considering PM understand, at least intellectually, that this is risk-reducing surgery, not a guarantee that cancer will not develop. There are no studies of women who have developed cancer following PM to determine the emotional impact of such a realization. The continuing cancer risk following PM means that women should understand the need for regular cancer checks, should have an awareness of other sorts of related risks such as risk of ovarian cancer for *BRCA1/2* carriers, and should have knowledge of what symptoms might indicate the presence of a malignancy in their chest.

To What Extent Do Women Opt for Prophylactic Mastectomy?

It is important to understand what leads some women to choose this option, even with little objective evidence of their cancer risk, whereas others with genetic test results indicative of high levels of risk foreclose early the possibility of ever having a PM. To date, PM has been the choice of a small minority of women at increased cancer risk. The recent efficacy studies and the increase in the number of women undergoing genetic counseling and testing, and thus receiving information about PM, is likely, however, to increase the number of women who consider this procedure. Cultural differences also appear to affect interest in and uptake of prophylactic mastectomy (Eisinger, Geller, Burke, & Holtzman, 1999; Evans, Anderson, et al., 1999; Julian-Reynier et al., 2001; Lerman et al., 1996; Wagner et al., 2000). Family and personal cancer history, risk perception, cancer worry, having children, physician recommendation, and age are other factors related to this choice.

Studies are somewhat difficult to compare because measures of level of "interest" are not standardized, and it is often hard to differentiate immediate, serious consideration from low-level consideration of undergoing PM at some future date. An Australian study found that 19% of 333 women attending their first breast cancer risk assessment clinical session answered yes to a question about whether they would consider PM if they were found to be *BRCA1/2* mutation carriers; 47% said they would not consider PM if found to be a carrier, and 34% said they were unsure (Meiser et al., 2000a). A recent U.S. study surveyed PM decisions made by 216 women from hereditary breast-ovarian families who were undergoing genetic testing (Lerman et al., 2000). Thirteen women came to the study having already had a PM, five of whom were later found not to be *BRCA1/2* mutation carriers. Of the 29 women who had never had cancer and were found to be *BRCA1/2* carriers, 36% said that they were considering PM at 1-month postdisclosure. Only one unaffected carrier (3%), however, actually had a PM in the first year following testing. Another U.S. study found higher rates of acceptance of PM, although the period of follow-up was not clearly stated (Morris, Johnson, Krasikov, Allen, & Dorsey, 2001). In that study, 60 patients underwent risk assessment counseling, with 37% ($n = 31$) initially considering prophylactic surgery, either PM or prophylactic oophorectomy. Fourteen patients (17%) chose to undergo PM, including one woman who had PM despite being told that her risk assessment showed she was not at high risk for breast cancer. Of the 31 patients judged by risk assessment alone to be high risk, 6 had bilateral mastectomies. Ten patients underwent genetic testing, and 4 of the 5 who were found to be positive (3 of whom had no personal cancer history) underwent PM. (The fifth woman found to be a mutation carrier had previously had both a prophylactic mastectomy and oophorectomy.) In addition, 3 patients who tested negative but who had previously had breast cancer went ahead with PM.

These studies illustrate that women opt for PM on the basis of a range of risk information and personal experience. Overestimation of risk has been prominently noted as a factor in leading women to opt for PM, with several studies strongly recommending psychotherapy for women to help them bring their perceived and actual breast cancer risk into closer agreement before proceeding to PM (Josephson, Wickman, & Sandelin, 2000; Meiser, Butow, et al., 2000).

What Do Women Who Have Undergone Prophylactic Mastectomy Say About the Experience?

The outcomes literature on PM remains small. A number of studies have asked women whether they regret having undergone PM or if they were satisfied with the experience. Somewhat predictably, the vast majority of women who choose this option do not later say that they regret it. In one study, 5% of women regretted PM (Borgen et al., 1998); in another study, 19% of the 639 women surveyed said they were dissatisfied, with much of the dissatisfaction centering on the surgical reconstruction of their breasts (Frost et al., 2000). Cognitive dissonance may play a role in minimizing expressions of unhappiness about such a major, irreversible decision. The majority of women, however, do express great relief at reducing their cancer risk via prophylactic breast surgery (Frost et al., 2000). Several studies also report, however, a reduced sense of feminine identity in a quarter to a half of the women following PM (Frost et al., 2000; Hopwood et al., 2000).

It remains difficult to clearly differentiate the women for whom PM represents a reasonable option, likely to improve overall quality of life by diminishing paralyzing cancer worry, from women for whom it is likely to lead to new problems of low self-esteem and poor feminine identity. Many women who seek PM (like other women) vastly overestimate their breast cancer risk. Genetic counseling can offer more realistic estimates of cancer risk, although for some women, these objective data do not appear to diminish their cancer-related anxiety (Watson et al., 1999). Women who opt for PM are frequently women whose mothers were diagnosed at an early age and who died of their breast cancer (Lloyd et al., 2000). The fear of dying young and leaving young children motherless appears to play a major role in propelling many women toward PM. Some have suggested that having a strong presurgical construct of womanliness not linked to one's breasts is a protective factor in aiding post-PM adjustment (Lloyd et al., 2000). Also, feeling that the decision was not coerced, but made independently after receiving answers to medical questions also appears critical in helping women adjust to PM. The opposite impression, feeling one has been coerced or "talked into" PM, contributes to the few reported negative outcomes (Lodder et al., 2002).

The nature of the anxiety a woman experiences clearly plays a role in decision making about PM and, possibly, in outcomes. Although anxiety has been linked to interest in PM, one study found that decliners of PM had higher trait anxiety than acceptors (Hatcher, Fallowfield, & A'Hern, 2001). Women who declined often used "detachment" as a coping style, rather than more problem-solving approaches. They appeared less likely to use their anxiety as a trigger for action and seemed more passive in the face of their worries. Over time (up to 18 months), the level of anxiety of women declining PM in this study was maintained, whereas women who underwent prophylactic mastectomies had significantly lower levels of anxiety 18 months later. Lodder et al. (2002) also found that women found to be mutation carriers who opted for prophylactic mastectomy were, on average, more anxious before receiving their genetic test result than were women mutation carriers who ultimately chose careful screening and watchful waiting following disclosure.

A range of sexual problems are reported in a significant number of women following PM surgery, ranging from relatively minor or temporary problems to disruption of sexual relations (Lodder et al., 2002). Women often blamed their own postsurgical disturbed sense of femininity, rather than their spouse or partner's hesitancy, for the sexual problems. Many women reported feeling isolated in not knowing others who had undergone PM and in feeling lack of support from others who opposed their decision (Lloyd et al., 2000).

Psychological and Social Support: New Roles for Psychologists

A few centers performing PM include psychological consultation as an essential component of the presurgical evaluation of prospective patients (Baron & Borgen, 1997; Hopwood et al., 2000). In most centers, a woman deciding whether to undergo PM would routinely see a breast surgeon (possibly for several visits) and a plastic surgeon to discuss reconstruction options, and she might undergo genetic counseling. Psychological consultation would not typically be included in the presurgical visits, although a referral might be suggested if the patient appeared markedly distressed or ambivalent.

Although many medical professionals acknowledge the major role of psychological factors in a woman's decision about PM, the depth of the issues aroused by consideration of PM is not fully understood. Surgeons and genetic counselors who might want to refer a patient considering PM may not know how to find a knowledgeable psychotherapist because understanding of the emotional issues related to prophylactic surgery is rare among mental health professionals, even some who work with cancer patients. The patients themselves are also often preoccupied with the "facts" related to the decision they are making, for example, the degree of risk reduction PM conveys, the time to recovery, and the pros and cons of various kinds of reconstruction. There is, in actuality, much factual information to be conveyed to potential PM patients, whose typically anxious state makes successful transmission of the information particularly challenging. But beyond the facts, there are many psychological aspects of the decision to be considered, including the accuracy of the woman's perception of her own cancer risk, the role of the woman's prior life experiences in her decision, the meaning she ascribes to undergoing this procedure, and the possible intimate and interpersonal ramifications the loss of her breasts may have, given her personality and social situation. Although both surgeons and genetic counselors usually raise questions about the anticipated personal impact with potential PM patients, their expertise and time pressures may not allow them to delve into the deeper emotional issues related to PM. Some patients may also be hesitant about seeking psychological help in preparing for surgery out of fear that the role of a psychologist would be to talk them out of PM, a procedure they feel is lifesaving. Overcoming these barriers, however, and enabling a woman to discuss the relevant psychological issues with a trained mental health professional as well as getting adequate answers to her medical questions from surgeons and genetic counselors (and possibly, access to CD-ROMs or other media aids) offers the best promise for enlightened decision making.

Many patients will have the possibility of PM raised to them and could benefit from the opportunity to discuss the possible psychological ramifications of the decision on their future well-being. Several examples follow.

* * *

Case Examples. Ms. A. accepted a referral from her oncologist for a presurgical psychological consultation a week prior to her surgery date for

PM to discuss her ambivalence about reconstruction. She started the session by saying that she thought it was most in keeping with who she was not to have reconstruction. She felt she would actually be most comfortable with no surgery beyond the prophylactic removal of her breasts. She had, however, seen a plastic surgeon who had suggested that she consider reconstruction. She was currently scheduled to have the reconstruction on the same day as her mastectomy. She came saying she was somewhat uneasy about whether this was truly what she wanted. The patient, age 34, had lost her mother to breast cancer at an early age. She felt sure she wanted PM and said she had known she would opt for PM for many years. Financial concerns had kept her from having genetic testing earlier, which she had done recently as a first step toward surgery. When she tested positive, the only issue remaining was the question of reconstruction. Talking with the psychological consultant over the course of an hour led to a discussion of her earlier experience with anorexia and bulimia. As the woman talked, she spoke of recent teasing from friends about the potential attractiveness of the breasts she could have following reconstructive surgery. In so doing, her facial expression changed from that of a very serious person to a happier, looser, almost girlish visage. More discussion led the patient to recognize that her feeling that she should not be choosing reconstruction came from the same tendency toward self-deprivation that had led to her previous anorexic and bulimic behaviors. She realized that she was really pleased by thinking of having new, perkier breasts and that reconstruction, far from being her reluctant choice, was her triumphant choice.

* * *

By contrast, there is a published case report of a woman in the Netherlands who used psychological consultation to resist family pressure and to confirm her decision not to undergo PM (de Vries-Kragt, 1998).

Mrs. Sandra van Dalen[1] was a 41-year-old *BRCA1* carrier. Her mother and the eldest of her three sisters had been diagnosed with metastatic ovarian cancer. Both had been treated and were well. Medical advice following the sister's diagnosis had led Sandra and the older of her healthy sisters to have procedures removing their ovaries (oophorectomy) and uterus (hysterectomy). When genetic testing later became available and was offered to her mother and affected sister, Sandra strongly advised them to be tested. When both were found to be carriers of the *BRCA1* mutation, the younger three sisters were tested. Sandra and her older sister were positive; her youngest sister was negative. The attending physician advised Sandra and her two

---

[1] Permission was granted to the article's author by the patient and her husband to publish their surname.

older sisters (one who had had cancer and one who had not but was a *BRCA1* carrier) to have bilateral prophylactic mastectomies. Sandra initially agreed but cancelled the surgery a week before she was to have her breasts removed. Despite earlier family discussion that each woman should make an independent decision, when Sandra decided not to have the PM surgery, her family members and friends voiced considerable disappointment. Even her husband, a physician, initially thought she should have the surgery. Another family emergency temporarily changed the focus of concern, but when that passed, family members returned to encouraging Sandra to do what they believed was best for the future of her family: to undergo PM.

A year and a half later, under considerable personal distress, Sandra entered psychotherapy to talk about her decision. She felt that her breasts mattered more to her psychologically after the removal of her ovaries and uterus, both in relation to her husband and in relation to her view of herself and her self-esteem. She was put off by seeing the "mutilation" her sister had undergone. She feared, however, that if she got cancer, people would blame her for not having had prophylactic surgery. She felt guilty for having encouraged the other family members to have genetic testing and felt that she did not think anyone in the family was happier because of the testing. She ultimately felt "that decisions like this are, in fact, inhuman." Sandra asked her doctors with some irony, why they didn't consider resecting the whole body, to prevent cancer. "Life," she said, " means taking risks." After looking at it from different angles, she remained firm in her decision not to have prophylactic breast surgery. With time, she not only became more comfortable with her decision but wanted her experience shared with professionals and potential patients. She wanted to convey the potential emotional risks that the decision to undergo genetic counseling had led to in her family. In her case, she retrospectively wished that she had not even been genetically tested (de Vries-Kragt, 1998, p. 78).

To recognize the isolation many women feel in making this decision and to respond to the wish many women express of wanting to talk with others who have undergone the procedure, the Clinical Genetics Service at Memorial Sloan-Kettering Cancer Center invited 19 women at high hereditary risk of breast cancer who had indicated an interest in PM to participate in a psychoeducational support group (Karp, Brown, Sullivan, & Massie, 1999). Four of the women agreed, and a fifth woman was subsequently added, comprising a group of five at-risk women. The group was led by a genetic counselor and two psychiatrists, one of whom had experience counseling women who were considering PM. All the group members had mothers who had had breast cancer; three of the mothers had died of their disease. Direct genetic testing was not available at the time the group was held. The group met for six weekly, 1.5-hour sessions, with an agenda determined, in large part, by the members. A woman who had had a PM was invited to one of the sessions. Another focus of the group content was revisiting the family experience with cancer. "The group members' memory of their mothers' course of the disease and outcome seemed to play a major role in the members' motivation for PM" (Karp et al., 1998, p. 168). A year after the completion of the group, the group leader telephoned the women for a follow-up report. None of the women had decided to undergo PM, and all felt that the group had encouraged them to feel more strongly that not having surgery was a reasonable decision for them. The authors felt that the women's positive view of the group's role supported their own belief about the utility of short-term groups for this new area of psychological concern. They emphasized the importance of having group leaders who are neutral about the value of prophylactic breast surgery, so that women can fully explore their own feelings and motivations (Karp et al., 1999).

Another paper from Memorial Sloan-Kettering Cancer Center (Massie, Mushkin, & Stewart, 1998) describes the intermittent, individual psychotherapy over a 9-year period of a 32-year-old woman who opted for PM. The woman was motivated to have PM because of her family history of breast cancer, including the death of her mother at age 44. The patient was described as being in "terror that she might die of breast cancer" after her sister was diagnosed with bilateral inflammatory breast disease. The therapy covered the period when the woman was anticipating and then undergoing prophylactic surgery and a subsequent period 4 years later (following the death of her sister) when she had genetic testing (which had not been available at the time of her surgery). Given the woman's feeling that she lacked other appropriate supports, the therapist accompanied the patient to the genetic test result disclosure session. At the session, the woman was told the test was negative for the *BRCA1* mutation, which had been found in the blood of her now-deceased sister. Her reaction was appreciation for the interim 4 years of respite she had had from the breast cancer worry that had been so pervasive in her life. She gave eager permission for her case to be shared with others, saying, "They simply have to understand how important it is for a woman to be able to make decisions about her own body."

SUMMARY

It is clear that psychological factors play an enormous role in women's motivation for PM. There are few medical interventions that promise a risk reduction rate of 90%. Nonetheless, a minority of high-risk women express interest in PM and fewer still undergo the procedure. It is likely that interest in PM will rise as increasing numbers of women are counseled about their hereditary breast cancer risk and increasing numbers are found to carry

BRCA1/2 mutations. It is also clear that many women carry exaggerated notions of what their risk is and often have outdated notions about the nature and efficacy of current breast cancer treatment, on the basis of their mothers' unsuccessful breast cancer treatment. Psychologists have major roles to play in helping to reduce anxiety based on such exaggerated fears. Psychological consultation should also be available for women with significant family history to discuss the personal and interpersonal impact that loss of their breasts might produce as well as the potential emotional benefits of undergoing surgery.

To be of help, however, psychologists working in cancer centers and those community psychologists and other mental health providers who want to offer these services must understand the driving force that many women feel in seeking PM to rid themselves of the cancer worry that impedes their everyday lives. The haunting memories of losing a mother at an early age lead many women to vow that they will not let this happen to their children. Having children was the only clear factor differentiating women who chose PM from those who did not in one study of high-risk women (Meijers-Heijboer et al., 2000). The drive toward PM leads some women to change doctors if their physician tries to dissuade them from the procedure because they feel their lives are in mortal danger without surgery. Although the majority report being satisfied with their decision about surgery after their breasts are removed, up to 50% report subsequent problems in feminine identification and sexual relationships (Lodder et al., 2002). It is clear that many of the women feel the price paid for reduced anxiety was high, but one they were willing to pay to increase the odds they would be able to raise their children to adulthood and enjoy their grandchildren.

Psychologists who provide PM interventions must be neutral about the value of PM. The purpose of the treatment is to reduce unrealistic fears or phobias, to enable the woman (and also possibly her spouse or partner) to contemplate actively the impact of the surgery and the meaning that loss of the woman's breasts will have for them as a couple. It should help the woman place this decision in a life context and to decide the extent to which this action is in keeping with her other beliefs and actions.

Once the decision is made to undergo PM, psychologists can help women prepare for surgery. Behavioral and psychodynamic treatment may be used to help patients cope with typical surgery-related fears, such as fears of anesthesia or pain. In addition, some women expressly want to mourn the anticipated loss of their breast. Some have devised rituals to help them take leave of their breasts (Josephson et al., 2000). Others prefer a rehearsal of events and emotions to come, especially anticipation of coping with their altered physical self.

More research and clinical training in this area are needed to guide practitioners in their psychological treatment of women considering or adjusting to PM. In addition, further outcomes research can inform physicians who offer advice and women who are making their decision about PM. "Given . . . the thousands genetically at risk who may soon visit our offices, there is a crucial role for psychological understanding and social support as we navigate the issues that arise out of a rapidly evolving genetic knowledge base" (Massie et al., 1998, p. 196).

PROPHYLACTIC OOPHORECTOMY

The other most commonly recommended form of prophylactic surgery for individuals with inherited breast/ovarian cancer susceptibility is prophylactic oophorectomy (PO), which is often accompanied by a hysterectomy (Paley et al., 2001). Prophylactic oophorectomy has been shown to reduce the risk of not only ovarian cancer but also of breast cancer, likely because of reduced hormonal levels (Rebbeck et al., 1999). Hence, it is considered of particular value to women who are carriers of *BRCA1/2* mutations who are subject to greatly increased risk of both breast and ovarian cancer. Estimates of the risk of developing ovarian cancer for women who have *BRCA1* mutations have been variably estimated to be between 16% (Struewing et al., 1997) and 60% (Easton, Ford, Bishop, & the Breast Cancer Linkage Consortium, 1995). Women who carry *BRCA2* mutations have ovarian cancer risks estimated to be between 20% and 27% (Breast Cancer Linkage Consortium, 1999; Ford et al., 1998).

Ovarian cancer remains the most lethal of the gynecological cancers. Because it is not easily detected, many women are only found to have ovarian cancer when it is in advanced stages. Available tests have marked imperfections, and there is no definitive, nonsurgical way of diagnosing it. Neither vaginal ultrasound nor CA-125 testing has been shown to reduce morbidity or mortality from ovarian cancer, and there is no proof of their efficacy in women who are mutation carriers (Rebbeck, 2000). These factors combine to make ovarian cancer a source of considerable fear among women whose family history includes ovarian cancer.

What Is Prophylactic Oophorectomy?

Prophylactic oophorectomy is the surgical removal of the ovaries to prevent cancer. It can be done laparoscopically as an outpatient procedure (Berchuck, Schildkraut, Marks, & Futreal, 1999) in many cases. The incidence of serious complications is low. Postsurgically, however, women undergoing PO experience immediate menopause, with side effects including loss of libido, hot flashes, urogenital atrophy, osteoporosis, and heart disease (Berchuck et al., 1999).

The surgically induced menopause that results from PO necessitates consideration of whether a woman should take hormone replacement therapy (HRT) to reduce the cardiac and osteoporosis risks, as well as consideration of the sexual and emotional ramifications. There is considerable controversy about the extent of breast cancer risk associated with use of HRT and little data about the effects in high-risk women (American College of Obstetricians and Gynecologists, Committee on Gynecologic Practice, 2001). One recent study suggests that whether a woman who undergoes PO uses HRT does not affect the likelihood that she will develop breast cancer (Rebbeck et al., 1999), but because of the study's small sample size, further research is needed. On the contrary, this study found that among women with known BRCA1/2 mutations, PO significantly reduced the risk of developing breast cancer, most likely because of a reduction in circulating estrogen.

Questions about the impact of length of HRT use make this issue one that young women concerned about increased hereditary breast cancer risk must revisit regularly, rather than a question resolved once and for all. As such, especially for women who are "monitors" (Miller, Fang, Manne, Engstrom, & Daly, 1999) of information about health risks, this decision and the lack of clear medical advice about HRT use can occasion continuing high anxiety, which must be considered in weighing the pros and cons of PO. The recent reversal of recommendations leading to dramatic reduction of HRT use among postmenopausal women in the general population is likely to influence HRT use among high-risk women, even though the studies do not address risk for this group (Writing Group for the Women's Health Initiative Investigators, 2002). Women undergoing PO usually have their uterus removed simultaneously and thus would not take the combination estrogen–progesterone that was studied in the Women's Health Initiative study, in which researchers found that women taking the combined regimen had significantly higher risks of breast cancer, with increasing risk the longer the hormones were used. In addition, studies have shown increased risk for stroke and pulmonary embolism among HRT users, which seems to outweigh other benefits (Beral, Banks, & Reeves, 2002). Many postmenopausal women in the general population have stopped taking HRT in the wake of these studies. Given this turning of the tide, it is likely that women at high hereditary cancer risk will be even more reluctant to take HRT. This may make decisions about oophorectomy more difficult for young at-risk women because they are typically 20 years or so younger when entering their surgical menopause following PO than are women who enter menopause naturally. New medications are being tested that can potentially relieve at least some of the side effects of surgically induced menopause in this population of women.

One option recently suggested for young women who are BRCA1 mutation carriers is that of tubal ligation, rather than PO at the conclusion of childbearing (Narod et al., 2001). Reductions in ovarian cancer occurrence were associated with tubal ligation for *BRCA1*, but not *BRCA2*, mutation carriers. This option would allow women who are *BRCA1* mutation carriers to postpone PO, and thus menopausal risks and symptoms, for a number of years, while offering a risk-reduction option at the conclusion of childbearing. Oral contraceptive use has also been shown to have a protective effect against ovarian cancer, and the combination of tubal ligation and past oral contraceptive was shown to be highly effective. The Narod study suggests that continuing oral contraceptive use following tubal ligation may further reduce the risk of ovarian cancer. This is an option young women may want to discuss with their physicians as part of their decision making regarding PO.

Histological examination of the ovarian tissue that is removed during PO surgery can reveal the presence of malignant or premalignant cells (Lu et al., 2000; Salazar et al., 1996), a circumstance that some patients may not anticipate. Obviously, when cancer is found, women are likely to feel they made the correct decision to have their ovaries removed but may, nonetheless, be shocked, especially given that they may then have to consider further treatment. This possibility should be discussed with women considering PO.

How Much Does Prophylactic Oophorectomy Reduce the Risk of Ovarian Cancer?

It is unfortunate that PO does not completely remove the risk of either ovarian or breast cancer. Women who have had their ovaries removed remain at risk of developing cancer in the underlying peritoneal (abdomen lining) tissues. Although there has not been a definitive study of the extent of risk reduction for ovarian cancer with PO, Struewing, Watson, Ponder, Lynch, and Tucker (1995) found that for women with a first-degree relative with ovarian cancer and a family history of breast and ovarian cancer, PO reduced the risk of ovarian cancer by about half.

A hypothetical model of risk reduction due to PO estimates that a 30-year-old woman who is a *BRCA1/2* mutation carrier can gain from 0.3 to 2.6 additional years of life expectancy as a result of PO (Schrag, Kuntz, Garber, & Weeks, 1997), although other researchers have questioned the assumptions that underlie this estimate (Rebbeck, 2000). Another study using a Markov model to estimate years saved by PO found benefit for *BRCA1/2*-positive women with affected first-degree relatives (2.6 years), but little or no benefit for women with lower levels of risk (0.4 years; Grann, Panageos, Whang, Antman, & Neugut, 1998). Benefit also declines with age at surgery and is minimal for women who are 60 years of age or older (Schrag et al., 1997).

Costs of Prophylactic Oophorectomy and Insurance Coverage

The cost of PO is considerably lower than the cost of PM and hence is likely to be less of an issue for a woman considering prophylactic surgery. There may still be some concern about alerting insurers to increased hereditary risk for ovarian cancer among unaffected women. Also, women who are *BRCA1/2* carriers from families with a family history only of breast cancer may find they need to provide medical explanations to the insurer about why they are at increased risk of ovarian cancer. A recent study (Kuerer et al., 2000) shows that only 20% of surveyed health insurance carriers had a specific policy of covering PO for women with a strong family history of ovarian cancer or who are *BRCA1/2* carriers. Twenty-eight percent of the surveyed companies had a policy of refusing coverage for family history, and 24% had a policy of not covering PO for *BRCA1/2* mutation carriers. Half had no stated policy.

Who Opts for Prophylactic Oophorectomy?

Screening guidelines for high-risk patients and *BRCA1/2* mutation carriers suggest PO for women who are older than 35 years who have completed childbearing (Burke et al., 1997). Permanently curtailing reproductive capacity and inducing menopause are major life steps to contemplate, especially for young women. Often these effects are minimized by professionals concerned about the risk to the patient's well-being and mortality posed by ovarian cancer and the threat of breast cancer. In the absence of alternative prevention techniques, or screening strategies, PO is often suggested as a reasonable option.

Studies have indicated that, as with PM, many of the women seeking PO are doing so based on exaggerated notions of the likelihood they will develop ovarian cancer and high levels of cancer worry (Meiser et al., 1999). Although many people in the general population are aware of the 1 in 9 likelihood of getting breast cancer, there is little general knowledge of the frequency of ovarian cancer among women in the general population, which is about 1% (Nahhas, 1997). Women from high-risk breast and ovarian cancer families often lack accurate knowledge of the risk to themselves (between 15% and 60%). Women from families that have experienced only breast cancer are often shocked to learn through genetic counseling that they also carry an increased hereditary risk of ovarian cancer. Following genetic counseling and the finding that they are at increased hereditary cancer risk, many women feel highly anxious and eager to do something quickly to reduce their cancer risk. Because the surgery itself lacks the complexity and visual impact of PM, many women find PO a more acceptable option and schedule an oophorectomy within a short time following disclosure of their test result or risk assessment.

Although PO is often considered more acceptable to high-risk women than PM, many women still do not accept this option. Many factors enter into the decision, including age, level of risk, reproductive status, and personality characteristics. Half of a group of Austrian women undergoing testing for *BRCA1/2* (but not yet aware of their result) said they would consider PO (Wagner et al., 2000), as did 33% and 76% of women in two American studies (Lerman et al., 1996; Lynch et al., 1997).

Actual uptake differs by time of follow-up and nationality, but rates in some centers are high. In an English study (Hallowell, 1998), 71% (*n* = 15) of 21 women recently counseled for hereditary susceptibility to breast and ovarian cancer to whom PO had been mentioned as an option reported that they would consider PO; 23% said they would not consider it. One year later, however, only four women had had PO. Women in that study expressed the sentiment that breasts were more central to their body image and sense of themselves than were ovaries. Many older women (mid- to late 40s) found it more acceptable to hasten the natural process of menopause through PO than to consider removal of the breasts. This was not universal, however, and some women felt strongly that even prophylactic oophorectomy went against the natural order of things, that it might not stop the onset of cancer, and that it could interfere with their obligations as wives and breadwinners.

> Well, they [ovaries] keep our hormone balance how it should be. I mean all women are different, and I think their hormones are for their body, and they keep that balance on the keel. Once you take those out, they go all over the place. I think when women stop having periods and go into the change, that's the natural cycle of things. I don't believe in interfering with the natural cycle of things if you don't have to. (Hallowell, 1998, p. 268)

Several studies have shown that a large number of women who undergo PO feel that they lacked some information they wish they had had, about the procedure itself, the remaining risk of cancer, or about sequelae of the surgery. A number of studies have suggested that more detailed or tailored genetic counseling or referral for psychological counseling or group therapy might be useful for women considering PO (Hallowell, 2000; Miller et al., 1999). Miller et al. hypothesized that differentiation of those women who are "monitors" (health-information seekers) from "blunters" (health-information avoiders) might lead to recommendations for different counseling approaches. They suggested that interventions for monitors might emphasize limitations of PO and teach strategies for reducing related

emotional distress, whereas blunters might be aided by interventions emphasizing the benefits of PO.

It seems clear that there will be an increasing population of women
who will need to decide whether PO is appropriate for them following risk
analysis during genetic counseling or disclosure of being a BRCA1/2 mutation
carrier. Thus, it seems important that mental health providers understand
both the pros and cons of PO surgery and that they feel prepared to help
women consider the issues. Particularly important may be finding ways to
help those women without high objective risk to consider treatment of their
anxiety, which does not involve surgery or its attendant risks and costs.

What Do Women Say Who Have Had Prophylactic Oophorectomy?

There are only two current studies of psychological outcomes following
PO. Both of these qualitative studies, one from the United Kingdom and
one from Australia, involve less than 25 participants, so it is not possible
to extrapolate results to the full cohort of women who have undergone PO.
Nonetheless, these studies provide the beginnings of an understanding of
the psychological impact of the procedure. Both report universal or nearly
universal relief in worry about ovarian cancer. Women in the Australian
study (Meiser et al., 2000b) emphasized that they felt more in control of
their lives following surgery. The English study (Hallowell, 2000) focused
on the women's lack of satisfaction with the information they were given
about the physical aspects of surgery and recovery and the emotional impact
PO would have. Women in that study had been between the ages of 31
and 45 at the time they underwent PO; only a minority had had specialized
genetic counseling. More than 20% of the women in that study felt that
they had not fully understood the endocrine function of the ovaries and
the fact that menopause would occur immediately. Half the women did not
recall discussion of menopause with their surgeons prior to PO.

Much of the dissatisfaction in both this and the Australian study
concerned the women's difficulty making decisions about whether to use
HRT, especially in light of concern that its use may exacerbate the risk of
developing breast cancer. The women in the English study felt that there
had been little or no discussion in most cases about the choice of types of
HRT or the length of time it was recommended that they take HRT. Two
women in that study reported that their consent had not been obtained for
the insertion of a hormonal implant, which had been done while they
were under anesthesia for PO. Most could not recall any discussion of the
menopausal symptoms they might experience following surgery, and thus,
in a number of cases, they had not recognized the symptoms as being related
to the removal of their ovaries. About a quarter of the women did not know
whether their cervix had been removed as part of the surgery. A few of the

women appeared not to know that PO did not completely reduce the risk of extra-ovarian peritoneal cancer. None recalled being given a numerical risk of ovarian cancer prior to surgery. Although the women felt well prepared for the physical aspects of the surgical experience itself, there were some complaints that the advice they received did not take into account their need to lift and take care of young children.

The Australian study emphasized differences between pre- and post-menopausal women undergoing PO and between premenopausal women who took HRT and those who did not following PO. The latter group did report loss of libido as a serious side effect of surgery, but the others largely reported no change in their sexual functioning following PO. One of the women reporting reduced libido stated after surgery that "everything sexual has been taken away from me," and she said that she regretted having had the surgery. Her preexisting depression apparently had worsened following PO. It is of interest that, except for this woman, the women in this group reported no decline in their sense of their own femininity following surgery. One woman reported increased libido following PO, which the researchers conjectured might have to do with reduced anxiety about developing cancer. Several of the women who had previously undergone a mastectomy positively compared the effects of losing their ovaries to the loss of their breast. The fact that ovaries are internal organs and thus not visible to others was cited as a major reason for the lesser emotional impact related to PO.

Women in the Australian group, most of whom had had genetic counseling and met with a gynecological oncologist, felt they had had sufficient information on which to base their decision, but half felt they had not had sufficient information about postsurgical issues. They felt they would have wanted more information about physical aftereffects and also felt emotionally unsupported by the medical staff following surgery. Patients suggested that a peer support group or newsletter would provide needed support and opportunities for sharing their experiences. Premenopausal women also felt strongly conflicted about the question of whether to increase their chance of developing breast cancer by taking HRT. Some who took HRT expressed guilt that they were now doing something that might lead to cancer, after have taken a major surgical step to reduce their odds but felt that their quality of life and that of their family was better when they took hormone replacement. One participant taking HRT reported "constant worry" about breast cancer. Several felt that conflicting reports and the lack of clear direction from physicians increased their discomfort with this decision.

Summary

Prophylactic oophorectomy offers significant reduction in worry about the risk of developing ovarian cancer for many women who are at increased hereditary risk and who find it an acceptable option. It also appears to convey significant reduction in the risk of breast cancer, which, in turn, could reduce worry for many at-risk women. It is not, however, a procedure to be entered into without thorough information and preparation. With increasing numbers of women being identified as *BRCA1/2* mutation carriers, PO will be offered to many women, including many premenopausal women. Particularly, but not exclusively, for those women, the choices related to PO should be reviewed with care and discussed at some length. Some physicians feel that women with *BRCA1/2* mutations who have a family history of ovarian cancer should be encouraged to undergo PO much more strongly than those without a family history. Postsurgical concerns, especially consideration of the pros and cons of HRT use, should be thoroughly discussed. It is only a moot victory if fear of breast cancer replaces worry about ovarian cancer after PO.

A number of critical psychological issues become part of this decision. Women who are very afraid of ovarian cancer, often because of their mother's experience, or women who discover their increased risk for ovarian cancer during genetic counseling and are encouraged to consider PO may feel they are in a great hurry to remove this fear by acting quickly. The first and most obvious issue is the question of the impact of consideration of PO on childbearing prospects. For many couples, the question of when they are finished with childbearing is a fluid one, resolved over the course of a number of years with mutual discussion and acceptance. A recommendation for PO can be experienced as something that must take precedence over any lingering thoughts about additional children. Although the threat of ovarian cancer is a very real one, the fact that it rarely occurs before age 40 should encourage women and their husbands to take the time they need to decide about the size of their family. Even without such considerations, questions about the use of HRT and the loss of libido and other menopause-associated issues (such as osteoporosis and increased cardiac risk) should encourage timely, thoughtful consideration of the appropriateness and timing of a decision for PO in younger women.

Literature on menopause is often written for much older women and may not address the sexual issues or feelings of young women about the abrupt end to their reproductive capacity that PO-induced menopause occasions. They may feel out of step with friends and may gain considerable support from a group or newsletter that enables them to share their family history and surgical experience with others who have similar experiences. Web sites such as the one for FORCE (Facing Our Risk of Cancer Empowered; http:// www. facingourrisk.org) can provide links to other women with similar issues and concerns. Although published studies show few women having a difficult time after PO or regretting their decision, there is some suggestion that women with a preexisting depression might be well advised to treat their depression before making a decision for PO.

For older, postmenopausal women, the psychological effects seem more limited. Here, too, however, it may be important to encourage the woman to get full information about what, if any, symptoms she may encounter as she recovers from surgery and to discuss fully the risk of residual disease and related worries.

RECOMMENDATIONS FOR PSYCHOLOGICAL CONSULTATIONS TO PATIENTS CONSIDERING PROPHYLACTIC OOPHORECTOMY OR PROPHYLACTIC MASTECTOMY

It should be clear from these summaries that many of the women who seek prophylactic surgery (or at least those who have sought it in the past) are passionate in their belief that surgery offers them the best chance for survival. The suggestion or requirement of psychological consultation as part of the presurgical workup must be carefully presented as a means of maximizing benefit. It is hoped that such a consultation could help by reviewing the many levels of relevant issues that have been known to arise for women undergoing the procedure and by discussing the particular patient's thinking about what the surgery will accomplish for her and how it will affect her life and relationships. It must be clear that the mental health professional offering the consultation is neutral about which decision the woman makes. The patient should feel that the therapists' only goals are to help her make the best decision about surgery and, if surgery is scheduled, to empower her to prepare for the surgical experience and the adjustments to follow.

Perhaps the first consideration is to review the medical indications and risk assessments the patient is using to make the decision about surgery. It is not the mental health professional's role to assign risks. Psychotherapists and psychological consultants in high-risk clinics use the risk information provided by medical or genetics professionals in determining or hypothesizing about the accuracy of the patient's personal risk estimates that he or she is using as the basis for decision making. It is clearly important for professionals to help patients view their risks, or the risk they believe they have, in light of scientific data that exist. Then, decisions about prevention or risk-reduction options can be made on the basis of appropriate basic assumptions. An example of a situation in which risk data may not have been used appropriately is the published report of a male *BRCA2* carrier who underwent a prophylactic mastectomy despite the fact that his breast cancer risk was only 2.5 %—less than half that of a woman in the U.S. general population

(Daltrey, Eeles, & Kissin, 1998). Many would conclude that this surgery was medically unnecessary and that preferable treatment would have been psychological counseling for the anxiety the man was apparently experiencing.

A well-trained psychologist or other mental health professional has the skills to evaluate the level of distress that a person considering prophylactic surgery reports and to initiate a discussion of the causes of the distress. It is important to establish what are the underlying psychological goals of surgery because it will only serve intended aims if the distress is due to factors that removal of the breasts or ovaries can accomplish. Unresolved grief reactions are frequently mentioned as components of the motivation for PM or PO, but there may well be aspects of that grief that are better served by psychotherapy than surgery. Many women say their motivation for prophylactic surgery is to avoid for themselves the premature deaths their mothers endured and to ensure that their children do not grow up without a mother. These powerful factors may actually make it difficult for some women to consider potential differences between their circumstances and their mother's. Taking such things into consideration might change the decision equation for them or the timing of their surgery. It may be that other aspects of the family experience related to the mother's death, such as estrangement from other relatives or survival guilt, are driving the decision. Resolution of these emotional issues through psychological consultation or psychotherapy can free the individual to make the decision about prophylactic surgery in as calm, rational, and effective a manner as possible.

Pervasive anxiety about fear of developing cancer is a frequent reason offered to justify prophylactic surgery, sometimes in the absence of objective cancer risk. Cancer phobia is often mentioned in the literature as a justification for the procedure. There are standard psychological treatments for phobic behaviors in other contexts, and it would not be unreasonable to attempt treatment of the anxiety related to cancer risk through cognitive behavioral or psychodynamic means first. Reconsideration of the decision about prophylactic surgery could occur following successful completion of the treatment. Without such intervening psychological treatment, the patient's cancer phobia might remain uncured and take other forms following prophylactic surgery.

Although the incidence of Munchausen syndrome in this context is low, it has been reported (Evans et al., 1996). If an individual is enrolled in a research program, medical records confirming a family history of cancer may have been done because it is often routine in such programs; clinical testing typically does not involve this step, however. Hence, if the mental health professional doing an evaluation of a patient considering PM or PO has reason to suspect that the family history supplied by the patient is fictitious or erroneous, it is advisable to suggest to the patient and the physicians involved that confirmation of family history of cancer would be useful prior to scheduling surgery.

With PM, major issues are aroused by the question of reconstruction, which can also be usefully reviewed for the emotional factors contributing to views of the various options. Some patients are firmly committed to a particular view. With assurance that the goal of reviewing their reasons is not to change the patient's mind, the patient may be willing to discuss her feeling about what is the right choice for her. Some women are overwhelmed by the information they have received through genetic counseling, medical consultation, or from other sources and are uncertain about what they really want. Others feel pressured to make a decision, either by family members with strong opinions or by the constraints of some of the surgical reconstruction options. TRAM flaps, for example, can only be done once per patient, so the woman with cancer considering PM must decide whether she wants both breasts removed at the time of her mastectomy for cancer with a TRAM flap to follow. A knowledgeable psychotherapist can help a woman even within a limited period of time, if necessary, to reach a decision that optimizes the match between her personality, social situation, and the medically available choices. When there is more time to make a decision (as is true for most bilateral prophylactic mastectomies), therapists can help women take the time they need to consider, thoughtfully and thoroughly, all the options in light of their own issues, history, and personalities.

The emotional impact of prophylactic surgery is felt not only by the patient herself but also by spouses and children, perhaps especially by daughters. Women in a Swedish study of psychosocial effects of PM suggested that their husbands and children be offered psychological support (Josephson et al., 2000). Hopwood et al. (2000) suggested that husbands be seen for at least one session of counseling prior to their wives' surgeries. Parents of women undergoing prophylactic surgery who are obligate or known carriers of *BRCA1/2* mutations may also experience guilt as the "cause" of the woman's need to have this surgery and could potentially benefit from discussion of their feelings.

Many women are surprised by the emotional upheaval they experience following prophylactic surgery, as well as by the physical pain they experience. Others find the short-term physical recovery to be relatively benign but suffer from multilayered grief or loss of self-acceptance related to their altered bodies. Unanticipated marital difficulties can surface, as sexual intimacy is redefined. Irritability may be related to the mood swings of menopause, the physical and emotional burdens of surgery, or depression. Although many aspects of the individual or couple therapy that may be initiated postprophylactic surgery may be similar to that in other settings, particular sensitivity may be needed to recognize the nuances of multilayered feelings and the mixture of relief and grief that may be expressed. Such mixed emotions may complicate the offering and receipt of social support within the couple, as well as within the therapeutic relationship. Psychological treatment can elucidate problems in interpersonal communication, possibly preventing long-term misunderstanding.

In conclusion, mental health providers have much to offer to high-risk women in providing a shared context to consider the burdens and challenges of evaluating the pros and cons of prophylactic surgery in light of the particular woman's experiences and wishes. Although it is crucial that women make their own decisions about this irreversible, risk-reducing option, psychologists and others trained to understand the range of issues that may be related to surgical removal of organs (ranging from maternal grief to sexual identification and self-image) may help define the central aims of the surgery and match them to the appropriate treatment. In addition, psychological consultation following prophylactic surgery may help women adapt optimally to the physical and emotional sequelae.

PROPHYLACTIC COLECTOMY

As briefly discussed in chapter 2, male and female familial adenomatous polyposis (FAP) and hereditary nonpolyposis colon cancer (HNPCC) mutation carriers are often advised to undergo surgical removal of their colon (colectomy) to avoid the development of colorectal cancer. The colorectal (CRC) cancer risk for individuals with FAP who carry APC mutations nears 100% and is about 70% for men and women with HNPCC mutations (Offit, 1998); this high risk level provides clear medical justification for colectomy for FAP and the recommendation, based on expert opinion, that colectomy be considered by persons with HNPCC who develop adenomatous polyps. It is estimated that prophylactic surgery in HNPCC mutation carriers increases life expectancy on average by 15.6 years (Syngal, Weeks, Schrag, Garber, & Kuntz, 1998). Psychological issues may be overlooked, given the high risk for cancer in carriers and the potential for surgery to reduce that risk drastically. As discussed in earlier chapters, HNPCC does carry with it additional cancer risks beyond CRC. Female HNPCC carriers are also likely to consider prophylactic oophorectomy and hysterectomy because ovarian and endometrial cancers occur with greater frequency in that population (Smith et al., 2001).

The options presented to individuals from FAP families who have developed polyps and mutation carriers from HNPCC families are total or subtotal colectomy. Total colectomy (colon removal) does not necessitate constant surveillance but has greater effects on bowel functioning. Subtotal colectomy, which allows for preservation of the rectum and more normal bowel function, necessitates regular screening of the rectum to ensure that cancer has not developed there (Lynch, Smyrk, & Lynch, 1997). There is a 12% risk of rectal cancer in mutation carriers, which typically occurs 4 to 6 years after prophylactic colectomy (Rodriguez-Bigas et al., 1997). Both surgeries carry significant psychological burdens because outcomes may affect self-esteem and confidence in everyday activities. There is remarkably little research on decision making regarding prophylactic colorectal surgery or about psychological outcomes of colectomy and coping with rectal surgery for cancer prevention (Holland, 1989; van Duijvendijk et al., 2000). This is clearly an area of growing importance because genetic testing for colon cancer predisposition genes will identify increasing numbers of people who will be advised to consider surgery. The psychological ramifications of genetic testing will be tied to issues about how the option of prophylactic surgery is presented, whether there are ways for patient-to-patient support networks to enlighten prospective surgical patients about the lifestyle changes or lack thereof that surgery necessitates, and whether psychotherapeutic consultation aids decision making. Because hereditary colon cancer affects both men and women, it will also be interesting to determine the extent to which gender affects outcomes and determines the efficacy of psychological interventions.

PROPHYLACTIC THYROIDECTOMY

Please see chapter 2 for a discussion of the rationale for prophylactic thyroidectomy in carriers of RET mutation carriers who are at increased hereditary risk for developing Multiple Endocrine Neoplasia type 2 (MEN2). This section of chapter 2 also reviews the limited psychosocial data in this area.

PROPHYLACTIC PROSTATECTOMY

There is no clinical recommendation for surgical removal of the prostate in members of high-risk prostate cancer families. Although researchers are actively pursuing leads toward what are likely to be several genes that predispose men to develop prostate cancer, genetic testing is not available for prostate cancer genes at this time (Karan, Lin, Johansson, & Batra, 2003).

REFERENCES

Al-Ghazal, S. K., Sully, L., Fallowfield, L., & Blamey, R. W. (2000). The psychological impact of immediate rather than delayed breast reconstruction. *European Journal of Surgical Oncology, 26,* 17–19.

American College of Obstetricians and Gynecologists, Committee on Gynecologic Practice. (2001, December). Committee opinion Number 62: Risk of breast cancer with estrogen-progestin replacement therapy. *Obstetrics & Gynecology, 98*, 1181–1184.

Anderson, R., & Kaczmarek, B. (1996). Psychological well-being of the breast reconstruction patient: A pilot study. *Plastic Surgical Nursing, 16*, 185–188.

Baron, R. H., & Borgen, P. I. (1997). Genetic susceptibility for breast cancer: Testing and primary prevention options. *Oncology Nursing Forum, 24*, 461–467.

Beral, V., Banks, E., & Reeves, G. (2002). Evidence from randomised trials on the long-term effects of hormone replacement therapy. *Lancet, 360*, 942–944.

Berchuck, A., Schildkraut, J. M., Marks, J. R., & Futreal, P. A. (1999). Managing hereditary ovarian cancer risk. *Cancer, 86*, 2517–2524.

Borgen, P. I., Hill, A. D. K., Tran, K. N., Van Zee, K. J., Massie, M. J., Payne, D., et al. (1998). Patient regrets after bilateral prophylactic mastectomy. *Annals of Surgical Oncology, 5*, 603–606.

Bostwick, J., III. (1995). Breast reconstruction following mastectomy. *CA: A Cancer Journal for Clinicians, 45*, 289–304.

Breast Cancer Linkage Consortium. (1999). Cancer risks in *BRCA2* mutation carriers. *Journal of National Cancer Institute, 91*, 1310–1316.

Burke, W., Daly, M., Garber, J., Botkin, J., Kahn, M. J. E., Lynch, P., et al. (1997). Recommendations for follow-up care of individuals with an inherited predisposition to cancer. II. *BRCA1* and *BRCA2. Journal of the American Medical Association, 277*, 997–1003.

Daltrey, I. R., Eeles, R. A., & Kissin, M. W. (1998). Bilateral prophylactic mastectomy: Not just a woman's problem. *Breast, 7*, 236–237.

de Vries-Kragt, K. (1998). The dilemmas of a carrier of *BRCA1* gene mutations. *Patient Education and Counseling, 35*, 75–80.

Easton, D. F., Ford, D., Bishop, D. T., and the Breast Cancer Linkage Consortium. (1995). Breast and ovarian cancer incidence in *BRCA1*-mutation carriers. *American Journal of Human Genetics, 56*, 265–271.

Eisen, A., Rebbeck, T. R., Wood, W. C., & Weber, B. L. (2000). Prophylactic surgery in women with a hereditary predisposition to breast and ovarian cancer. *Journal of Clinical Oncology, 18*, 1980–1995.

Eisinger, F., Geller, G., Burke, W., & Holtzman, N. A. (1999). Cultural basis for differences between US and French clinical recommendations for women at increased risk for breast and ovarian cancer. *Lancet, 353*, 919–920.

Evans, D. G. R., Anderson, E., Lalloo, F., Vasen, H., Beckmann, M., Eccles, D., et al. (1999). Utilisation of prophylactic mastectomy in 10 European centers. *Disease Markers, 15*, 148–151.

Evans, D. G. R., Kerr, B., Cade, D., Hoare, E., & Hopwood, P. (1996). Fictitious breast cancer history. *Lancet, 348*, 1034.

Ford, D., Easton, D. F., Stratton, M., Narod, S., Goldgar, D., Devilee, P., et al. (1998). Genetic heterogeneity and penetrance analysis of the *BRCA1* and

BRCA2 genes in cancer families. *American Journal of Human Genetics, 62,* 676–689.

Frost, M. H., Schaid, D. J., Sellers, T. A., Slezak, J. M., Arnold, P. G., Woods, J. E., et al. (2000). Long-term satisfaction and psychological and social function following bilateral prophylactic mastectomy. *Journal of American Medical Association, 284,* 319–324.

Gail, M. H., Brinton, L. A., Byar, D. P., Corle, D. K., Green, S. B., Schairer, C., et al. (1989). Projecting individualized probabilities of developing breast cancer for white females who are being examined annually. *Journal of the National Cancer Institute, 81,* 1879–1886.

Grann, V. R., Panageos, K. S., Whang, W., Antman, K. H., & Neugut, A. (1998). Decision analysis of prophylactic mastectomy and oophorectomy in *BRCA1*-positive or *BRCA2*-positive patients. *Journal of Clinical Oncology, 16,* 979–985.

Hallowell, N. (1998). "You don't *want* to lose your ovaries because you think 'I might become a man.'" Women's perceptions of prophylactic surgery as a cancer risk management option. *Psycho-Oncology, 7,* 263–275.

Hallowell, N. (2000). A qualitative study of the information needs of high-risk women undergoing prophylactic oophorectomy. *Psycho-Oncology, 9,* 486–495.

Harcourt, D., & Rumsey, N. (2001). Psychological aspects of breast reconstruction: A review of the literature. *Journal of Advanced Nursing, 35,* 477–487.

Hartmann, L. C., Schaid, D. J., Woods, J. E., Crotty, T. P., Myers, J. L., Arnold, P. G., et al. (1999). Efficacy of bilateral prophylactic mastectomy in women with a family history of breast cancer. *New England Journal of Medicine, 340,* 77–84.

Hatcher, M. B., Fallowfield, L., & A'Hern, R. (2001). The psychosocial impact of bilateral prophylactic mastectomy: Prospective study using questionnaires and semistructured interviews. *British Medical Journal, 322,* 1–6.

Holland, J. C. (1989). Gastrointestinal cancer. In J. C. Holland & J. H. Rowland (Eds.), *Handbook of psychooncology: Psychological care of the patient with cancer* (pp. 208–218). New York: Oxford University Press.

Hopwood, P., Lee, A., Shenton, A., Baildam, A., Brain, A., Lalloo, F., et al. (2000). Clinical follow-up after bilateral risk reducing ("prophylactic") mastectomy: Mental health and body image outcomes. *Psycho-Oncology, 9,* 462–472.

Hughes, K. S., Papa, M. Z., Whitney, T., & McLellan, R. (1999). Prophylactic mastectomy and inherited predisposition to breast carcinoma. *Cancer, 86,* 2502–2516.

Josephson, U., Wickman, M., & Sandelin, K. (2000). Initial experiences of women from hereditary breast cancer families after bilateral prophylactic mastectomy: A retrospective study. *Journal of Surgical Oncology, 26,* 351–356.

Julian-Reynier, C. M., Bouchard, L. J., Evans, D. G., Eisinger, F. A., Foulkes, W. D., Kerr, B., et al. (2001). Women's attitudes toward preventive strategies for hereditary breast or ovarian carcinoma differ from one country to another: Differences among English, French and Canadian women. *Cancer, 92,* 959–968.

Karan, D., Lin, M. F., Johannsson, S. L., & Batra, S. K. (2003). Current status of the molecular genetics of human prostatic adenocarcinomas. *International Journal of Cancer, 103,* 285–293.

Karp, J., Brown, K. L., Sullivan, M. D., & Massie, M. J. (1999). The prophylactic mastectomy dilemma: A support group for women at high risk for breast cancer. *Journal of Genetic Counseling, 8,* 163–173.

Kuerer, H. M., Hwang, S., Anthony, J. P., Dudley, R., Crawford, B., Aubry, W. M., & Esserman, L. J. (2000). Current national health insurance coverage policies for breast and ovarian cancer prophylactic surgery. *Journal of Surgical Oncology, 7,* 325–332.

Lerman, C., Hughes, C., Croyle, R. T., Main, D., Durham, C., Snyder, C., et al. (2000). Prophylactic surgery decisions and surveillance practices one year following *BRCA1/2* testing. *Preventive Medicine, 31,* 75–80.

Lerman, C., Narod, S., Schulman, K., Hughes, C., Gomez-Caminero, A., Bonney, G., et al. (1996). *BRCA1* testing in families with hereditary breast-ovarian cancer: A prospective study of patient decision making and outcomes. *Journal of the American Medical Association, 275,* 1885–1892.

Lloyd, S. M., Watson, M., Oaker, G., Sacks, N., Quercidella Rovere, U., & Gui, G. (2000). Understanding the experience of prophylactic mastectomy: A qualitative study of ten women. *Psycho-Oncology, 9,* 473–485.

Lodder, L. N., Frets, P. G., Trijsburg, R. W., Meijers-Heijboer, E. J., Klijn, J. G. M., Seynaeve, C., et al. (2002). One year follow-up of women opting for presymptomatic testing for BRCA1 and BRCA2: Emotional impact of the test outcome and decisions on risk management (surveillance or prophylactic surgery). *Breast Cancer Research and Treatment, 73,* 97–112.

Lu, K., Garber, J. E., Cramer, D. W., Welch, W. R., Niloff, J., Schrag, D., et al. (2000). Occult ovarian tumors in women with *BRCA1* or *BRCA2* mutations undergoing prophylactic oophorectomy. *Journal of Clinical Oncology, 18,* 2728–2732.

Lynch, H. T., Lemon, S., Durham, C., Tinley, S. T., Connolly, C., Lynch, J. F., et al. (1997). A descriptive study of *BRCA1* testing and reactions to disclosure of test results. *Cancer, 79,* 2219–2228.

Lynch, H. T., Severin, M. J., Mooney, M. J., & Lynch, J. (1995). Insurance adjudication favoring prophylactic surgery in hereditary breast-ovarian cancer syndrome. *Gynecologic Oncology, 57,* 23–26.

Lynch, H. T., Smyrk, T., & Lynch, J. (1997). An update of HNPCC (Lynch syndrome). *Cancer Genetics and Cytogenetics, 93,* 84–99.

Massie, M. J., Mushkin, P. R., & Stewart, D. E. (1998). Psychotherapy with a woman at high risk for developing breast cancer. *General Hospital Psychiatry, 20,* 189–197.

Meijers-Heijboer, E. J., Verhoog, L. C., Brekelmans, C. T. M., Seynaeve, C., Tilanus-Linthorst, M. M. A., Wagner, A., et al. (2000). Presymptomatic DNA testing and prophylactic surgery in families with a *BRCA1* or *BRCA2* mutation. *Lancet, 355,* 2015–2020.

Meijers-Heijboer, H., van Geel, B., van Putten, W. L. J., Henzen-Logmans, S. C., Seynaeve, C., Menke-Pluymers, M. B. E., et al. (2001). Breast cancer after prophylactic mastectomy in women with a *BRCA1* or *BRCA2* mutation. *New England Journal of Medicine, 345,* 159–164.

Meiser, B., Butow, P., Barratt, A., Friedlander, M., Gattas, M., Kirk, J., et al. (1999). Attitudes toward prophylactic oophorectomy and screening utilization in women at increased risk of developing hereditary breast/ovarian cancer. *Gynecologic Oncology, 75,* 122–129.

Meiser, B., Butow, P., Friedlander, M., Schnieden, V., Gattas, M., Kirk, J., et al. (2000a). Intention to undergo prophylactic bilateral mastectomy in women at increased risk of developing hereditary breast cancer. *Journal of Clinical Oncology, 18,* 2250–2257.

Meiser, B., Tiller, K., Gleeson, M. A., Andrews, L., Robertson, G., & Tucker, K. M. (2000b). Psychological impact of prophylactic oophorectomy in women at increased risk for ovarian cancer. *Psycho-Oncology, 9,* 496–503.

Miller, S. M., Fang, C. Y., Manne, S. L., Engstrom, P. F., & Daly, M. D. (1999). Decision making about prophylactic oophorectomy among at-risk women: Psychological influences and implications. *Gynecologic Oncology, 75,* 406–412.

Mock, V. (1993). Body image in women treated for breast cancer. *Nursing Research, 42,* 153–157.

Moran, S. L., Herceg, S., Kurtelawicz, K., & Serletti, J. M. (2000). TRAM flap breast reconstruction with expanders and implants. *AORN Journal, 71,* 353–368.

Morris, K. T., Johnson, N., Krasikov, N., Allen, M., & Dorsey, P. (2001). Genetic counseling impacts decision for prophylactic surgery for patients perceived to be at high risk for breast cancer. *American Journal of Surgery, 181,* 431–433.

Nahhas, W. A. (1997). Ovarian cancer: Current outlook on this deadly disease. *Postgraduate Medicine, 102,* 112–118.

Narod, S. A., Sun, P., Ghadirian, P., Lynch, H., Issacs, C., Garber, J., et al. (2001). Tubal ligation and risk of ovarian cancer in carriers of *BRCA1* or *BRCA2* mutations: A case-control study. *Lancet, 357,* 1467–1470.

Offit, K. (1998). *Clinical cancer genetics: Risk counseling and management.* New York: Wiley-Liss.

Paley, P. J., Swisher, E. M., Garcia, R. L., Agoff, S. N., Greer, B. E., Peters, K. L., et al. (2001). Occult cancer of the fallopian tube in *BRCA-1* germline mutation carriers at prophylactic oophorectomy: A case for recommending hysterectomy at surgical prophylaxis. *Gynecologic Oncology, 80,* 176–180.

Rebbeck, T. R. (2000). Prophylactic oophorectomy in *BRCA1* and *BRCA2* mutation carriers. *Journal of Clinical Oncology, 18*(Suppl.), 100s–103s.

Rebbeck, T. R., Levin, A. M., Eisen, A., Snyder, C., Watson, P., Cannon-Albright, L., et al. (1999). Reduction in breast cancer risk following bilateral prophylactic oophorectomy in *BRCA1* mutation carriers. *Journal of National Cancer Institute, 91,* 1475–1479.

Rhodes, D. J., Hartmann, L. C., & Perez, E. A. (2000). Breast cancer prevention trials. *Current Oncology Reports, 2,* 558–565.

Rodriguez-Bigas, J., Vasen, H. F. A., Mecklin, J. A., Myrhoj, T., Rozen, P., Bertario, L., et al. (1997). Rectal cancer risk in hereditary non-polyposis colorectal cancer. *Annals of Surgery, 225,* 202–207.

Rowland, J. H., Diosso, J., Holland, J. C., Chaglassian, T., & Kinne, D. (1995). Breast reconstruction after mastectomy: Who seeks it, who refuses? *Plastic and Reconstructive Surgery, 95,* 812–822.

Rowland, J. H., Holland, J. C., Chaglassian, T., & Kinne, D. (1993). Psychological response to breast reconstruction: Expectations for and impact on post-mastectomy functioning. *Psychosomatics, 34,* 241–250.

Salazar, H., Godwin, A. K., Daly, A. B., Laub P. B., Hogan W. M., Rosenblum N., et al. (1996). Microscopic benign and invasive malignant neoplasms and a cancer-prone phenotype in prophylactic oophorectomies. *Journal of the National Cancer Institute, 88,* 1810–1820.

Schain, W. (1991). Breast reconstruction: Update of psychosocial and pragmatic concerns. *Cancer, 1*(Suppl.), 1170–1175.

Schain, W., Wellisch, D. K., Pasnau, R. O., & Landsverk, J. (1985). The sooner the better: A study of psychological factors in women undergoing immediate versus delayed breast reconstruction. *American Journal of Psychiatry, 142,* 40–46.

Schrag, D., Kuntz, K. M., Garber, J. E., & Weeks, J. C. (1997). Decision analysis—Effects of prophylactic mastectomy and oophorectomy on life expectancy among women with BRCA1 or BRCA2 mutations. *New England Journal of Medicine, 336,* 1465–1471.

Smith, R. A., von Eschenbach, A. C., Wender, R., Levin, B., Byers, T., Rothenberger, D., et al. (2001). American Cancer Society Guidelines for the Early Detection of Cancer: Update of early detection guidelines for prostate, colorectal, and endometrial cancers. *CA: A Cancer Journal for Clinicians, 51,* 38–75.

Struewing, J. P., Hartge, P., Wacholder, S., Baker, S. M., Berlin, M., McAdams, M., et al. (1997). The risk of cancer associated with specific mutations of BRCA1 and BRCA2 among Ashkenazi Jews. *New England Journal of Medicine, 336,* 1401–1408.

Struewing, J., Watson, D. F., Ponder, B. A., Lynch, H. T., & Tucker, M. (1995). Prophylactic oophorectomy in inherited breast/ovarian cancer families. *Journal of the National Cancer Institute Monorgraphs, 1995,* 33–35.

Syngal, S., Weeks, J. C., Schrag, D., Garber, J. E., & Kuntz, K. M. (1998). Benefits of colonoscopic surveillance and prophylactic colectomy in patients with hereditary nonpolyposis colorectal cancer mutations. *Annals of Internal Medicine, 129,* 787–796.

van Duijvendijk, P., Slors, J. F. M., Taat, C. W., Oosterveld, P., Sprangers, M. A. G., Obertop, H., & Vasen, H. F. A. (2000). Quality of life after total colectomy with ileorectal anastomosis or proctocolectomy and ileal pouch-anal anastomosis for familial adenomatous polyposis. *British Journal of Surgery, 87,* 590–596.

Wagner, T. M. U., Moslinger, R., Langbauer, G., Ahner, R., Fleishman, E., Auterith, A., et al. (2000). Attitude towards prophylactic surgery and effects of genetic counselling in families with BRCA mutations. *British Journal of Cancer, 82,* 1249–1253.

Ward, C. M. (1981). Breast reconstruction after cancer—Aesthetic triumph or surgical disaster? *British Journal of Plastic Surgery, 34,* 124–127.

Watson, M., Lloyd, S., Davidson, J., Meyer, I., Eeles, R., Ebbs, S., et al. (1999). The impact of genetic counselling on risk perception and mental health in women with a family history of breast cancer. *British Journal of Cancer, 79,* 868–874.

Watterson, P. A., Bostwick, J., III, Hester, T. R., Jr., Bried, J. T., & Taylor, G. I. (1995). TRAM flap anatomy correlated with a 10-year clinical experience with 556 patients. *Plastic Reconstructive Surgery, 93,* 96–106.

Writing Group for the Women's Health Initiative Investigators. (2002). Risks and benefits of estrogen plus progesterone in healthy postmenopausal women. *Journal of the American Medical Association, 288,* 321–333.

7

A FAMILY MATTER

The family unit ought to be preserved and guarded, and certainly not harmed.

(DudokdeWit et al., 1997, p. 70)

Genetic medicine is family medicine. By its very nature, genetics seeks to define why particular families share markedly increased disease predispositions that present with the hallmarks of genetic disease and that are not the burden of the rest of the population. One of the major features that differentiates genetic medicine from traditional medicine is the direct relevance of one person's genetic status for the health risks of other relatives. It is the family connections that raise much of the psychological and ethical ante regarding genetic counseling and testing for cancer genes. Each step in the process of counseling and testing is affected by family relationships and, in turn, exerts an effect on family dynamics.

"Family" in a biological sense means blood relatives linked by common chromosomes. The social-psychological meanings of family encompass many kinds of connections. Some are marked by the clearly demarcated groupings and interrelationships such as "family of origin" or "nuclear family"; others are colored subjectively by the quality and nature of the connections forged between people in multiple generations. Differences between the biological and social definitions of family contribute to the complexity of work in genetic counseling and testing (Alby, 2003). These differences also speak to the need for mental health professionals with proficiency in understanding issues implicit in both conceptions of family.

The intertwining of the social and medical sciences in genetics is exemplified by the necessary introduction of family material, both biological and psychological, into discussions between geneticists or genetic counselors and their patients. Although an internist on an initial visit is likely to take a family history, asking the patient who in his or her family has had which diseases at which age, the physician is unlikely to inquire about the social connection between family members, for example, "How do you get along with your sister?" That aspect of the relationship is usually considered irrelevant to the medical issues that concern the internist. Discussion with a genetic counselor may repeat many of the health-related questions the internist has asked in taking a family history. Medical questions may be even more specific, including questions about age of onset of the disease, and specific disease characteristics (such as possible bilaterality of breast cancer or associated features of a cancer genetic syndrome). In addition to the increased diagnostic detail, however, the genetic professional is likely to focus on the emotional aspects of family relationships. If the patient is unaffected (i.e., has not had cancer), this discussion might initially arise in the process of ascertaining whether an affected relative might be responsive to a request that he or she undergo testing so that a familial mutation can potentially be identified. Discussion of the social qualities of the relationship between the two would be germane to a judgment about the willingness of the affected relative to be tested, for example. Focus on the subjective nature of the family relationships might also occur in discussion about the potential dissemination of the genetic information to others in the family for whom it would have medical relevance. The complexity of social relationships within families is legion. It is not unusual to hear, "I don't speak to my sister," "My mother and my aunt have fought for years, ever since my grandmother died," " I don't know where my first cousin lives or even what her name is now," or "My aunt has been pushing me to have my ovaries out for years now, but I'm not ready." Unlike psychotherapy, however, the emotional issues between relatives are not the ultimate focus of the discussion. In genetic counseling, the discussion of patients' social relationships is in the service of ascertaining how best to serve the needs of the patient in answering his or her questions about disease risk and how to handle the dissemination of information within the family.

Genetic counselors receive training in counseling skills to help them manage the range of emotions that discussion of such personally relevant, charged information can elicit. They are also trained to help patients decide whether to inform family members and how to convey the necessary genetic information. In the genetic counseling session, patient and counselor will consider whether additional health information is needed from other family members and whether asking a relative to be tested for the benefit of others in the family is necessary or acceptable to the patient. Genetic counselors do not have time nor are they prepared (without separate, additional training) to serve as psychotherapists to help patients specifically with the resolution of emotional conflicts or interpersonal difficulties with family members. Referral of the patient for psychotherapy is common when it becomes clear that deeper underlying issues cannot be resolved in the context of genetic counseling. Sometimes it is recommended that at least initial sessions of psychotherapy occur before further pursuit of genetic testing because some degree of resolution of issues with relatives may be a prerequisite for further planning for testing. The emotions attached to conflicts with relatives or unresolved grief that is experienced in the context of genetic testing may also require more long-term therapy.

Therapists who are sufficiently familiar with genetic issues to help families struggling with these issues will increasingly be a welcome oasis for members of those cancer families who wish to discuss the implications of what is called, "risk notification" (McDaniel & Speice, 2001). Individuals already in therapy and those who seek therapeutic help as part of their decision making around genetic counseling and testing will find it useful to discuss the many family conflicts and potential changes in family dynamics that genetic testing threatens to initiate. Because genetic issues affect others in the family, individuals who usually rely heavily on family members for social support may be particularly eager to seek help outside the family for problems related to genetic testing, perhaps because they may not want to share with relatives their ambivalence, hesitation, or other feelings about decisions that have direct implications for the relatives. Therapists in the community and those in hospitals or affiliated with primary practitioners or genetic counseling programs can be of great help to these individuals in sorting out the medical concerns and family issues related to the presence of cancer and cancer predisposition in the family. The issues are intertwined and complex, and the services of professionals trained in understanding the diversity of family relationships and knowledgeable about stress reduction and the relationship of psychological variables to health will have important roles to play in supporting patients and in offering consultation to physicians and counselors involved in genetic counseling and testing (McDaniel & Campbell, 1999).

FAMILY INTERACTION PRIOR TO TESTING

The labeling of a family as a "cancer family" when a predisposing mutation has been identified in affected members can have very different impacts on individuals within that family. The effect is a reflection of the relationships prior to the illness, family members' expectations and assumptions about the role of the illness in the family, and the way in which news of the mutation is introduced to them. Some family members say that they had "known" by observing the frequent occurrence of cancer in their family beginning early in their lives (often in middle childhood or adolescence) that the increased susceptibility to cancer must be inherited. They had often had to defy others in the science classroom, family, or hospital who belittled the association, saying, "Cancer is not a hereditary disease," or "It was different cancers that your family members had, not the same one. Those cancers are not related to each other." These patients now say that they felt certain the frequency of cancer in their family and extended family must have had a common cause. For these individuals, including some who have had cancer themselves, the finding that there is, indeed, a "cancer gene" in the family is often greeted as a kind of triumph, as verification of their earlier beliefs. Many of these individuals view knowledge as the beginning of possible paths to prevention or cure. "Knowledge is power" is a phrase often heard from these people. For others, especially those who have had little awareness of the many cancers in the family, because of either their place in the family or, possibly, their avoidance of discussions of family health history, this information can come as a shock and, in some cases, as an unwanted intrusion into their ongoing ways of managing their emotions in the face of elevated health risks.

One of the least understood aspects of genetic testing is that it is not a crystal ball that one may consult in all circumstances to determine whether someone is or is not at increased risk of developing cancer or another disease. It is, in its most clearly predictive form, a relatively primitive ability to match a mutation (or small set of mutations) found either in a family or an ethnically homogeneous community that has been shown to be correlated with the development of disease, with the presence or absence of that mutation in at-risk members of the family or community. If a mutation is identified in one or more family members who have had cancer and then testing is done on their relatives, it can be the means to discover either the welcome news that a relative does not carry mutation or that they do carry the worrisome mutation. In the case of "good news," testing provides information that can relieve stress and worry about an individual's disease risk, as well as provide the news that one cannot pass on the high familial risk to children. When the mutation in the tested individual "matches" the mutation in family members who have had the associated type of cancer or when the presence of certain mutations is associated with disease in that religious or ethnic community, testing can indicate that frequent, targeted screening for early detection of the disease is warranted. Risk-reducing measures also will likely be offered for consideration.

Requesting that another individual in one's family, often in one's extended family, undergo a medical test at some cost and potential social and emotional risk to themselves and their family is not a small favor. Nonetheless, from the perspective of the person making the request for "just a tube of blood," it can seem inconceivable that a sister, brother, mother, aunt, or cousin would not see the enormous impact that their willingness to undergo testing could have. Many individuals willingly undergo testing for the sake of a relative, even if their preference would have been to "let sleeping dogs lie" and not be tested. Refusal also is not uncommon. Geller, Doksum, Bernhardt, and Metz (1999) described a study in which 7 out of 10 family members declined the request of a relative that they undergo genetic testing for a cancer predisposition gene.

FAMILY ILLNESS EXPERIENCE AFFECTS
KNOWLEDGE OF FAMILY HEALTH HISTORY

Family experience with illness may itself affect what information is known about the family health history. In families in which the prevalence of cancer among younger adults is high, resulting in the early deaths of parents, children may have incomplete or distorted knowledge of the family history of illness. Remarriage of a parent may further distance the child from relatives on the side of the family in which the cancer predisposition exists. When asked to gather such data from relatives in connection to genetic counseling to assess their own risk, the individual being counseled may be reluctant to approach certain relatives for fear of arousing painful memories, because of the lack of an ongoing, close relationship, or because of enmity between branches of the family. There may also be concern about whether the inquiry might be interpreted as blaming the family members for transmission of the deleterious characteristic. Denial may also play a role. In a study by Glanz, Grove, Lerman, Gotay, and LeMarchand (1999), 25% of individuals who were known from verified medical records to have a first-degree relative who had had colon cancer said that none of their first-degree relatives had had colon cancer.

How do people put together the family history information that genetic counselors and physicians want to know when questions of inherited cancer risk come up? Often they ask their mother, if she is alive. Women have been referred to as the "kin-keepers" (Green, Richards, Murton, Stratham, & Hallowell, 1997) of the family, and it is the women in the family who are much more likely to be asked about the family medical history. In a 1997 study (Green et al.), women seeking breast cancer genetic testing who needed to provide family history data were asked how they had gotten the information they provided. All of the women with living mothers had asked their mother or asked no one. Less than a quarter of the women whose mothers had died questioned any male relative about the family history. Half of the women in this study felt that they could not or would not contact at least one potential informant, with reasons given focusing on not wishing to upset a relative who was too old or ill by the request or not feeling close to the potential informant. Some informants or other relatives specifically asked the women seeking testing not to discuss her plans with certain relatives, which sometimes interfered with asking family history questions of those individuals. In one case, a woman used a ruse to ask her mother family history questions, fearing that raising the issue directly would be upsetting because the woman's sister had recently died.

Gaps in family health history, due to either incomplete or incorrect knowledge or reporting of family history, compound the difficulty of identifying individuals at increased genetic risk.

> Where the issue is whether or not a "genetic" disorder may be present, the pedigree is pivotal because it is the raw data with which the counselor has to work in order to assess the likelihood that there is a Mendelian disorder in the family. Gaps or inaccuracies in the information supplied by the proband about other family members, or misunderstanding of this by the geneticist, can result in critical differences in the geneticist's assessments and so counseling. Thus, the information that probands are able to obtain about their family histories from other family members is crucial and family communication is of key importance. (Green et al., 1997, p. 48)

K. A. Schneider (personal communication, May 1999) reported that 37% of individuals attending a counseling program for *p53* testing in families with Li–Fraumeni syndrome (see chap. 2 for discussion of this disorder) did not provide sufficient family history to enable a physician to recognize the presence of the syndrome. This means that in about one third of the cases, individuals who were eligible for genetic testing might not have been offered the option had the decision rested with their physician's recognition of their at-risk status rather than, as was the case, with identification of the family through a cancer registry. As discussed in chapter 5, some people have offered false family histories of cancer when seeking genetic testing or to qualify for programs restricted to at-risk individuals (Kerr et al., 1998). In some of those cases, the falsified family history was provided by a relative to the proband, suggesting some disturbance in their relationship.

INTRAFAMILIAL PRESSURE RELATED TO TESTING

A major tenet of the ethics of informed consent is autonomy, and nowhere is this more relevant than with regard to genetic testing. However, there are many reports of pressure—subtle in some families and quite direct in others—for at-risk family members to take particular steps (e.g., to be tested, to have prophylactic surgery). Empathy for differing views about the value of genetic information within families often seems to be lacking. Rather, the fear of future generations repeating the illnesses of the past generation can lead to strong encouragement, sometimes bordering on coercion, from a parent to an adult child, from sister to sister, from sister to brother, and so on. A 27-year-old woman may opt to carry out biannual breast screening and mammograms, transvaginal ultrasounds, and the full screening regime recommended for mutation carriers rather than being tested because she is not ready to know whether she is a mutation carrier. Her mother may find it difficult to accept that the young woman could be tested, with 50–50 odds of finding out that such measures were unnecessary, but refuses to do so. A young man may put off going for genetic counseling about the hereditary colon cancer that killed his father in his early 50s. He doesn't want to hear about colectomy; he is not ready. A 34-year-old woman with three cousins, all found to be *BRCA2* carriers and all of whom chose prophylactic mastectomy, does not want to be pushed to have a prophylactic mastectomy at every family gathering and in every phone call. She does not want to hear how great it is to worry less and does not want surgery. It is not for her, not now, not ever, she thinks, but her cousins just do not seem to hear her.

It seems difficult for many at-risk family members to imagine how others in the family configure risk. They have a difficult time imagining a different way of coping with the familial risk, leading others to different conclusions than their own about screening or prevention options. Pressure between family members can interrupt or alter longstanding, close relationships. Although lip service is often paid to the need for everyone to make up his or her own mind, the opposite sentiment is often played out as well-meaning relatives plague others who disagree about the benefits of approaching these problems in particular ways.

On the other hand, some people who take the responsibility to motivate others to undergo testing experience considerable guilt when the results become known. If it turns out that the "motivator" is negative and others in the family test positive, especially if the person testing positive has a difficult time adjusting to the news, the "motivator" may rethink the wisdom of his or her actions. The guilt is lessened somewhat if there are tangible actions that can be taken to improve the odds that the person will not develop cancer and if the person testing positive takes advantage of the knowledge to appropriately adjust a screening regimen. Such improvements help to justify the emotional pain that disclosure occasions in the originally unwilling relative. Yet if there is relatively little to do to prevent cancer or to improve the likelihood of early detection and if the person testing positive remains upset for an extended period, the guilt of the "motivator" for having pushed so hard may be intense.

NONPATERNITY

One fact that can be uncovered in a search of family or medical records is nonpaternity, cases in which people learn through genetic analysis that the person they have always believed to be their father is not. Although nonpaternity or, more accurately, misassigned paternity, is a relatively rare event, estimated to occur between 5% and 10% of the time (Richards, 1996), when it occurs, it can have a powerful effect on family reaction to genetic testing and may occasionally raise questions for the professional about whether to reveal the finding of nonpaternity. Discovery of nonpaternity may result from a mother's direct revelation when whole families have access to the genetic practitioner, or it may come from other knowledgeable relatives. In one family, for example, the older sisters knew that their brother had a different father from theirs and informed the genetic counselor of this. Because in this case the paternal line was the one carrying the deleterious mutation, this meant that the man seeking testing was not at risk for the familial mutation affecting his siblings. The dilemma for the genetic counselor was whether to go ahead with the testing and to reveal only that the man was not a carrier of the mutation or to reveal the nonpaternity, thus making testing unnecessary, but potentially causing significant emotional distress and possible family disruption. Revelation of this family secret would likely spur resentment that the information had been kept from the man but revealed to his sisters. Many factors would play a role in this decision, including the ethical stance of the counselor, the financial issues involved, and the counselor's knowledge of and sensitivity to the psychological damage such a revelation might initiate.

FAMILY COMMUNICATION FOLLOWING GENETIC TEST RESULT DISCLOSURE

Once test results are delivered to a family member, the issues of who in the family will be privy to that knowledge and how such information will be disseminated become predominant. Whether genetic information is shared within the family and the ways in which family members respond to news about the presence or absence of a familial mutation have tremendous medical and social implications.

Who Is Told?

To date, research suggests that in most cases, information about a test result is shared with relatives rather quickly after it is disclosed. Julian-Reynier et al. (1996) reported that a week after breast and ovarian cancer gene result disclosure, 70% of 161 cases had shared their result with relatives, as had been recommended; 16% intended to but had not yet done so; and 13% did not intend to inform any relatives for reasons including lack of a significant relationship or lack of belief that informing relatives would lead to any positive change. Eighty-five percent of tested individuals who did inform their relatives felt the response had been positive; six percent felt the interaction about the result had gone "very badly."

A French study (Bonadona et al., 2002) of family communication among 23 cancer patients who were mutation-positive for BRCA1/2 and colon cancer gene tests had similar findings at six weeks post-disclosure. All participants had told at least one close relative. This included 83% who had told their spouse or partner, 78% who told one or more siblings, and half who told a parent. All parents with a child over age 18 told their child, and none of those with children under 18 told their child.

In a U.S. study, within a month following BRCA1/2 testing, 81% of 201 male and female mutation carriers disclosed their result to a sister and 60% told a brother (Lerman, Peshkin, Hughes, & Isaacs, 1998); 77% told adult children, 47% told a child who was 14 to 18 years of age, and 37% told a child under age 13. Female carriers were more likely to tell sisters (89%) than were brothers (56%) and were more likely to tell teenage children (54% of female mutation carriers vs. 17% of male carriers). It was unclear whether the children might have been informed by their mothers about their father's mutation status. Men were more likely to disclose their status to relatives if they were not mutation carriers, leading the authors to suggest that men are more comfortable sharing good news than bad with family members.

Hughes et al. (2002) reported a more in-depth study of disclosure of BRCA1/2 test results to sisters by 43 affected (breast or ovarian cancer) women. In this study, 96% of the carriers communicated their result to their sisters versus 76% of those with uninformative results. One quarter of the sisters were informed the same day, and 70% within a week of disclosure. Primary motivations for not sharing results were not feeling close to a sister or not wanting to upset her.

In a study of the disclosure of hereditary nonpolyposis colon cancer (HNPCC) genetic testing, 83% of the 30 participants told at least one relative within the first week following the receipt of their test result. Parents were told 80% of the time; 65% of respondents told their spouse, 27%

informed their children (age not specified), and 75% told one or more extended family members (Esplen et al., 2001).

SPECIAL RELATIONSHIPS, SPECIAL ISSUES

Siblings

It comes as a surprise to many adults that they share more genetic characteristics with siblings than they do with their children (Richards & Ponder, 1996). Because siblings have the same parents contributing to their genetic makeup, they theoretically can share up to 100% of their genes. In contrast, parents and children typically share 50% of their genes, because 50% is contributed by each parent. Many people confuse their genetic similarity with their emotional closeness to a relative. The social relationships between children and parents are typically closer than those between adult siblings. Adult siblings vary enormously in the range and depth of their ongoing relationships. Some retain much of the closeness of childhood, staying in daily or weekly contact and relating closely with each other's families. Others have more distant relationships, being typically out of contact for months at a time and interacting only a few times a year. Still others are completely estranged. Genetic testing for a familial cancer mutation highlights the biological connections between siblings, regardless of the social relationships. It brings the sibling relationships into stark relief in ways that few things, other than the illness or death of a parent, can do. Some siblings become much closer through the experience, many maintain their usual relationships, and others find that opposing views about how to integrate, communicate about, and act on genetic information creates or fortifies chasms in their relationship. Because genetic testing results also raise issues for subsequent generations, tension between some siblings has to do with differences in opinion about the importance or timing of informing the next generation about the genetic risks attributable to a cancer-predisposing mutation in the family.

It is interesting that the closeness of family members does not necessarily predict how they will choose to deal with genetic information. One set of sisters who came for testing were very close and spoke daily. The sister who first came for cancer genetic counseling decided she did not want to share with her sister that she was undergoing testing. Both sisters came for counseling and testing but did not tell each other. One sister tested positive and one negative, but each remained ignorant of the other's status. Their frequent communication on other matters continued without discussion about testing or test results.

Siblings who are close are often supportive of each other through the testing process. Some serve as companions during the counseling sessions, and some want to go through testing at the same time. It is generally recommended that siblings who are simultaneously tested bring another support person to the disclosure session and that the test result be given separately to each sibling. This provides time for each to absorb, cognitively and emotionally, their own result before dealing with the comparison of their results.

In-depth studies of the changes in the social relationships and communication patterns of adult siblings from high-risk cancer families are needed. Such studies will be of great interest in describing the social and emotional impact on 21st-century families of highlighting biological links through genetic counseling and testing.

Adoption

Adoption is an area in which the ethical issues related to genetic testing approach Solomon-like proportions. Adoptive parents wish to know all they can about the health risks of the child they may adopt. Genetic testing will increasingly be able to provide information about the child's likelihood of developing many serious diseases. Although genetic testing stands to free some children from the curse of a negative family history when they have not inherited a deleterious familial mutation, it also stands to condemn others to unadoptability based on increased hereditary risk of future illness. Decisions about the conditions under which genetic testing of preadoptive or adopted children is legitimate and about what genetic information should be shared with prospective parents could make monumental differences in the ultimate life plan of the child. The framing of the genetic information given to parents is also of great importance. It is one thing to say "There is a family history of colon cancer in the father's family" and another to say "There is a 50% chance that this baby has inherited an *APC* mutation and a strong likelihood that he may need to have his colon removed before reaching adulthood." It makes a difference for a prospective parent to be told, "The mother's mother had breast cancer" versus "This baby girl has a *BRCA2* mutation and therefore has an 85% risk of breast cancer beginning in her 30s and a 20% to 60% chance of getting ovarian cancer." Parents with other options may decide not to adopt the child, relegating him or her to a kind of "second-tier of diminished adoptability" (J. F. Smith, 2000), although he or she is completely healthy at present.

To date, ethicists have sided with the decision not to test preadoptive children to answer questions about the child's risk for adult-onset, untreatable conditions. Wertz, Fanos, and Reilly (1994) wrote, "Testing for untreatable, adult-onset disorders prior to adoption makes the child into a commodity undergoing quality control" (p. 880). It may become more difficult to define "untreatable," however. What if a gene that predisposes one to early smoking behavior were to be definitively located? Should a preadoptive child be tested for mutations in that gene so that he or she could receive targeted interventions as a teen? What if links to childhood leukemia or diabetes could be found in a child's genetic information, even though the predictive value was low that the child would actually develop the disease? What information is in the best interest of the child for prospective adoptive parents to know, so that later they are not overwhelmed by the medical challenges the child and family face? When might such disclosure not be in the child's best interest? These are weighty issues with no clear answers and no empirical evidence on which to base decisions.

For an adopted child, the possibility of inherited risk for cancer or other serious disease may increase anxiety about what, in some cases, may seem an unbridgeable gap between biological family and adoptive family. Although some medical information is usually available to adopted children about their parents, it is usually not sufficient to be used for determination of cancer risk. With increasing openness about adoption and links between birth mothers and their children, medical information about hereditary risk may become more available to adopted individuals. The information available from the mother may still be incomplete, however, because the mother may not have access to the father or know his updated family medical history. It is possible that the desire to have medical information may be used as a spur to find one's birth mother or for biological parents to feel strongly that the knowledge they have gained about genetic cancer risks should be provided to a child given up for adoption.

Parents: Passing on the Nightmare

Little or no in-depth study exists of the impact on a parent of passing on a cancer predisposing mutation, but there is much anecdotal clinical information about the deep guilt parents have when they learn that a son or daughter has inherited a cancer predisposition gene that they carry. After all, parents take great pride when they see in children or grandchildren evidence that the child inherited positive characteristics—"She has your pretty blue eyes" or "He has your noble head." Some people in the current first-generation of information about inherited risk for cancer can remain sanguine about the fact that they did not, of course, know when their child was conceived that they carried such a deleterious mutation because the child was born before these genes were found. In the future this "excuse" will not be available, but what will be the emotional consequences for parents who know the risk of passing on a cancer predisposing mutation when they conceive their children? Will it feel even more guilt-producing when a child develops cancer? The decision not to have any children is an extreme one, especially when the onset of the disease for which the hereditary predisposition exists is in adulthood and when there is some promise that prevention or treatment might be much improved by the time the child develops the disease. To try to select only embryos without the deleterious mutation suggests complications in the reproductive process that may appeal to some part of the at-risk population but are beyond the financial reach of most. Some ethicists may also argue that this kind of attempt to manipulate offspring toward perfection is unwarranted (Wagner & Ahner, 1998). It seems clear only that parental guilt is strong with regard to inherited disease predisposition and that the emotional intertwining of generational risk raises the potential for parental guilt that is likely to become more complex with further genetic advances.

Obligate Carriers

Obligate carriers are people who are assumed to carry a predisposing mutation because the same mutation is present in their parent and their child or twin. When an individual's parent and child share the same genetic mutation, it is clear by logical deduction that that individual was the genetic conduit by which the mutation in the grandparent was given to their child. An identical twin can also be an obligate carrier; if one twin is found to be a carrier, it can be assumed that the other twin also carries the mutation. This testing-by-logic leads to the conclusion that an individual who has not been tested must be a mutation carrier. Obligate carriers present some of the most difficult questions about autonomy that arise in the context of cancer genetic testing. Should the proband not be tested to spare parents from knowledge that they do not wish to have about their own genetic makeup or of having passed on a "bad" gene? Typically, genetic counselors try to deal individually with each person's situation and to give precedence to those seeking information to prevent or minimize the impact of disease. This can be seen as potentially doing harm to the individual whose genetic makeup is revealed by the deduction that they are obligate carriers, however.

* * *

Case Example. Joan is a 38-year-old married woman with three children, a son who is 10 and daughters aged 12 and 17. Her mother died of breast cancer when Joan was 15. Her aunt had ovarian cancer and has also died. Joan's older sister was found to carry a *BRCA2* mutation and has informed all of the siblings, five in all, of their own potential risk. Joan has decided to be tested. She wants to know to be able to determine whether to have her ovaries removed and to be able to talk to her daughters about what genetic risk might mean for them. Joan is an identical twin. Her sister, Meredith, is not married and thinks it likely that she will never have children. She is a lawyer in a very competitive firm, specializing in health law. Meredith hopes to become a partner. She is quite sure she does not want to know her *BRCA2* status. She is careful about her health, eats wisely, and sees her gynecologist at least once a year for breast exams. She has even had a transvaginal ultrasound to look for any signs of ovarian cancer. Her health insurance coverage is through her work. She does not want there to be any opportunity for her employer to uncover any genetic vulnerability that might be used to counter her rise to partnership, nor does she want to be in a position in which she would either have to reveal her status or lie if asked on an insurance form whether she had any reason to think she was at increased genetic risk of cancer. Meredith has told Joan how strongly she hopes that Joan will not get tested. Joan is angry at her older (by 2 minutes) sister; she feels it unfair that, in addition to her own concerns about testing, she has to take Meredith's feelings into consideration. She feels she has to choose between feeling guilty toward her sister and guilty toward her daughters. She even worries about her son, because *BRCA2* mutations predispose men to higher rates of breast cancer as well. She really wants to know. Her mother wasn't there to help her struggle with issues about growing up, and she wants to know how to guide her own daughters. She worries a lot about the possibility that she could get sick. Although she knows that treatment for breast cancer is better now than when her mother was diagnosed, it still makes her blood run cold to hear anything on television about breast cancer. Her anxiety gets in the way of doing breast self-exams, and sometimes she puts off going to see the doctor for a year or more because she thinks he might find cancer in her breast. Joan thinks that maybe if she knew for sure she had the mutation her mother had, it would help her to take better care of herself. If she didn't have the mutation, she could rejoice and reassure her kids. When she talks to her husband about all this, it only gets more complicated. He tends to think she should do what she wants and simply try not to worry so much about Meredith's feelings. This is harder for Joan to do than she likes to admit. She always looked to Meredith as the authority on what is "right" to do, yet Joan is worried about her children. She has considered not telling Meredith the result, but she knows that this would never work. Her actions, her concerns about her children—or her lack of concern—would tell Meredith right away, without Joan having to say a word. They know each other too well. It is all part of a very old pattern of either deferring to Meredith and her wishes or feeling that she is not doing things the right way.

* * *

IN SICKNESS AND IN HEALTH:
THE MARITAL IMPACT OF GENETIC TESTING

In cancer families, the focus is usually on the blood relatives, those who share the potential genetic predisposition for illness. Spouses are in a particularly awkward and difficult position, with dual interests. They are concerned about the future health of their husband or wife and are also concerned about their children. Their role is supportive with respect to their spouse, but central in concern for their children. Their spouse's family of origin and extended family may exert a strong influence on the husband or wife's decision making. The primacy of their marital relationship can feel challenged at times by the intense, shared interest among the spouse's siblings and other blood relatives about testing and, if positive, about subsequent decisions regarding surgery and other issues. Spouses sometimes feel left out of major discussions. Although husbands and wives usually do talk together about testing, often at length, and spouses are frequent companions at genetic counseling sessions, the final decision rests with the husband or wife alone. If the husband or wife is particularly distressed by the testing experience, it is their spouse who is likely to feel the impact most acutely, and he or she may wonder if the decision was the right one.

There may also be present in the spouse some anger about the introduction, however unwillingly, of genetic "damage" into the family. In many cultures in the world today, there is overt discrimination against anyone whose damaged health might make him or her a less fit spouse or who might expose his or her children to unusual disease risk. There may be feelings of anger experienced by both parents at the Hydra of hereditary illness, threatening many central aspects of the family's stability simultaneously. Spouses also may feel some conscious or unconscious anger at their husband or wife for being the bearer of this threat.

Spouses' style of dealing with health-related threats may be different from that of their husband or wife that, in turn, may make them view genetic testing decisions through a quite different lens. If a spouse thinks testing is not worthwhile, his or her views may be experienced as uncaring or as insensitive to the cancer worry experienced by the husband or wife who wants to be tested. If the spouse is the anxious one about health issues in general, and about the hereditary cancer risks in the husband or wife's family in particular, hesitation about testing may seem unbearable. Pushing for the testing to get done may be experienced as nagging.

Family relationships may change as bloodline relatives with little prior relationship suddenly have a common concern of great magnitude. This, in turn, changes the family dynamics in ways that could ignite enmities or create discomfort for those who are not a part of the central action. Although in some families this common genetic concern leads family members to coalesce, in others it may fuel ongoing battles. Relationships with in-laws may be altered by their willingness or unwillingness to support the desire to be tested of other family members. Conversely, it may be the pressure exerted by some family members for testing that proves upsetting. The emotional links between blood relatives may intensify their relationship in ways that are not completely shared by the non-blood relatives.

The relationship between the at-risk relatives often intensifies over the notification of a predisposing mutation in the family. How, in turn, do these issues, of direct relevance to one's spouse and children but not to oneself, affect the marital relationship and balance of power within nuclear families? Who decides how or if children are informed of a parent's genetic status? What if your wife's sister deals differently with her children, informing them about the positive tests in her family, and giving her children information you do not want your children to have? What are your rights as a spouse or as a co-parent? Whose information is it? What if you and your wife or husband differ about whether to encourage genetic testing in young adult children? How do parents who are not themselves at risk for the deleterious mutation that has been found in their husband or wife's family feel about the genetic testing of their children? Are they relieved not to be the parent concerned about having passed this dangerous inheritance on to their children? Are they able to be empathetic to their spouse about the guilt that is aroused? Or does the carrier spouse feel that the husband or wife's enthusiasm to tell the children is a sign of not understanding the guilt they are feeling as the person who may have conveyed this threatening mutation to their sons or daughters—"It's not his genes"?

There is remarkably little research in this area. One study by Coyne and Andersen (1999), conducted before breast cancer genetic testing was actually available, suggested that, at least in the self-selected members of a cancer registry they studied, spouses were at least as important and influential as sisters in decisions made about testing for breast and ovarian cancer predisposing mutations. Women who received good support from spouses were more likely also to have good support from female relatives than women whose spouses were unsupportive. Their findings suggest the likelihood that perception of support and skills in achieving good social support is a function of the personality of the person supported, rather than a characteristic of the supporter, a view held by experts in social support theory (Sarason, Pierce, & Sarason, 1990). The low distress levels of the women studied were attributed in large part to the presence of supportive spouses.

Divorce significantly changes the equation between spouses and is likely in many circumstances to make communication around risk to children much more difficult. There may even be concern in some families that a parent's genetic cancer risk could be used as a reason to award physical custody to the other parent to ensure continuity for the children in the event that the at-risk parent develops cancer and dies at an early age. Concern regarding genetic testing as a possible threat to health insurability may also be heightened in such cases.

Spouses may be asked to carry out one additional role with regard to genetic testing. A widowed spouse whose husband or wife had cancer and was from a family suspected of carrying a deleterious mutation may be asked permission as next of kin to allow a preserved, paraffin tissue sample from the deceased spouse's tumor to be used to gather DNA for genetic analysis. Hospitals keep such samples after surgical removal of malignant tissue. The next of kin has the right to request that the hospital release the sample for medical or research purposes. Samples vary in the way they have been preserved, so it is not always clear that a paraffin sample will provide adequate DNA, but it is often the only tissue available that could provide enough DNA for testing to be possible. A sibling, child, niece, or nephew of the deceased might make such a request. As can be imagined, this request can arouse strong emotions. Some who might want to make such a request may hesitate to do so, fearing that they would upset the surviving spouse. Others may persevere in the hope that a mystery that could not be solved during the lifetime of the deceased relative can now be resolved, with potential to provide useful information for future generations. Many factors play a role in the decision of surviving spouses who face this situation, including their orientation toward science, relationship with the person making the request, feelings about what their spouse would have wanted them to do, and ability to comprehend what is being asked of them. Because of the importance of the request, in some families this issue could be a trigger for seeking family therapy.

If individuals or couples seek therapy around these family issues, discussion may focus on some of these topics: changing family boundaries and allegiances; a spouse's sense of alienation, loneliness, detachment, or resentment; misunderstanding of the partner's guilt, dealing with anger about the intrusion of these hereditary issues into family life; pressures from extended family; rearousal of grief about deceased family members, and so on. This is especially true because the spouse or partner may be unaware of the full range of mixed emotions aroused by the potential use and implications of genetic technology. It may be difficult for nonblood relatives to acknowledge, for example, the relief at not sharing the burdens of genetic predisposition and for those at-risk to understand the complex worry of family members who do not share their personal risk but remain much affected by the outcome of genetic testing in children and other family members.

GENDER AND MARITAL STATUS

Unmarried Women

Single women must also cope with finding support through the process of deciding about and undergoing genetic counseling and testing. Women without current partners express concern about how future partners will react to knowledge of the presence of a heightened cancer risk in their family or, more specifically, in themselves if they were tested and found to be carriers. This fear may be the reason a number of young women in very high-risk families prefer to put off the experience of testing, choosing instead to conduct regular screening as would be recommended for a female mutation carrier. Concern about genetic breast and ovarian cancer risk can make unmarried, young women more concerned about finding a mate and having children early rather than feeling that they have until age 40 or older to consider childbearing. Again, there are little data in this area. In the Coyne and Andersen study (1999), unmarried women had distress scores below those of unhappily married women, but means on distress scores for all groups were at normal levels. Contrary to what many may think, unmarried women in that study received less support from female relatives than did married women.

There are a number of special issues that lesbians who undergo cancer genetic testing may encounter. Lesbians with a family history of breast and ovarian cancer have been found to have high levels of cancer worry and interest in cancer genetic testing (Durfy, Bowen, McTiernan, Sporleder, & Burke, 1999). The first task they may face (as would gay men undergoing testing as well) is ensuring that their partner is accorded an invitation to participate as a spouse in the counseling and disclosure sessions. Second, family communication issues arising from the testing may be complicated by family relationships in some families already strained by parental or sibling difficulty in accepting the patient's sexual orientation. Family members or patients may confuse issues of the heritability of cancer risk with more complex questions about the heritability of sexual orientation. This confusion may confound open discussion about informing extended family members who are at risk. Lesbian couples' concerns about heightened cancer risk might also affect planned decisions about having children and could alter decisions about which partner will be impregnated. These practical decisions could have deep ramifications for the couple's emotional relationship. More long-term concerns about domestic partner insurance coverage, especially if the mutation carrier were to become ill or unemployed, may be an additional burden. One positive note is that in the event that it is the noncarrier partner who is the biological mother of any children the couple shares, the couple would be spared worry about having passed the deleterious mutation on to the next generation. This could, however, be a cause of envy from the parent's siblings who are mutation carriers, who would be worried about their own children's inherited cancer risks.

Men

Women have tended to dominate the world of cancer genetic testing to date. Women are the kin keepers, the knowledgeable ones about family history. They are also at risk for the cancers caused by the first major cancer predisposition genes, BRCA1 and BRCA2, and some genetic testing programs for these genes have limited enrollment to women. The predominance of patients seeking BRCA1/2 have been from families in which the transmission is through the maternal line, because these families are easier to identify. Although men are at some increased risk for breast cancer if they are carriers of BRCA2 mutations, their medical risks pale in comparison to the level of risk that female carriers have of developing cancer as a result of their hereditary predisposition. Men with BRCA2 mutations are at about a 7% lifetime risk of developing breast cancer, whereas women in BRCA1/2 families have an 85% risk. Although this is certainly a dramatic difference, it is also worth noting that the men's 7% risk of breast cancer is only a few percentage points lower than the risk of breast cancer for women in the general population, which is 11% to 12%.

Men and women are at risk for colon cancer, but there is little work to date illustrating the differences in the ways men and women cope with knowledge of colon cancer risk. In the future, men will be tested for prostate cancer risk, and the tables will be turned. Women will only be transmitters of risk to their sons, although there is the possibility that a mutation in a prostate cancer predisposition gene may put them at some increased risk for associated cancers.

Men find it particularly difficult to talk about issues related to breast and ovarian genetic testing. They are often reluctant to talk to their sisters or mothers both because the female relatives carry greater cancer risks and because the cancer risk concerns female sexual and reproductive organs, topics adult male and female siblings do not typically discuss. Men from cancer families are also, however, unlikely to find male companions outside the family with whom they are comfortable talking about issues related to breast or ovarian cancers. Nonetheless, when interviewed about their feelings, men reveal deep emotions about hereditary BRCA1/2 risk.

> At first sight, males seem neither interested nor concerned about predictive testing. The denial-avoidance behaviour and minimization in the males at-risk may lead to an underestimation and consequently

underdiagnosis of the psychological distress. This behavior can cover underlying conflicts that are fed by fear, guilt, or unresolved grief and loyalty conflicts. (DudokdeWit et al., 1996, p. 256)

Clinical interviews with men in the context of genetic testing, and the few research reports that exist (all largely dealing with *BRCA1/2* testing), illustrate some stylistic differences between men and women but also reveal the strong emotions that many men express about the impact of hereditary cancer on their female relatives and fears for the well-being of their female offspring. Many men do not seem to have the same preoccupation with cancer risk that burdens their female relatives. Some men appear to minimize or deny the impact of such risk on their lives, but this may be more a matter of a style for handling stress rather than a lack of concern or worry. Men in breast cancer families tend to focus their concerns on the well-being of female relatives, but this does not preclude deep feelings about the vulnerabilities involved for all. Men worry not only about their daughters, but also about the impact of genetic information on other men in the family. One man, a physician, from a breast and ovarian cancer family felt that his father would be so upset if he was found to be a mutation carrier (with implications for his children) that he decided he would have to lie to his father if that were the outcome of testing. As he considered the prospect of lying to his father, he decided it made him so uncomfortable that he would forego genetic testing.

Men and women typically differ in their approach to health care generally, in how they view family relationships, and in how they view technological advance. Although bravado and denial may help some men cope with fear about cancer in the short run, it may be useful to develop psychological interventions that allow for more direct expression of emotion. For example, a Web site for men with breast cancer provides an opportunity to discuss issues of common concern (http://interact.withus.com/interact/mbc/). It may well be that future research will help develop approaches to genetic counseling or versions of written genetic materials targeted particularly to the issues around which men focus their concerns.

CULTURAL ISSUES

Individuals' attitudes toward advances in medicine are often guided, at least in part, by cultural or ethnic beliefs about the value of medicine. Different cultures have had different experiences with "genetics" and are likely to respond differently to the promise of new technologies that can test one's blood for genetic variances. Blue-blooded Yankees are likely to view family history and genetic connections as indications of belonging to a powerful social group. Mormons study genealogy and find within it a sense of strength and purity that is of central importance to their cultural and religious teachings. Their books on genealogy have been invaluable to researchers who have used the founder effects within the Mormon community to isolate mutations that convey high levels of cancer risk. African Americans tend to be fearful of medical projects based on genetics because of discrimination black Americans faced in the past. How people feel about genetics is likely to influence how and what they communicate about genetic information offered to them. As previously mentioned, the study by Hughes et al. (1999) found that 27% of at-risk women in African American families had informed their spouses and parents about their involvement in genetic testing, compared with 66% of the Caucasian women who discussed genetic testing with their husbands and 40% who discussed testing with a parent. It is not clear whether this means that African American women discussed their concerns about testing with other women, either in the family or outside of the family, sought support through their church, or were simply less likely to discuss the matter.

Little is currently known about cultural differences as they relate to family communication in genetic testing. One study of women seeking genetic testing for BRCA1/2 showed that only 27% of African Americans discussed genetic testing with their spouse, and 27% told a parent, compared with 66% of Caucasian women who discussed testing with their spouse and 40% who talked about testing with a parent (Hughes, 1999).

A population-based sample of 200 Jewish women showed a strong reliance on the belief that "knowledge is power" as reflected in their nearly universal belief that relatives should be informed about the presence of a deleterious genetic mutation in their family. More than 97% believed their genetic information should be shared among relatives if the disease was preventable, and 85% believed in sharing genetic information about nonpreventable diseases (Lehmann, Weeks, Klar, Biener, & Garber, 2000). Other cultures with less belief in the benefits of scientific knowledge might be considerably more skeptical about the importance of universally spreading awareness of genetic traits through the family. It may also be that there are differences between hypothetical responses about family communication and individuals' reactions when confronted with the question of whether to share actual personal genetic information with relatives.

Cancer genetics research to date has focused largely on the well-educated, high-income groups that are overrepresented in family cancer registries. This is likely a function of the kind of organized, high-level health care that has been sought by families who are more comfortable within the medical system and less financially burdened. As our knowledge of cancer genetics expands, the individuals seeking testing will represent a far more culturally and socially diverse group. It will be a challenge to psychologists, both clinically and in research settings, to understand the meanings that these individuals assign to genetic testing and the values that they put on the kind of abstract, but still potentially useful, information achieved through testing. We have much to learn about how variation in socioeconomic status, education, culture, gender, and the framing of genetic information affects willingness to be tested, understanding and acceptance of the results, and communication of genetic information within families of diverse cultural and ethnic origins.

SUMMARY

It is within the context of the family that the impact of genetic medicine will have some of its most fascinating ramifications. Emphasis on the biological links between family members has the potential to bring families together in hopes of improving the health outlook for present and future generations. In so doing, some demarcation is created from those unlucky members of past generations whose suffering now serves to spotlight the family as one with a possible hereditary predisposition for disease. As it becomes increasingly routine to need to know one's family medical history in detail, perhaps new ways will be found, beyond word of mouth, to keep track of and disseminate such information. Interaction about illness and family predisposition to cancer will not be easy or routine, however, in many families. Cultural and demographic factors will play some role in determining how families integrate genetic information and how inter-relationships are affected by genetic test results that convey differential risks for serious diseases, like cancer, to family members. It is clear only that the wrenching memories of the past, the unsettling news of the present, and the hopes and fears for the future that families will experience in the context of genetic counseling and testing will call out for intervention and support from mental health professionals.

REFERENCES

Alby, N. (2003). *The new psychological and ethical problems arising from oncogenetic counseling.* Unpublished manuscript.

Bonadona, V., Saltel, P., Desseigne, F., Mignotte, H., Saurin, J. -C., Wang, Q., et al. (2002). Cancer patients who experienced diagnostic genetic testing for cancer susceptibility: Reactions and behavior after the disclosure of a positive test result. *Cancer Epidemiology, Biomarkers, & Prevention, 11,* 97–104.

Coyne, J. C., & Andersen, K. K. (1999). Marital status, marital satisfaction, and support processes among women at high risk for breast cancer. *Journal of Family Psychology, 13,* 629–641.

DudokdeWit, A. C., Tibben, A., Frets, P. G., Meijers-Heijboer, E. J., Devilee, P., Klijn, J. G. M., et al. (1997). *BRCA1* in the Family: A case description of the psychological implications. *American Journal of Medical Genetics, 71*, 63–71.

DudokdeWit, A. C., Vaseu, H. F., Meijers-Heijboer, H., Ford, D., van Vliet, M., van Tilborg, A. A., et al. (1996). Males at risk for the *BRCA1* gene: The psychological impact. *Psycho-Oncology, 5*, 251–257.

Durfy, S. J., Bowen, D. J., McTiernan, A., Sporleder, J., & Burke, W. (1999). Attitudes and interest in genetic testing for breast and ovarian cancer susceptibility in diverse groups of women in Western Washington. *Cancer Epidemiology, Biomarkers, & Prevention, 8*, 369–377.

Esplen, M. J., Madlensky, L., Butler, K., McKinnon, W., Bapat, B., Wong, J., et al. (2001). Motivations and psychosocial impact of genetic testing for HNPCC. *American Journal of Medical Genetics, 103*, 9–15.

Geller, G., Doksum, T., Bernhardt, B. A., & Metz, S. A. (1999). Participation in breast cancer susceptibility testing protocols: The influence of recruitment source, altruism, and family involvement on women's decisions. *Cancer Epidemiology, 8*, 377–385.

Glanz, K., Grove, J., Lerman, C., Gotay, C., & LeMarchand, L. (1999). Correlates of intentions to obtain genetic counseling and colorectal cancer gene testing among at-risk relatives from three ethnic groups. *Cancer Epidemiology, Biomarkers, & Prevention, 8*(4/2), 329–337.

Green, J., Richards, M., Murton, F., Statham, H., & Hallowell, N. (1997). Family communication and genetic counseling: The case of hereditary breast and ovarian cancer. *Journal of Genetic Counseling, 6*, 45–60.

Hughes, C., Lerman, C., Schwartz, M., Peshkin, B. N., Wenzel, L., Narod, S., et al. (2002). All in the family: Evaluation of the process and content of sisters' communication about *BRCA1* and *BRCA2* genetic test results. *American Journal of Medical Genetics, 107*, 143–150.

Hughes, C., Lynch, H., Durham, C., Snyder, C., Lemon, S., Narod, S., et al. (1999). Communication of *BRCA1/2* test results in hereditary breast cancer families. *Cancer Research, Therapy, and Control, 8*, 51–59.

Julian-Reynier, C., Eisinger, F., Vennin, P., Chabal, F., Aurran, Y., Nogues, C., et al. (1996). Attitudes towards cancer predictive testing and transmission of information to the family. *Journal of Medical Genetics, 33*, 731–736.

Kerr, B., Foulkes, W. D., Cade, D., Hadfield, L., Hopwood, P., Serruya, C., et al. (1998). False family history of breast cancer in the family cancer clinic. *European Journal of Surgical Oncology, 24*, 275–279.

Lehmann, L. S., Weeks, J. C., Klar, N., Biener, L., & Garber, J. E. (2000). Disclosure of familial genetic information: Perceptions of the duty to inform. *American Journal of Medical Genetics, 109*, 705–711.

Lerman, C., Peshkin, B., Hughes, C., & Isaacs, C. (1998). Family disclosure in genetic testing for cancer susceptibility. *Journal of Health Care Law and Policy, 1*, 353–372.

McDaniel, S. H., & Campbell, T. L. (1999). Genetic testing and families. *Family Systems and Health 17*, 1–3.

McDaniel, S. H., & Speice, J. (2001). What family psychology has to offer women's health: The examples of conversion, somatization, infertility treatment, and genetic testing. *Professional Psychology: Research and Planning, 32*, 44–51.

Richards, M. (1996). Families, kinship, and genetics. In T. Marteau & M. Richards (Eds.), *The troubled helix: Social and psychological implications of the new human genetics* (pp. 249–273). Cambridge, England: Cambridge University Press.

Richards, M., & Ponder, M. (1996). Lay understanding of genetics: A test of a hypothesis. *Journal of Medical Genetics, 33*, 1032–1036.

Sarason, B. R., Pierce, G. R., & Sarason, I. G. (1990). Social support: The sense of acceptance and the role of relationships. In B. R. Sarason, I. G. Sarason, & G. R. Pierce (Eds.), *Social support: An interactional perspective* (pp. 97–128). New York: Wiley.

Smith, J. F. (March 10, 2000). *Genetic testing of adoptive children: Ethical and policy issues*. Paper presented to the Colloquium on the Ethics of Genetic Testing in Adoption, University of Massachusetts, Boston.

Wagner, T. M. U., & Ahner, R. (1998). Prenatal testing for late-onset diseases such as mutations in the breast cancer gene (*BRCA1*). *Human Reproduction, 13*, 1125–1128.

Wertz, D. C., Fanos, J. H., & Reilly, P. R. (1994). Genetic testing for children and adolescents: Who decides? *Journal of the American Medical Association, 272*, 875–881.

8

CHILDREN AND GENETIC TESTING

Children figure heavily in the motivation of many adults who seek cancer genetic testing (Lerman, Daly, Masny, & Balshem 1994; Lerman et al., 1996). Because of the young age of onset of many hereditary cancers, many individuals being tested for mutations in cancer predisposition genes are in the 20- to 45-year-old range and have young children or are contemplating starting a family. Consequently, many are concerned not only about the threat to their own mortality that a positive genetic test poses but also about their ability to raise their children to adulthood. Parents of all ages worry about the possibility of passing or having passed a hereditary cancer risk to their children. For those who do test positive, heightened concern about the risk to children often precipitates questions about whether children who are minors can be tested. Parents who are mutation positive are eager to know which way the genetic die has been cast for their children. Concern also arises in families of tested adults with children about the involvement of the children in discussions about their parents' test results.

The topic of children's involvement in genetic testing arouses strong reactions on both sides. We have little firsthand knowledge about what children in "cancer families" experience as they learn about the family medical history and the possibility of genetic testing generally, and as their parents undergo testing. Anecdotal clinical reports suggest that many children in cancer families are well aware of the threat of cancer to family members from at least middle childhood and worry about whether they or their parents will get cancer or die from cancer. There is only limited data about whether children are told about parents' genetic test results when parents are tested for adult-onset cancer predisposition genes. We do not know what actually transpires in conversations between parents and children of different ages and cultural backgrounds about testing generally or about parental test results. We know little in a systematic way about the worry children in cancer families have about cancer and about genetic testing.

Children of individuals undergoing cancer genetic testing are a challenging group for researchers to study. They are usually not present at the test center, and parents are often reluctant to have researchers talk to their children about hereditary predisposition, especially those parents who are not planning to share information directly with their children. In addition, differences in cognitive understanding about the meaning of a genetic test result between children of different ages and from diverse family experiences would require large sample sizes and would complicate findings.

ADULT-ONSET CONDITIONS

For adult-onset conditions such as breast and ovarian or colon cancer, the prevailing philosophy is that genetic testing should be postponed until adulthood when individuals can decide for themselves whether they want to know their genetic status. Some advance counterarguments about why the genetic testing of children for adult-onset cancer predisposition genes should be permissible and why the routine avoidance of such testing is unnecessarily paternalistic. I discuss both the pros and cons of testing children for adult-onset diseases in this chapter and present the policies put forth on this issue by various professional organizations.

Clearly, there are many factors to consider in thinking about children's involvement in cancer genetic testing. A primary question is whether there are potential benefits—medical or psychological—to children of being informed about hereditary cancer risks or being tested to see if they are mutation carriers. Psychological issues for older children include their cognitive ability to handle complex, personally relevant information and to make informed decisions independently. Ethical concerns center on informed consent. Another issue is the potential influence that knowledge of genetic information about family members may have on family equilibrium and the child's well-being. The implications of knowledge of risk information on children's developing self-esteem and self-image are relevant, as are the potential implications of secrecy for family relationships. Issues of family communication as well as communication between children and professional providers bear on the topic of whether it is advisable to discuss concerns about cancer genes with children and, if so, how such communication should proceed. Because of the absence of direct research on the impact of genetic testing on children in cancer families, therapists who see such children, either individually or in the context of their families, may be among the first to learn of the impact of cancer genetic risk information on children.

HISTORICAL PERSPECTIVE

In considering questions of whether and what children should be told about a familial cancer predisposition and the possibility of genetic testing, it is useful to consider how discussions of serious illness with children have been dealt with in other contexts. It is, of course, only in the last 20 to 30 years that U.S. children with life-threatening diseases like cancer have been told the nature of their illness and the prognostic implications of their condition (Powazek, Payne, Goff, Paulson, & Stagner, 1980). This recent openness represents a dramatic change in recognizing the negative impact of parent–child and provider–child secrecy about a child's illness. It was previously believed that children could be protected from fears of dying or anxiety about unpleasant procedures if they were not told that such events were going to happen. In the 1960s and early 1970s, various researchers and clinicians used inventive techniques to conduct research on seriously ill children's understanding of their condition. It became apparent that children were excellent interpreters of their parents' behavior, especially their nonverbal behavior (Vernick & Karon, 1965; Waechter, 1968). As a result, children knew their condition was grave and surmised, in many cases, that they had cancer. They often followed their parents' lead, however, in not bringing up concerns about their illness, leaving many children traumatized and alone, unable to verify or modify their worries.

Viewing honesty as a benefit to the emotional well-being and adjustment of very ill children occurred, probably not coincidentally, with improvements in the treatment of childhood cancer. Beginning in the 1970s, combination chemotherapies made major improvements in the life expectancy of children diagnosed with leukemia and many other forms of childhood cancer. This, in conjunction with research on the ill effects of secrecy, led to a seeming revolution in the idea that children should be informed about their diagnosis and the treatment plan, with opportunities provided for children to ask questions, of both parents and providers, about their condition. Subsequent research and writing showed better adaptation in children from families in which open communication about illness was the norm (Koocher & O'Malley, 1981; Sourkes, 1982).

INFORMING CHILDREN ABOUT GENETIC TEST RESULTS

The studies we have to date tell us that, at least in the United States, some, but not all, children under 18 are informed about the cancer predisposition in their family and are told by their parents about the parent's genetic status. We know little about how decisions regarding telling or not telling children are made, less about exactly what children are told or understand, and virtually nothing about the range of reactions children have to receiving this information. Table 8.1 summarizes factors that can influence decision making about the sharing of family genetic information with children.

There are, of course, important differences between informing children about their own cancer (or other serious illness) and informing them about a parent's result on a genetic test of cancer predisposition. The threat to the child who is ill is immediate and may well be apparent to them from changes in bodily function or appearance, obvious emotional distress in parents and other informed family members, and, possibly, change in family dynamics. They will also shortly begin treatment, often aggressive treatment for their disease. Information about a cancer genetic test result is abstract, and although there may be a threat to the child's ultimate well-being, at least with adult-onset disorders, the threat is not immediate. In fact, the test result given to a parent who tests positive is not a diagnosis in the parent either, but information about the increased likelihood that cancer will occur in the future, or a possible explanation of why it has occurred in the past. Little may be visibly different about the child's or the family's life as a result of testing, although it is not unlikely that the parent who tests positive (and possibly other informed relatives) may be experiencing emotional distress. Uninformed children may have few clues about why their parent appears distressed but, at least in some families, will likely be aware of increased anxiety, parental medical visits, and other changes in their daily lives. Especially in families heavily burdened by cancer, the child may become apprehensive about whether cancer has occurred again and wonder who (including him- or herself) is ill. Not being told about the reason for the increase in parental distress could lead some children to become more anxious, especially if there are not opportunities to ask parents about what has occurred. In some other families, the worry about inherited cancer risk may be relatively well concealed, with children having little or no sense of a major change in the family. Nonetheless, it is likely that not disclosing something as central to the life of the family as cancer genetic testing results raises the possibility that the child may inadvertently overhear or otherwise come upon the information unprepared.

On the other hand, in a family that has experienced many cancer diagnoses (and possibly cancer deaths), learning a parent has a high likelihood of getting cancer (or getting cancer again) could indeed be a source

TABLE 8.1
Factors in Children's Understanding of Genetic Information

Child Factors	Parent Factors	Family/Social Factors	Illness/Genetic Characteristics of Cancer Family History
Developmental/cognitive level of the child • Age • Developmental level • Cognitive deficit or skill • Understanding of illness	Parental ability to communicate about genetic information • Availability of parent (parent illness, death, or other factors) • Empathy, skill in parent–child communication • Parent's own understanding of the genetic information • Parent's own childhood experience of cancer in family members	Ethnic, cultural, or religious attitudes about discussion of health information • Openness of health-related communication versus secrecy • Fear of effect of talking about cancer • Fear of discrimination or stigma	High penetrance of inherited predisposition versus multifactorial etiology • Adult onset versus childhood onset • Treatment available versus no treatment
Child stress related to family cancer experience • Parental illness or death • Illness or death of other relatives • Possible illness experience of the child themselves		Gender • Girls may be more open to discussion of heredity • Mothers may involve children, especially girls, more in discussions of heredity than fathers	
Child emotional status • Depression, anxiety related to family illness experience or other factors • Shame, guilt about family illness experience • Willingness to communicate with parents	Parental emotional status • Depression or high anxiety related to personal or family cancer history • Stress related to caretaking for ill relatives	Access to accurate genetic information • Health insurance coverage for genetic counseling • Availability of appropriate genetic counseling, at least for parents	

of extreme worry for many children. In addition, if a child learns that he or she is also at increased risk for cancer, it may further increase fears, especially if the child believes that this cancer could strike at any time. The complexity of genetic information creates a fertile field for misunderstanding, even in adults, particularly in making a distinction between discovery of mutation status and diagnosis of illness.

Although honesty is preferable to deception, it is not always easy to determine how much to say to a child about whether cancer predisposition truly does "run in the family." As with many other issues, children can often help adults to define what they want to know. Children's questions can be a good starting place for discussion and a guide to understanding the scope of the child's interest and concern. If an 8-year-old child asks, "Why is there so much cancer in our family?" a parent can tell the child that this is a good question that many grown-ups and their doctors are interested in, too. The parent could usefully ask the child if he or she has any theories about why the cancers occur. The answers may provide insight into whether the child is worried about him- or herself or parents, or whether the child has a theory that requires some correction or reassurance (e.g., that cancer is punishment for bad behavior, "God doesn't like us," etc.).

Depending on the parent's willingness and the child's interest, parents might go on to offer information about how the doctors are trying to learn more about what causes cancer to happen in families. A parent might explain that there is a way to tell whether some people in the family might need to take special tests or have doctor visits more often to try to prevent cancer. Children may want to know concrete details. If the child wants to know more, the parent could describe how blood is taken and then tested with special machines. The parent could inquire whether the child has questions or wants to know more, and then encourage the child to ask questions in the future as well. Some parents may share with their children that they may undergo testing or have been tested. They might go further and ask if he or she wants to know the test result. An interested child would be likely to ask whether he or she can be tested too, and a parent would have to think carefully about the answer, offering reassurance, in most situations, that they are too young and do not need these tests now, but that they may choose to be tested when they are older.

It is hoped that such a conversation could take place with a parent who is calm, available to the child, and reassuring in tone and demeanor, because those characteristics convey as much or more than words to the child. The conversation is bound to have emotional ramifications for many parents, however. Some may take advantage of psychotherapy, if available, to prepare for such a discussion with their children, and others may want to use psychological resources to help them with the emotions aroused by sharing personal and family vulnerabilities with their children.

WHAT DO CHILDREN NEED TO UNDERSTAND
ABOUT GENETIC TESTING

The information provided during cancer genetic testing sessions is often challenging to comprehend even for well-educated, medically savvy adults. Children are not typically included in genetic testing sessions. The information they receive usually comes from parents who are not professionals trained in the communication of complex, genetic information. Parents are experts in understanding their children, but they may also be experiencing their own emotional difficulties in telling their children about a familial cancer predisposition and about the implications of their own test result, which no doubt adds a layer of complexity to the communication. Surely children do not require the same level of understanding as adults who may have to understand complex risk information to make decisions about treatment or about risk-reducing surgeries or other interventions. What is it that children, especially young children, need to hear to make sense of a parent's test result?

Richards (1996) pointed out that children, from early ages, have intrinsic concepts of inheritance and kinship based on family resemblance, but that these are often quite different from Mendelian genetic concepts. He recommended using the child's own conceptualizations and fitting the information to be conveyed into that framework, rather than teaching the child basic Mendelian genetics. He called this a "bottom-up" approach, noting that language and concepts must be age appropriate. Richards commented further that many adults use words like "gene" or "DNA" quite successfully with only a general idea of the actual definitions of those terms.

Basic ideas to be conveyed include the following:

1. Who is at risk for having an increased likelihood of disease?
2. How can people learn whether they are at increased risk?
3. What is the disease(s) to which the gene conveys risk?
4. What should be done to reduce risk if the child or his or her parent does have an increased risk?
5. What are the implications of not having the increased risk?

FACTORS IN CHILDREN'S UNDERSTANDING
OF GENETIC PREDISPOSITION AND GENETIC TESTING

Many factors influence the child's understanding of genetic information. With increasing age, children understand more of what adults mean by genetics and heredity. Children who have lived with cancer in their families have a greater understanding of what cancer is, understand much of the "lingo" around cancer diagnosis and treatment, and are more likely to understand (and worry about) what it means to have a risk of developing cancer. On the other hand, family experience with cancer causes stress that can interfere with cognitive understanding. If cancer has occurred in parents and, especially, if the parent has died or is seriously ill, it may be stressful for the child to consider discovering with certainty that he or she is also likely to get cancer, even if the diagnosis is decades away. If the child suffers from depression or other psychological symptoms, due, at least in part, to the family experience with illness, that, too, may interfere with understanding and listening ability. If it is a parent who is explaining the hereditary risk for cancer in the family, the parent's affect and style of presentation, as well as the parent's comprehension of the facts, will also affect what the child hears and how much sense of threat is communicated. Cultural factors, including the belief in some cultural and ethnic groups that talking about cancer can make it happen, can also influence how the information is conveyed. The degree of threat posed by the genetic predisposition will also affect the child. A cancer that could occur any time, such as in Li–Fraumeni syndrome, is different from one that will only occur after age 25 or 30, although both are frightening for children and parents to contemplate. The information required to make an informed decision about genetic testing is complex, and many parents may not fully understand what they were told by the genetic counselor. There is much room for confusion and misunderstanding among both adults and children.

COMMUNICATION OF PARENTAL CANCER GENETIC TEST RESULT TO CHILDREN

BRCA1/2

A definitive study has yet to be done on the impact of communication of a parent's *BRCA1/2* test result. There are, however, a number of studies that are relevant to some part of the process of parent–child communication of test results.

Parent Communication and Distress

Tercyak et al. (2001) observed parental patterns of communication in relation to parental distress. Among 133 adults tested for *BRCA1/2*, about half shared their test results with a minor child. It appeared that factors unrelated to cancer history or test result predicted parent–child communication. Neither parental history of cancer nor test result was related to parents' decision about communication with their children. In most families, either all or none of the children were told, even when there were both adolescent and preadolescent children, suggesting that personality qualities of the parent or preexisting family style appear to govern openness of communication. Mothers were more likely to tell children than fathers. General distress, as measured by the Center for Epidemiological Studies—Depression Scale (CES–D; Radloff, 1977), was significantly associated with parental decision to communicate results to children. Cancer-related distress was not related to the decision to communicate. Communicating with children did not alter parental distress, again supporting the notion that the desire to communicate is related to general, preexisting psychological vulnerability in parents.

Hypothetical Child Interest and Response

A pilot study at Georgetown University Medical Center questioned 20 children, aged 11 to 17, whose mothers were tested for *BRCA1/2* about their health beliefs and worry about cancer and opinions about genetic testing (Tercyak, Peshkin, Streisand, & Lerman, 2001). Children knew their mothers were undergoing genetic testing, but were assessed before test results were available. Their anxiety and depression were measured using the State–Trait Anxiety Inventory for Children (Spielberger, 1973) and the Reynolds Adolescent Depression Scale (Reynolds, 1987). Behavior problems were measured using the Achenbach Youth Self-Report (1991). Sixteen of the children had mothers who had had cancer, mostly breast cancer.

The children almost universally thought they were in good or excellent health, but about half worried at least a fair amount that they or a family member would develop cancer some day. Ninety percent showed at least a fair amount of interest in knowing about their personal cancer risk. Although most thought about the possibility that their mother's cancer might recur, only about 20% described their worry as interfering with their daily activities. Anxiety, depression, and internalizing and externalizing behavior problem rates were within normal levels. Qualitative data included the report of cancer anxiety in a teenage girl, which was triggered by a talk with her mother about the fact that if the mother were to test positive, she would be at increased risk for both ovarian and breast cancer. This finding is similar to that in many women who are surprised to learn in genetic counseling that being positive for *BRCA1/2* exposes one to elevated risk for cancers beyond breast cancer.

Colon Cancer

There are as yet no research studies of parent–child communication about parental hereditary nonpolyposis colon cancer testing. See "Genetic

Testing of Children With Medical Benefit in Childhood" later in the chapter for a discussion of testing children for familial adenomatous polyposis.

GENETIC TESTING OF CHILDREN FOR ADULT-ONSET CANCER PREDISPOSITION

Parents have a great interest in knowing whether their children carry a cancer predisposition gene. A study of mothers of children with cancer reported that 42% would test healthy siblings of the child with cancer for a cancer predisposition gene if a test were available, even if there were no medical benefit to knowing (Patenaude, Basili, Fairclough, & Li, 1996). In another study, a third of high-risk women thought it legitimate to test a 13-year-old daughter of the carrier of a mutation predisposing to breast and ovarian cancer (Geller et al., 1998). In a study of unaffected first-degree relatives of women with breast or ovarian cancer, 88% thought it permissible for parents to consent to cancer genetic testing for their minor children (Benkendorf et al., 1997).

Many individuals who are found through genetic testing to be carriers of cancer predisposing mutations say they want to know whether their children inherited the deleterious mutation. Because current practice disavows testing of children under age 18 for adult-onset conditions (see "Who Decides?" later in the chapter), however, it is unclear how many parents would actually seek testing for their minor children if it were deemed appropriate by genetics professionals. In the course of genetic counseling for adult-onset cancer susceptibility genes, the rationale for the prohibition on testing children for adult-onset disorders is typically discussed. Nonetheless, Hamman et al. (2000) found that four to seven months following genetic counseling and disclosure of BRCA1/2 test results, 26% of the 218 adult participants stated their general belief that children under age 18 should have the option of genetic testing, even after being told that the current professional recommendation was not to test children under age 18. Of the 104 participants who had children under 18, 17% said they would want their own children tested; 83% said they would not want their children tested.

PROS AND CONS OF TESTING CHILDREN FOR ADULT-ONSET CANCER

Arguments about the values, pro and con, of testing children for adult-onset hereditary cancer predisposition raise many challenging points about

TABLE 8.2
Pros and Cons of Genetic Testing of Children for Adult-Onset Conditions

Pros	Cons
Reduces parental anxiety	Unclear at what age to test
Removes worry about cancer risk from children who do not carry familial mutation	Child's knowledge of genetic status could affect self-esteem and emotional well-being; could precipitate development of behavioral problems
Parents better able to support or plan for child if genetic risk status is known	Prevents individual from exercising right to know genetic status in adulthood
Parents better able to plan whether to have more children	Decisions about testing child should be based on actual competence, not presumed incompentence
Knowing risk status may motivate child to avoid smoking and other health risks possibly related to cancer development	May be difficult to assure privacy of genetic information
Allowing adolescents the autonomy to make their own decision about testing may enhance self-esteem and encourage adherence to recommendations	Possible discrimination or stigma related to employment, armed services selection, marriage, and so on
	Misinterpretation could lead to not getting appropriate health screening
	Could disrupt familial equilibrium; differential treatment of siblings in education goals, emotional involvement, and financial consideration could result
	Children may not fully understand implications of testing
	Possible uninsurability could result

what constitutes the best interest of the child (see Table 8.2). Some argue that reduction in parental anxiety is a legitimate goal of testing because it benefits both the parents and children (Fryer, 1995). Others focus on the need for data about the competence of children to make these decisions and about the impact of cancer genetic testing on children and adolescents (Michie & Marteau, 1998). They argue that decisions about testing children should be empirically based rather than based on arguments that presume to understand the emotional and social consequences of learning one's test result in childhood. Others assert that adolescents should be distinguished sharply from younger minor children in considerations about genetic testing (Elger & Harding, 2000). They cite research stating that by the age of 14, children are as competent as adults to make informed consent decisions (Melton, 1983; Weithorn & Campbell, 1982). Others point out that, although this may be true, it is, at least in part, due to the poor understanding many adults have of genetic concepts and of their own susceptibility to disease (Patenaude, 1996; Ponder, Lee, Green, & Richards, 1996). Elger and Harding also argued that many adolescents, especially in European countries, are making critical educational decisions between ages 14 and 17 as they elect the nature of baccalaureate degree they will pursue. In fact, in England, the Gillick provisions of the law determine that children age 16 and over who are mature enough to understand the consequences of their actions can make health care decisions for themselves (*Gillick v. West Norfolk and Wisbech Area Health*, 1985). Elger and Harding argued further that there is little difference in social risk between giving results to a 17-year-old and an 18-year-old and that there may well be important benefits to supporting the autonomy of adolescents. They cited research stating that adolescents' coping and treatment compliance are improved when the adolescents have greater participation in decision making about their care (Clarke & Flinter, 1996; Lewis, 1983).

On the other side, many argue that to "do no harm," parents and clinicians should avoid testing children for cancer genes if there is not immediate potential medical benefit. Kodish (1999) argued that the earliest age at which a child should be tested for a cancer susceptibility gene is the earliest age of onset at which the disease occurs, thereby, he believes, maximizing the benefits and minimizing the risks. Others feel it is unethical to "acquire knowledge that a child will be affected by as an adult unless there is early treatment available" (Dalby, 1995). They believe that not to test the child is to respect the child's right to decide as an adult when and if he or she will be tested. Not testing a child also avoids the potential problem of uninsurability, especially because children are unlikely to have lifetime health, life, or disability insurance at the time they are tested if tested as children.

Stigmatization, both within the family and in the larger social context, of those children in the family who are mutation carriers is less likely to occur if the child is not tested. Not testing also avoids the difficult issue of separating siblings into those with and without the mutation, with potential differential effects on parental attention and investment. Future research will help us to understand the pros and cons of not testing at-risk children under 18 and thus not differentiating siblings with and without genetic mutations versus testing in childhood and knowing who is and who is not a carrier of a genetic mutation conveying increased cancer predisposition.

WHO DECIDES?

A number of professional organizations and individuals have come forward with strong recommendations against the testing of children for adult-onset disorders (American Medical Association, 1995; American Society of Human Genetics and American College of Medical Genetics, 1995; Clinical Genetics Society, 1994; Collins, 1996; Kommission fur Offentlichkeitsarbeit und ethische Fragen der Gesellschaft fur Humangenetik E. V., 1995). The reasons cited for not testing children for adult-onset disorders include potential harms of stigmatization, lowering of self-worth in the child, guilt in unaffected siblings and parents, and social risk of discrimination in employment and insurability (Wertz, Fanos, & Reilly, 1994).

The Huntington disease (HD) gene was one of the earliest for which testing was possible. Some of the professional statements on the testing of minor children came about to inform clinicians and laboratories about the inadvisability of testing children for HD (Went, 1990). Some clinicians and researchers feel that the incurable and untreatable nature of HD has too blackly colored our views about the advisability of testing children and adolescents for cancer and other conditions where treatments exist (Cohen, 1998). The American Society for Clinical Oncology and other groups, both in the United States and abroad, have nonetheless issued recommendations that minor children not be routinely genetically tested for adult-onset cancer predisposition genes when there is no treatment or medical intervention in childhood that is likely to influence the course of a disease. Some room has been left in a number of these statements for exceptions to the rule, although it is made clear that these should be used sparingly.

Many parents hold different views, believing that the decision should be up to them about whether to have their child tested. Many object to what they feel is unnecessary paternalism in not leaving the choice about testing—a decision related to their child's health—in their hands. Some professionals also believe that it is "appropriate paternalism" for parents to make decisions about genetic testing of minor children, with progressive involvement of older children. Kurtz (1998) advised that when parents feel strongly about wanting to test children, against the advice of numerous medical professional groups, their motivations for testing should be explored and consideration given to the question of whether testing will truly resolve their concerns. They stated that, if parents continue to insist on testing, it should be an option open to them. Others believe that a decision about the testing of adolescent children should be a joint one, made by both the child and the parent, and not carried out unless consensus can be reached (Friedman, 2000). It is known that professional and laboratory practice varies significantly in willingness to process testing of samples from children (Wertz & Reilly, 1997), with some acquiescing more or less easily to parents' wishes.

Others question why competent adolescents shouldn't decide for themselves about being tested (American Society of Human Genetics, 1995;

Binedell, 1998). Some feel that waiting until children are adults could lead to resentments within families (Cotton, 1995). Decisions on the basis of the adolescent's competence to make a decision with such lifelong consequences involve individual evaluation of each case on its own merits, however. It also should include an exploration of whether the decision about testing is actually masking other issues, including unresolved family conflicts that would be better referred for psychotherapeutic treatment. Such a careful assessment is costly and time-consuming, however; many feel that the general prohibition against the testing of children for adult-onset is a reasonable guide in the majority of cases.

Much future research is needed to evaluate to what extent, if any, the findings from studies of the psychosocial impact of genetic testing on adults are applicable to the impact on children and adolescents. The relatively low percentage of adults who have elected cancer genetic testing among invited samples may or may not imply that adolescents, given the same choice, would decide the same way. On the other hand, few of the adults who have received test results from cancer genetics tests have expressed regret, and many have expressed relief, even those who tested positive. Would that be the same with tested adolescents, or would many mutation carriers tested as children later be sorry that they knew from such an early age about the high likelihood they would develop cancer? To what extent is it different to contemplate getting Huntington's disease, which is incurable, compared with knowing that one is likely to develop breast or colon cancer, both illnesses for which treatment is available and cure is possible? Would the current restrictions on testing children for adult-onset disorders be markedly different in the future if there are great advances in the treatment for breast, ovarian, and colon cancer, rendering them more likely to be chronic than life-threatening disorders?

In the meanwhile, families with strong histories of cancer in many relatives will have to live with the anxiety of knowing which of their young members are at increased risk and which are not, and deciding when, if at all, genetic testing should be used to try to answer that question. For some parents, the taboo on testing children may actually be helpful, allowing them not to make a difficult decision about whether to allow their children to undergo testing.

Psychotherapy may well help many parents live with the discomfort, guilt, anxiety, and depression that may accompany worry about children's cancer risk. Especially valuable will be therapists who have some conception of the challenging issues involved, the opinions offered by professional organizations, and the presence of an opposing group who favor informed decision making by parents or, in some cases, by adolescents with a good grasp of the pros and cons.

Psychotherapists' skills can also be valuable to the genetics professional team working with parents who want to test their minor children for adult-onset cancer predisposition genes. This is especially the case in considering testing children who are too young to be able to voice a competent view of their own. Even the professional prohibitions against testing children for adult-onset disorders leave room for considerations of exceptional cases in which testing may be justified. There are, however, no guidelines for deciding in which cases it may do more harm than good not to test a minor child. Kessler (1998) argued that parents who wish to reduce their own anxiety by testing their children should more properly be referred for personal counseling. The ability of mental health professionals, especially those with family therapy training, to elicit and integrate the views of all relevant parties and to explore the full range of possible effects on the family that testing a child might have can be of great use. The mental health profession-al's well-reasoned recommendation about potential psychological effects on the parents, child, and family system is likely to be of great value in helping the genetics professional make a decision about whether to honor the parents' request for testing (Chapple, May, & Campion, 1998).

GENETIC TESTING OF CHILDREN WITH MEDICAL BENEFIT IN CHILDHOOD

When there is immediate, potential medical benefit to the child who undergoes genetic testing for cancer predisposing mutations, the ethical conflicts are severely reduced. "Potential medical benefit" implies that there are interventions or intensive screening for cancer that begin in childhood. When there is medical benefit, parents are fully legally empowered to make decisions about genetic testing, and ethical concern would be likely to be raised only when parents reject the possibility of screening or testing their child, putting him or her at high risk of early malignancy. Nonetheless, the process of genetic testing, even with potential benefits to the child, is not without psychological impact on the child and family.

Genetic testing is routinely carried out in children under 18 when there are screening procedures or risk-reducing interventions that should begin in childhood. Familial adenomatous polyposis (FAP) and multiple endocrine neoplasia 2 (MEN2) are the most prominent examples of such conditions. For FAP, screening for intestinal polyps begins at approximately age 10; in MEN2, thryoidectomy may be recommended as early as the first year of life if a child is known to be a mutation carrier. In Von Hippel–Lindau disease, a hereditary disorder characterized by benign brain or eye tumors and often associated with renal cancers, symptoms can begin to develop in adolescence or even sometimes in childhood (Laxova, 1999). Because of the range of symptoms, screening involves an extensive annual battery of tests that can be avoided if a child is found by genetic testing not to be at increased hereditary risk for cancer. Genetic testing for mutations in the *Rb* gene is also done in some children who have unilateral retinoblastoma to see if it is of a hereditary etiology, which carries with it a 50% risk of developing a second malignancy. Testing is also done in some research settings for children with Wilm's tumor to see if they have mutations in their *WT1* gene.

Few data are available on how children react to undergoing genetic testing for conditions that are manifest in childhood or for which preventive interventions need to be started in carriers before age 18, and most of the literature concerns children with FAP. A study from the United Kingdom and Australia found that children (*n* = 60; 31 positive and 29 negative) who were tested remained, on average, in the normal range for anxiety, depression, and behavioral symptoms (Michie, Bobrow, & Marteau, 2001). The children, who were aged 10 to 16, appeared to understand the implications of their testing. Mutation-positive children had significantly higher risk perception and worry about FAP and felt more threatened following disclosure than mutation-negative children. There was no significant difference in self-esteem between mutation-negative and mutation-positive children, and they also did not differ in perceptions of their current health; 30 of 31 mutation-positive children and 26 of 29 mutation-negative children rated their current health as "good" or "excellent." A tenth of the mutation-positive children, however, expressed regret about knowing their genetic status.

A U.S. study also found that mean scores for children tested for the *APC* gene that predisposes to FAP remained in the normal range on measures of anxiety, depression, and behavioral functioning following test result disclosure (Codori, Petersen, Boyd, Brandt, & Giardello, 1996). Results from that study of 43 children from 23 families in which one parent had FAP and about half of the children were mutation positive illustrates the interdependence of family members' reactions to disclosure and to illness. Some patients did show increased distress after testing, however, with three children moving from normal to clinical ranges on anxiety following result disclosure. It is interesting that two of these three children were mutation negative. The reactions of the children in this sample were different, depending on which parent had FAP. Having an ill mother was associated with significantly higher depression scores in children who were themselves mutation carriers and a trend toward higher anxiety scores following disclosure in both mutation positive and negative children. The authors suggested that a mother's reaction to illness may color children's perceptions and especially children's reaction to testing positive themselves. It was not clear in these families why children whose test results were both positive and negative and who had fathers who were ill showed reductions in anxiety and behavior problems after disclosure. In families in which some children tested positive and some negative, the parent who was not ill had significantly increased depression after the children's test results were disclosed. There was also a trend toward increased depression in healthy (non-FAP) parents when all children tested positive and a similar trend for parents with FAP when any of their children tested positive. It may be easier for the parent who did not contribute the genetic cancer predisposition to express the sadness, depression, and disappointment in response to learning that their children as well as their spouse have the disease than it is for the affected spouses, for whom the sadness may be mixed with guilt.

In a long-term (23–55 months) follow-up of 48 tested child FAP patients and their parents from this Johns Hopkins Hereditary Colorectal Cancer Registry sample, the association between child depression and anxiety scores and gender of the ill parent was not sustained at significant levels (Codori et al., 2003). There was a nonsignificant increase in depression scores at follow-up for mutation-positive children with affected mothers. The children's mean scores on depression and anxiety scales remained at normal levels following result disclosure and did not differ significantly by mutation status. There were five children who had normal-range psychological scores at baseline who showed clinically elevated scores at one or more follow-up points. The most striking finding of this study was, however, the significant impact of sibling scores. Children who carried APC mutations and who had a sibling who was also positive had significantly increased depression scores at one year following disclosure. Mutation-positive children who had no siblings who carried the mutation had significantly decreased depression scores at one year. Of the five children with clinically elevated scores at follow-up, three were mutation-negative with at least one mutation-positive sibling, and two of the five were mutation-positive with at least one mutation-negative sibling. Increases were greater for anxiety than for depression, especially for mutation-negative children. None of the five children with elevated scores were from families in which all the children were positive. Among parents, depression was significantly higher at one year for parents whose children had mixed positive and negative results compared with parents whose children were all mutation-positive. Parents whose depression scores showed the greatest increase from baseline (one standard deviation rise or a change from normal to clinical level scores) tended to be from mixed-result families (3 of 5) and to be the unaffected parent (4 of 5). The authors concluded that mutation-negative children with positive siblings were "particularly vulnerable to clinical levels of anxiety symptoms after testing." They hypothesized that this effect may be similar to the effects on healthy siblings of children who have cancer and may also reflect erroneous conceptions of illness that the children hold. (Other research has suggested that children may not distinguish between a positive genetic test result and diagnosis with the illness to which the gene predisposes carriers [Fanos, 1996, 1997].) Codori et al. (2003) suggested further that parents may be overwhelmed by the needs of the mutation-positive children and may be perceived as being unavailable to help the mutation-negative child with their feelings of guilt, anger, and loneliness. They hypothesized further that mutation-positive children with mutation-positive siblings may feel responsible for not only their own status, but also that of their sibling who also carries a mutation. They recommended that future research in this area combine quantitative and qualitative methods and larger samples to further explore reasons underlying these findings. The authors advised,

> At the very least, our data suggest that the mixed families and those where more than one child tests positive are in need of support long after disclosure of the test results. This support should ideally include contact with the entire family by a psychologist, pediatrician, family therapist, or anyone with training in developmental psychology and parent-child relationships. Although mechanisms to facilitate longitudinal follow-up may currently be impractical in clinical settings, our findings should call for a multidisciplinary approach to the genetic testing of children. (Codori et al., 2003, p. 127)

The findings of the Johns Hopkins group, like those of the Smith, West, Croyle, and Botkin (1999) study of adult siblings being tested for BRCA1/2, suggest that the impact of a genetic test result changes depending on the family's experience with illness and the test results of other family members. Although this finding is not surprising to clinicians, understanding the complexity of this relationship will be a challenge to researchers. Methodologists with a strong background in understanding family dynamics will be essential in designing studies that can tease out important categories of impact to explain the outcomes, some surprising, that occur when multiple family members undergo genetic testing. There is still much we do not know about children's true feelings regarding genetic testing that cannot fully be gleaned from standard measures. It is hoped that there will be psychologists and other mental health providers available to offer services to children who undergo testing to help them cope with family pressures, the implications of the illness of their parent, and the emotions of learning their own result, whether positive or negative. Qualitative research would also be valuable in helping us to understand the meaning to a child of being tested for a predisposition to a disease that their parent has or is likely to develop. This research also points to the need for support of parents, both the ill parent and the healthy parent, particularly when siblings have received divergent genetic testing results.

There is also a clear need for development and evaluation of genetic counseling protocols for the delivery of cancer genetic information to children and adolescents. Children have different levels and ways of understanding heredity and illness in their families and different styles of responding to threatening information. Future research should attempt to uncover optimal means of delivering genetic information to children, as well as educating parents to help their children understand the complexities of familial predisposition to cancer and other serious diseases.

REFERENCES

Achenbach, T. M. (1991). *Manual for the Youth Self-Report and 1991 Profile*. Burlington: University of Vermont, Department of Psychiatry.

American Medical Association, Council on Ethical and Judicial Affairs. (1995). *Testing children for genetic status* (Code of Medical Ethics, Report 66). Chicago: Author.

American Society of Human Genetics and American College of Medical Genetics. (1995). Points to consider: Ethical, legal, and psychosocial implications of genetic testing in children and adolescents. *American Journal of Human Genetics, 57*, 1233–1241.

Benkendorf, J. L., Reutenauer, J. E., Hughes, C. A., Eads, N., Williston, J., Powers, M., et al. (1997). Patients' attitudes about autonomy and confidentiality in genetic testing for breast-ovarian cancer susceptibility. *American Journal of Medical Genetics, 73*, 296–303.

Binedell, J. (1998). Adolescent requests for predictive genetic testing. In A. Clarke (Ed.), *The genetic testing of children* (pp. 123–132). Oxford, England: BIOS Scientific Publishers.

Chapple, A., May, C., & Campion, P. (1998). Predictive and carrier testing of children: Professional dilemmas for clinical geneticists. In A. Clarke (Ed.), *The genetic testing of children* (pp. 195–210). Oxford, England: BIOS Scientific Publishers.

Clarke, A., & Flinter, F. (1996). The genetic testing of children: A clinical perspective. In T. Marteau & M. Richards (Eds.), *The troubled helix: Social and psychological implications of the new genetics* (pp. 164–176). Cambridge, England: Cambridge University Press.

Clinical Genetics Society. (1994). Report of the working party on the genetic testing of children. *Journal of Medical Genetics, 31*, 785–797.

Codori, A.-M., Petersen, G., Boyd, P., Brandt, J., & Giardello, F. M. (1996). Genetic testing for cancer in children: Short-term psychological effect. *Archives of Pediatrics and Adolescent Medicine, 150*, 1131–1138.

Codori, A.-M., Zawacki, K. L., Petersen, G. M., Miglioretti, D. L., Bacon, J. A., Trimbath, J. D., et al. (2003). Genetic testing for hereditary colorectal cancer in children: Long-term psychological effects. *American Journal of Medical Genetics,* *116A,* 117–128.

Cohen, C. B. (1998). Moving away from the Huntington's disease paradigm in the predictive genetic testing of children. In A. Clarke (Ed.), *The genetic testing of children* (pp. 133–144). Oxford, England: BIOS Scientific Publishers.

Collins, F. S. (1996). BRCA1—Lots of mutations, lots of dilemmas. *Journal of Medicine, 334,* 186–188.

Cotton, P. (1995). Prognosis, diagnosis, or who knows? Time to learn what gene tests mean. *Journal of the American Medical Association, 273,* 93–95.

Dalby, S. (1995). Responses to the Genetics Interest Group of the Clinical Genetics Society report: "The Genetic Testing of Children." *Journal of Medical Genetics, 32,* 490–491.

Elger, B. S., & Harding, T. W. (2000). Testing adolescents for a hereditary breast cancer gene (*BRCA1*). *Archives of Pediatric and Adolescent Medicine, 154,* 113–119.

Fanos, J. (1996). *Sibling loss.* Mahwah, NJ: Erlbaum.

Fanos, J. (1997). Developmental tasks of childhood and adolescence: Implications for genetic testing. *American Journal of Medical Genetics, 71,* 22–28.

Friedman, L. R. (2000). Genetic testing of adolescents: Is it in their best interests? *Archives of Pediatrics and Adolescent Medicine, 154,* 850–851.

Fryer, A. (1995). Genetic testing of children. *Archives of Disease in Childhood, 73,* 97–99.

Geller, G., Bernhardt, B. A., Doksum, T., Helzsouer, K. J., Wilcox, P., & Holzman, N. A. (1998). Decision-making about breast cancer susceptibility testing: How similar are the attitudes of physicians, practitioners, and at-risk women? *Journal of Clinical Oncology, 16,* 2868–2976.

Gillick v. West Norfolk and Wisbech Area Health, 3 All ER, 402 (1985).

Hamman, H. A., Croyle, R. T., Venne, V. L., Baty, B. J., Smith, K. R., & Botkin, J. R. (2000). Attitudes toward the genetic testing of children among adults in a Utah-based kindred tested for a *BRCA1* mutation. *American Journal of Medical Genetics, 92,* 25–32.

Kessler, S. (1998). Family processes in regard to genetic testing. In A. Clarke (Ed.), *The genetic testing of children* (pp. 113–121). Oxford, England: BIOS Scientific Publishers.

Kodish, E. D. (1999). Testing children for cancer genes: The rule of earliest onset. *Journal of Pediatrics, 135,* 390–395.

Kommission fur Offentlichkeitsarbeit und ethische Fragen der Gesellschaft fur Humangenetik E.V. (1995). Stellungnahme zur Entdeckung des Brustkrebsgens *BRCA1* [Commission for public consideration of the ethical questions of the Society of Human Genetics (1995). Position on the discovery of the *BRCA1* breast cancer gene.]. *Medikal Genetik, 7,* 8–10.

Koocher, G. P., & O'Malley, J. E. (Eds.). (1981). *The Damocles syndrome: Psychological consequences of surviving childhood cancer.* New York: McGraw-Hill.

Kurtz, Z. (1998). Appropriate paternalism and the best interests of the child. In A. Clarke (Ed.), *The genetic testing of children* (pp. 237–243). Oxford, England: BIOS Scientific Publishers.

Laxova, R. (1999). Testing for cancer susceptibility genes in children. *Advances in Pediatrics, 46,* 1–38.

Lerman, C., Daly, M., Masny, A., & Balshem, A. (1994). Attitudes about genetic testing for breast-ovarian cancer susceptibility. *Journal of Clinical Oncology, 12,* 843–850.

Lerman, C., Narod, S., Schulman, K., Hughes, C., Gomez-Caminero, A., Bonney, G., et al. (1996). BRCA1 testing in families with hereditary breast-ovarian cancer: A prospective study of patient decision-making and outcomes. *Journal of the American Medical Association, 275,* 1885–1892.

Lewis, C. E. (1983). Decision making related to health: When could/should children act responsibly? In G. B. Melton, G. P. Koocher, & M. J. Saks (Eds.), *Children's competence to consent* (pp. 75–91). New York: Harcourt Brace Jovanovich.

Melton, G. B. (1983). Children's competence to consent: A problem in law and social science. In G. B. Melton, G. P. Koocher, & M. J. Saks (Eds.), *Children's competence to consent* (pp. 1–18). New York: Harcourt Brace Jovanovich.

Michie, S., Bobrow, M., & Marteau, T. M. (2001). Predictive genetic testing in children and adults: A study of emotional impact. *Journal of Medical Genetics, 38,* 519–526.

Michie, S., & Marteau, T. M. (1998). Predictive genetic testing in children: The need for psychological research. In A. Clarke (Ed.), *The genetic testing of children* (pp. 169–179). Oxford, England: BIOS Scientific Publishers.

Patenaude, A. F. (1996). The genetic testing of children for cancer susceptibility: Ethical, legal, and social issues. *Behavioral Sciences and the Law, 14,* 393–410.

Patenaude, A. F., Basili, L., Fairclough, D. L., & Li, F. P. (1996). Attitudes of 47 mothers of pediatric oncology patients toward genetic testing for cancer predisposition. *Journal of Clinical Oncology, 14,* 415–421.

Ponder, M., Lee, J., Green, J., & Richards, M. (1996). Family history and perceived vulnerability to some common diseases: A study of young people and their parents. *Journal of Medical Genetics, 33,* 485–492.

Powazek, M., Payne, J. S., Goff, J. R., Paulson, M. A., & Stagner, S. (1980). Psychosocial ramification of childhood leukemia: One year post-diagnosis. In J. L. Schulman & M. J. Kupst (Eds.), *The child with cancer: Clinical approaches to psychosocial care research in psychosocial aspects* (pp. 143–156). Springfield, IL: Charles C. Thomas.

Radloff, L. S. (1977). The CES–D scale: A self-report depression scale for research in the general population. *Applied Psychological Measurement, 1,* 385–401.

Reynolds, W. M. (1987). *Reynolds Adolescent Depression Scale: Professional manual.* Odessa, FL: Psychological Assessment Resources.

Richards, M. P. M. (1996). Families, kinship, and genetics. In T. Marteau & M. P. M. Richards (Eds.), *The troubled helix: Social and psychological implications of the new human genetics* (pp. 249–273). Cambridge, England: University Press.

Smith, K. R., West, J. A., Croyle, R. T., & Botkin, J. R. (1999). Familial context of genetic testing for cancer susceptibility: Moderating effects of siblings' test results on psychological distress one to two weeks after *BRCA1* mutation testing. *Cancer Epidemiology, Biomarkers, & Prevention, 8,* 385–392.

Sourkes, B. M. (1982). *The deepening shade: Psychological aspects of life-threatening illness.* Pittsburgh, PA: Pittsburgh University Press.

Spielberger, C. D. (1973). *Manual for the State–Trait Anxiety Inventory for Children.* Palo Alto, CA: Consulting Psychologists Press.

Tercyak, K. P., Hughes, C., Main, D., Snyder, C., Lynch, J. F., Lynch, H. T. R., & Lerman, C. (2001). Parental communication of *BRCA1/2* genetic test results to children. *Patient Education and Counseling, 42,* 213–224.

Tercyak, K. P., Peshkin, B. N., Streisand, R., & Lerman, C. (2001). Psychological issues among children of hereditary breast cancer gene (*BRCA1/2*) testing participants. *Psycho-Oncology, 10,* 336–346.

Vernick, J., & Karon, M. (1965). Who's afraid of death on a leukemia ward? *American Journal of Diseases of Children, 109,* 393–397.

Waechter, E. H. (1968). *Death anxiety in children with fatal illness.* Unpublished doctoral dissertation, Stanford University.

Weithorn, L. A., & Campbell, S. B. (1982). The competency of children and adolescents to make informed treatment decisions. *Child Development, 53,* 1589–1598.

Went, L. (1990). Ethical issues policy statement on Huntington's disease molecular genetics predictive test. *Journal of Medical Genetics, 27,* 34–38.

Wertz, D. C., Fanos, J. H., & Reilly, P. R. (1994). Genetic testing for children and adolescents: Who decides? *Journal of the American Medical Association, 272,* 875–881.

Wertz, D. C., & Reilly, P. R. (1997). Laboratory policies and practices for the genetic testing of children: A survey of the Helix network. *American Journal of Human Genetics, 61,* 1163–1168.

9

SOCIAL AND ETHICAL ISSUES: DUTY TO WARN, AUTONOMY, PRIVACY, AND DISCRIMINATION

Genetic information, by virtue of its ability to predict the likelihood of future illness and the relevance it has for many individuals in a family, requires careful handling. When the Human Genome Project was initiated, the creation of a branch to study the ethical, legal, and social implications of genetic advances reflected the fact that there was concern about privacy protection and social impact as genetics comes to play an increasingly larger role in medicine and society.

In the context of the psychotherapy office, the ethical policies that guide the handling of genetic information will be reflected in the interactions that patients report having with genetics professionals. The concerns that patients bring to their therapists for discussion will often involve their comfort or discomfort with those interactions and with the ethical policies in place. For that reason, we review here some of the prominent ethical issues that may impact patients with genetic concerns.

DUTY TO WARN

Professionals' Duty to Warn

In 1998, the American Society of Human Genetics (ASHG) issued a policy statement about the rights and responsibilities of physicians to override usual patient–doctor confidentiality to inform a patient's at-risk relatives about the presence of a familial, hereditary disease-predisposing mutation in exceptional cases (ASHG Social Issues Subcommittee on Family Disclosure, 1998). Physicians were directed to contact the patient's at-risk relatives when the patient refused to do so, when the risk conveyed was for a serious disease (not defined) and when remediation or early detection might reduce the morbidity or mortality of the disease for that person.

In 1996, a New Jersey Superior Court (*Safer v. Estate of Pack*, 1996) held the estate of a physician liable for not informing family members that a patient's cancer was indicative of familial adenomatous polyposis, which, as noted in previous chapters, is a hereditary disorder conveying a high risk of developing colon cancer (Liang, 1998). The court concluded that the physician's duty included a "duty to warn those at risk of avoidable harm for a genetically transmissible condition."

There are many questions about who "owns" genetic information and what the responsibilities of providers and family members are to inform relatives about the hereditary risks for serious illness, especially if there are effective treatments or prevention strategies that can be initiated as a result of that knowledge. Cancer genetics is a field in which there are a number of recommended preventive or risk-reducing behaviors, some of which have been proven to be effective in preventing cancer or reducing mortality, but many of which still lack definitive proof. Depending on the degree of proof required, however, some would argue that there is sufficient evidence to suggest the potential medical benefit of informing relatives when a familial mutation is found in a cancer predisposition gene. Knowledge of the mutation might lead family members to begin screening at earlier ages or to be more aggressive with regard to screening or risk-reducing surgery. This information might be particularly valuable to individuals from branches of cancer families who are unaware of the hereditary risks. This might be the case, for example, in a branch of a family with breast and ovarian cancer in which the mutation was inherited through the paternal side and where there had been few female children born for several generations. Members of this branch of the family might not be attuned to hereditary risk for breast and ovarian cancer because there would have been few at-risk female family members to develop breast or ovarian cancer and to come to the attention of medical professionals. Similarly, a prostate cancer family with few male children might avoid notice for several generations. There would be no excess numbers of prostate cancer cases to lead clinicians to suspect the hereditary predisposition that was nonetheless being passed on to future generations. Information about hereditary risk would be especially valuable if passed on from parts of the family in which the cancers had more aggressively penetrated and in which the early age of onset of at least some of the cancers would have brought relatives to the attention of genetics professionals.

A genetic counselor or physician would typically encourage an individual found to be a mutation carrier to notify other relatives who might also be at increased hereditary risk. Even when a patient is not genetically tested but undergoes genetic counseling, the counselor is likely to recommend that the individual pass on the knowledge gained to relatives, with the suggestion that they, too, might benefit from personalized counseling. The question addressed by the ASHG policy, however, is what the genetics professional or physician should do if the patient, for one reason or another, refuses to pass on the information. This policy statement takes the rather bold step of deciding that the transmission of genetic risk information should be similar to mandates for the reporting of contagious diseases, such as syphilis or HIV. In those cases, when a partner refuses to inform contacts, the responsible physician, if aware of how to reach at-risk individuals, would make contact and inform them of their disease risk.

Some patients are reluctant to contact relatives either because of fear of upsetting them or feelings of guilt (e.g., the guilt of passing a cancer predisposition to one's child). In other cases, it is the belief that the knowledge would not be understood or that knowledge of a hereditary predisposition would make no positive difference, either because the person was already doing all that could be done preventively or because they would not be likely to act on the information. In other cases, it is the longstanding estrangement of relatives that inhibits contact about genetic matters. Some individuals find it uncomfortably personal or intrusive to reveal one's risk for cancer or other serious disease and the particulars of difficult family history information to someone they do not know or know well who is nonetheless a blood relative.

A policy such as that advocated by the ASHG and similar policies put forth by the President's Commission for the Study of Ethical Problems in Medicine and Biomedical and Behavioral Research (1983) and the Institute of Medicine (1994), however, fail to take into consideration the tangled web of interconnectedness that is the modern family or the possible negative consequences on doctor–patient relationships. The intrinsic message the physician brings in such an informing scenario is "Your negligent relative wouldn't tell you about this, so I am mandated to do so." The person receiving the call is likely to be unprepared for and perhaps uncomfortable with the genetic information the physician imparts. The information would come not from the person's instigation, but at the will and on the timetable of the informing physician. Does the relative have a right to informed consent to receive or avoid the incoming information? The relationship between the relatives, if one existed, may be permanently harmed. In some cases, the relatives may be virtual strangers, in which case the call from a physician may seem even more intrusive and bizarre. How much knowledge is the physician mandated to impart? Does he or she have to be certain that the information was correctly received and acted on? How far does the responsibility go? The possibly irreparable harm that could come in the emotional upset of such a communication is not considered. The factor of time is not considered; how quickly should the patient be required to inform relatives before the physician feels he or she must step in? Does the relative's age or the immediacy of risk matter? This policy does not recognize the untenable position the physician is put in, informing people who are most likely not his patients about a risk that is often not immediate, but abstract and uncertain, without the benefit of any relationship to the person being informed. Little consideration is given to questions of how such policies erode trust between patients and physicians and may, in the long run, do more harm than good. Without patient–doctor trust, patients may be reluctant to discuss their concerns about hereditary predisposition to illness with a physician, and more lives may be lost as a result.

Because it has become clear from the low uptake of Huntington's disease genetic testing and cancer genetic testing research projects that many individuals from high-risk families do not want to know about their personal disease risk (Harper, Lim, & Craufurd, 2000; Patenaude et al., 1996), it is likely that many relatives contacted by an unknown physician and told of a familial cancer predisposing mutation would be displeased to receive the information. Although such a call might help some individuals to seek appropriate genetic services, the intrinsic emotional risks are high, and the demands on the physician go well beyond usual professional expectations. Practical issues such as liability and billing cast further doubt on the wisdom of such an approach.

Most clinicians disagree with this policy and prefer to maintain their relationship with their own patient and any relatives whom the patient chooses to involve. They hope that the continuing relationship with their patient will ultimately be more successful in convincing him or her to inform relatives than would an artificial communication by the physician over the patient's objections. Nonetheless, in the presence of professional policy statements such as the 1998 ASHG statement on confidentiality, the physician's position is a vulnerable one. That statement has generated much discussion and concern among physicians who feared its existence could make them subject to legal suit if they failed to override the wishes of a patient reluctant to talk to relatives, as in the New Jersey case. Of interest, is that in June 2003, the American Society of Clinical Oncology (ASCO), the professional organization for adult oncologists, including those who see cancer genetics patients, issued an update of its policy about genetic testing for cancer susceptibility (ASCO, 2003). Its position espouses a view of provider confidentiality much more in line with standard practice and the wishes of genetics providers. This new policy recommends that providers should "remind" patients of the importance of spreading genetic information and test results to family members. It states further that "ASCO believes that the cancer care provider's obligations (if any) to at-risk relatives are best fulfilled by communication of familial risk to the person undergoing testing, emphasizing the importance of sharing this information with family members so that they might also benefit" (p. 2401).

There are other duty to warn issues for professionals to consider. Given the rapidly advancing knowledge in the field of cancer genetics, questions also arise about the role of health care providers to contact those at-risk when new information about additional risks associated with the mutations found in their family becomes available. If it is found, for example, that the gene for breast-ovarian cancer also conveys a somewhat increased risk for prostate cancer in male carriers, should all who have been previously counseled be contacted to make sure that they understand this new risk? How big a risk would be needed to justify such a step? To what lengths should providers go to reach former patients in this highly mobile society? What about informing 18-year-olds about familial risk that they may not have learned about from their parents? It is often stated that in genetic conditions, "the patient is the family," but there are potential professional practice conflicts inherent in that concept within the relationship of an individual medical provider and his or her patient and, certainly, when the relationship is between an individual patient seeking psychotherapy services and a psychotherapist. There remain serious (and interesting) questions about the privacy of genetic information and about the limits of professional responsibility in updating medical information related to hereditary predisposition for patients and their family members that will need to be addressed professionally, ethically, and legally in coming years.

Psychotherapists are trained to understand the far-reaching complexity of family relationships. They are likely to understand how disruptive and distressing a physician's well-meaning message about the presence of hereditary risk might be to the person told, as well as to the original patient. Much of the silence on the part of mutation carriers is, at least consciously, well meaning, reflecting the shame, fear, or concern of the mutation carrier. Waiting until one can talk in person with a relative, waiting until a child has finished exams, is over the latest boyfriend breakup, is out of college, and so on are rationales for postponing communication that speak to the fear that the information itself may seriously interfere with the relationship or that the pain of conveying or receiving such threatening news will be intense. In some circumstances, it is the absence of any emotional relationship with a relative one has never known that makes it difficult to think of speaking of such personal matters. Getting to the root of the psychological reasons why one family member refuses to convey potentially lifesaving information to a relative is more likely to effect a change in the family communication standoff than is a policy that places the physician in an untenable role between his patient and an unknown relative. Psychotherapeutic intervention, possibly involving multiple family members, is a more appropriate venue for resolving problems of family communication than is the mandated communication by physicians. Such discussions are not likely to fit into the timetable of the busy geneticist, genetic counselor, or internist. Nor is the focus of their training on the resolution of family conflicts. Useful professional links can be forged between genetics professionals and psychotherapists to encourage early referral of patients for family therapy or individual therapy geared to resolution of conflicts related to family communication of genetic information. As physicians gain skill in recognizing cancer genetic predisposition syndromes and counseling patients about the advisability of informing at-risk relatives, they may also be increasingly able to recognize circumstances in which a timely referral for psychotherapy or family therapy may be the most useful "preventive" action that can be taken.

Parents' Duty to Warn

Are parents morally obligated to share genetic information with their children? Although parents do have certain obligations in caring for their minor children, the legal considerations usually involve the provision of basic needs.

> Parents must provide basic nutrition, not caviar; a roof over one's head, not a mansion. Parents must also ensure that children receive demonstrably effective medical treatment needed to avert serious imminent harm, such as antibiotics for meningitis. No state would deem neglectful a parent who failed to talk with her children about genetic risks. (Clayton, 1988, p. 380–381)

Ellen Wright Clayton (1998), a medical-legal expert in this field, has said that most states would be highly unlikely to view parents as liable for actions involved in the normal rearing of children, including failure to communicate the sorts of health concerns conveyed by genetic test results.

When parents are reluctant to share genetic information with their children, it is most often because they wish to spare themselves, their children, or both the distress of considering the consequences that could occur as a result of the disease predisposition. The motivation is usually avoidant rather than angry, but in some cases, it may be difficult not to interpret the action as withholding and malevolent. An example is a circumstance in which a terminally ill father with colon cancer refuses to give a blood sample for genetic testing to benefit his healthy adult children. They and other relatives are worried about their risk of developing cancer and are requesting the valuable information that the testing could provide. The emotions aroused in such cases are strong; the father's action can be seen as dooming the children and other relatives to possibly unnecessary and unpleasant screening for a lifetime and to continuing uncertainty about hereditary cancer risk. Considerable therapeutic work might help a child cope with his or her parent's unwillingness to give the "tube of blood" that could provide answers to questions of personal cancer risk for generations to come. It is also possible, although by no means assured, that therapeutic work with the parent or with parent and children together might help the parent to reconsider the children's request.

A therapist could also encounter a case in which a terminally ill patient refused to let family members learn his or her test result while he or she was alive but was willing to have the test result revealed after death. Or, if there is currently no known mutation in the family, there could be a case in which a patient leaves a blood sample with a researcher with specific instructions that if or when additional genes are found that could explain the hereditary origins of the patient's cancer, the patient gives permission for the blood to be tested and the results given to named relatives in the event that he or she is not alive. These options can be discussed with patients and relatives who are struggling with issues about the sharing of genetic information within the family. The arrangement would usually be worked out through the patient's internist or oncologist. If a patient has made any of these arrangements, it would be useful to have his or her intentions in writing.

AUTONOMY

Prenatal Genetic Testing for Adult-Onset Cancers

It is technologically possible to determine whether a fetus is carrying a mutation in an adult-onset cancer predisposition gene. As previously discussed, many individuals from high-risk cancer families are eager to avoid for themselves and their children the trauma they experienced and observed with the illness, and often death, of a parent from the same cancer they now fear. Many individuals from such families express an interest in prenatal diagnosis, even for adult-onset cancer predisposition. Prenatal diagnosis, they believe, would offer such parents the opportunity to know in advance of their child's birth about the genetic makeup of their child and to plan accordingly. They could enjoy the knowledge, if it were the case, that the child did not inherit the deleterious mutation. Or, if the child does carry a mutation, parents willing to consider abortion would have the option to prevent the birth of the child bearing a mutated gene, thus stopping the line of inheritance of the cancer syndrome. Although the prospect of stopping generations of repeated cancers has appeal to many who have wondered if there is any way to block the disease pattern in their family, there are, obviously, many intrinsic problems in the use of prenatal diagnosis for adult-onset cancer predisposition. Abortion is morally or religiously unacceptable to many and is a difficult experience to undergo for those who find it acceptable. Many are concerned that the kind of genetic engineering that would be represented by prenatal testing for adult-onset breast or colon cancer syndromes with abortion of fetuses carrying a mutated gene would be a step toward the "slippery slope" of "designer" children, with dire social consequences.

If the fetus is identified as having a deleterious mutation, but the parents opt not to abort, the knowledge of the resulting child's mutation status could cause problems within the family. The parents would be knowledgeable from before the child's birth about his or her increased genetic risk for cancer. This might well lead to the child's being treated differently from how he or she would have been or differently from siblings without the predisposition. Even if the parents withhold the information from the child until later in life, the child's status would be likely to be intuited from the parental behaviors. This disturbance in family relationships would not be matched by any medical benefit in childhood, because, for most adult-onset cancer predisposition syndromes, little or nothing could be done to prevent cancer until the child reached adulthood. Prenatal diagnosis of the child would, however, have robbed that individual of any say in whether his or her genetic status became known. For these reasons, there is today a widely accepted policy of not testing children for adult-onset genetic disorders. "To safeguard its progress against an ethically controversial application and the dangers of careless misuse, its [molecular genetic medicine's] use in prenatal diagnosis should not be extended to include diseases such as hereditary breast cancer" (Wagner & Ahner, 1998, p. 1128).

In particular cases, some individuals traumatized by their own family history of cancer who approach childbearing with trepidation may need help in accepting the limitations on prenatal testing for adult-onset cancer predisposition in most centers.

PRIVACY AND DISCRIMINATION

Insurance

Individuals at increased hereditary risk for cancer greatly fear loss of insurance because of genetic discrimination. Few things are more frightening to such individuals than imagining that they are diagnosed with one or more cancers, in need of expensive, specialized care over many years, and are without the means to pay for it because of having been rendered uninsurable on the basis of hereditary predisposition. Fear of uninsurability is a reason that individuals may give for their reluctance to be tested for a hereditary mutation (although, in some cases, this may be a more socially acceptable cover for reluctance tied to a more personal rationale). One recent study (Peterson, Milliron, Lewis, Goold, & Merajver, 2002) found that a little more than a quarter of individuals seeking counseling for hereditary breast and ovarian cancer risk and eligible for BRCA1/2 testing declined testing, citing concerns about cost, confidentiality, and discrimination (all related to insurance coverage) as their reasons. Based on the fact that about 52% of their sample of tested individuals had positive BRCA1/2 results, the authors estimated that 14% of those who declined testing would be positive for BRCA1/2 and would not learn of their genetic status because of concerns related to insurability.

Insurance companies have made clear their fear of "adverse selection" (Lowden, 1992). Adverse selection is the situation that occurs when individuals, knowledgeable about their own hereditary cancer risk, take out large life insurance policies and generous health insurance plans based on information about their health that is not available to the insurer. This would be the case when someone who tested positive for a familial cancer gene did not inform the insurance company about his or her genetic risk status before purchasing large policies at average rates. Put more simply, insurers think it unfair for people to know more about their own health and health risks than the insurers do. When this is the case, they say, their actuarial tables are not accurate in predicting future health care needs, and thus the cost the subscriber is charged is woefully inadequate and robs the insurer of the profit they need to make on policies. They argue that the cost to all policyholders will increase as a result of adverse selection because insurers would have to recoup their losses by raising premiums generally. Their ultimate threat is that if they cannot make a reasonable profit, the insurance companies would go out of business, leaving individuals with fewer insurance options.

What individuals with hereditary predispositions for disease fear is that insurers, if informed that a person carries a hereditary disease-predisposing mutation for a serious illness, would make insurance prohibitively expensive or deny insurance altogether. Genetic counseling for cancer predisposition typically includes advice to purchase any needed additional insurance prior to learning one's results, but this may be financially difficult for many at-risk individuals to do. Many people seeking cancer genetic testing who have not previously had cancer pay for the testing themselves to avoid giving the insurance company access to their result. Genetic counselors do typically caution patients that, although they are not required to volunteer genetic information to insurers, they cannot lie to the insurance company. If a lie is discovered on the insurance application, the insurance company is not obligated to provide coverage and is likely to void the policy. Insurers do, of course, have access to the applicant's family history of illness (which also must be accurately reported), but for a variety of reasons, family history is often not used to set premiums or deny coverage. On the other hand, individuals without cancer but with a significant family history of cancer who are found on testing not to carry a familial mutation might actually want to inform their insurance company to make clear that they should be assessed only general population rates, because they do not have increased hereditary risk for cancer.

Individuals who have previously had cancer often ask their insurance company to pay for genetic testing. Their insurability has been considerably more altered by their cancer diagnosis than it is likely to be by the test result, and determination of the hereditary etiology of the cancer may help in prevention of additional cancers. Proof that the individual is at increased hereditary risk can often be used as rationale for asking the insurance company to pay for increased screening or risk-reducing surgeries.

Patients with significant family history of cancer can often get risk-reducing surgeries or increased screening paid for on the basis of family history, especially with medical backup from genetics professionals or oncologists (Lynch, Severin, Mooney, & Lynch, 1995; Peterson et al., 2002). Discussion during genetic counseling or a visit to a medical or surgical oncologist about how to approach an insurance company to pay for risk-reducing procedures is recommended.

There have been many fewer reported problems with insurability for carriers of cancer predisposition genes than was anticipated (Peterson et al., 2002). This has led some to claim that the risks of insurance discrimination on the basis of genetic status has been overstated and that patients and professionals should drop their guard. Others believe the lack of many cases to date reflects insurers' uncertainty of where to set the bar for refusing coverage or raising rates for individuals who carry mutations in their cancer predisposition genes. Those who favor continued vigilance caution that genetic information is permanent and unalterable and, in fact, affects subsequent generations. They believe caution in the release of the information is warranted until it become clearer how the insurers will deal with the threat of adverse selection.

Legal Protections

There is not at yet (and may never be) full legal protection of genetic privacy. The federal Health Insurance Portability and Accountability (HIPAA) Act of 1996 was the first law at a national level to address the handling of genetic information. This law was hailed as an important initial step in the evolution of federal legislation (Rothenberg, 1997), but it also provided only some of what advocates feel is needed to protect fully those throughout the society who seek and will seek genetic information. The HIPAA legislation prohibits discrimination in a group health insurance plan based on any "health status–related factor," including genetic information. Genetic predisposition cannot be viewed as a "preexisting condition" and cannot alone serve as the basis for denial of coverage. This federal legislation applies mainly to those who have group health insurance and does not offer any protection for those without health insurance. It also does not preclude insurers from excluding coverage for certain procedures, such as prophylactic surgery, nor does not make it compulsory for insurers to get permission before releasing genetic information.

On December 20, 2000, President William J. Clinton issued federal rules to protect the privacy of medical records that have some bearing on genetic information. The rules were subsequently accepted by President George W. Bush and support the necessity of informed consent from patients for release of their medical information for treatment or payment purposes and health plans and health plan providers from sharing medical information with employers, an attempt to limit workplace discrimination. The standards for the disclosure of psychotherapy notes under these rules is stricter than for other health information, and the rules say that health plans cannot determine eligibility or lack thereof on the basis of a patient's unwillingness to give permission for disclosure of psychotherapy notes. Nonetheless, there are many aspects of genetic privacy that are not covered by existing laws, so it is wise for patients and providers alike to be cautious about storing or disclosing information about hereditary risk status and, particularly, about insisting that written permission is given before information about genetic status is released.

Many states have introduced laws to try to ensure that genetic information is not used to deny health insurance coverage or raise premiums through classification at a higher risk level or ensure that an employer cannot insist that applicants or employees take genetic tests as a basis for employment. Some states prohibit the release of genetic information without informed consent. The laws differ greatly state by state, and a provider may need help to interpret exactly what is and is not covered. Local genetic counselors or genetics advocacy groups are usually able to provide updated information about the protections offered in one's local area. Another source of information about state laws related to genetic privacy is a Web site maintained by the Health Privacy Project at Georgetown University, which summarizes relevant state regulations and includes the definitions of terms used in the state laws (http://www.healthprivacy.org). The latter is important because the definitions may determine what is or is not thought to be a genetic condition under the law. Another useful source for updated information about state laws is the Web site of the Genetic Technologies Project (http://www.ncsl.org/programs/health/genetics/ndishlth.htm). Therapists treating patients with genetic concerns are well advised to understand the laws about genetic privacy in their state. The presence of good legal privacy protections for genetic information may lessen the importance of special efforts to keep genetic information out of patients' medical records or the therapist's psychotherapy notes.

It is important to remember that although there may be some protection regarding the availability of health insurance, there is considerably less certainty that there will be protections against genetic discrimination for those seeking to buy life or disability insurance. Many view life insurance as an aspect of financial planning, not a social right. There has been some experimentation in Europe with plans by which minimum levels of life insurance could be purchased without reference to health status or genetic information, but it is not clear that these have found wide approval. Disability insurance often has the strictest requirements because it can result in the biggest expenditure by an insurance company over a period of many years. For this reason, this may well be an area in which the requirements regarding genetic status may ultimately be the most stringent. It is well to advise patients considering genetic testing who can afford to maximize their life and disability insurance to do so prior to testing, so that they can honestly deny knowing their genetic status if asked about it on an insurance physical.

Therapist for the Genetic Age:
Writing Patient Notes and Other Communications

Consideration for the privacy of genetic information of those who seek psychotherapy to discuss issues related to their own and family members' genetic test results creates dilemmas for the psychotherapy provider. Usual patient–client privilege applies, of course, but it is not absolute. Should a therapist avoid all mention of the genetic test result in personal patient notes or, if working in a hospital or clinic, in the patient's medical record? Because the patient's test result might be important for other clinicians working with the patient to understand, is it reasonable to record it as part of the explanation of the reality concerns to which the patient is reacting? Or is it preferable to avoid at all costs any direct mention of the patient's genetic status?

There is no published guidance on this matter. A social work article shares the same dilemma for social work providers and reports that creation of a "shadow chart," a record outside of the medical record of the genetic counseling information and the genetic test result, was used in at least one circumstance (Freedman, 1998). It is not clear what the legal status of such a chart would be.

It is probably best to share with the patient or client the dilemma and to discuss the pros and cons of recording genetic information. It may be appropriate to request permission in writing from the patient to record genetic information in private notes or in the medical chart, if that is what the patient prefers. Assuming the patient prefers only general reference to his or her cancer risk, the therapist's notes could more generally refer to the patient's concern with the history of cancer in his or her family or cancer worries relative to specific cases of cancer that occurred in the family. Discussion with the patient should also include consideration of the wording of communications with insurance companies about justification for psychotherapeutic sessions, including designation of diagnoses and so on. It is likely that communication about the patient's affective state should not in most cases include specific mention of the genetic testing the patient had or its result. More general wording such as, "adjustment reaction to illness in family members," "anxiety related to family cancer history," for example, might be preferable.

CONCLUSION

The relationship between a therapist and patient is typically based on trust and privacy. Genetic information does not, by itself, change the therapeutic relationship. The broad relevance of genetic information and the changing legal environment regarding privacy protection for such information places an additional burden on the therapist seeing patients with genetic concerns. Although the content of sessions dealing with genetic issues might be new, the therapeutic issues that arise in discussions of genetic predisposition are just what they have always been. An attentive therapist has much to offer to patients burdened by a family "past" that includes a significant history of cancer, by awareness of their own heightened hereditary risk of cancer, by challenges in family communication about genetic issues, and by concerns for the cancer risk of future generations. Attention to how specific information about genetic testing results is or is not recorded, stored, and released will ensure that the patient's trust and freedom to communicate openly with the therapist can be maintained. This is not different from responsibilities a therapist typically takes on. Patient anxiety may be heightened, however, with regard to genetic information and the changing legal status of patient medical records, and awareness of ethical dilemmas may require some additional prudence from the therapist with regard to genetic test results to reassure his or her patients.

REFERENCES

American Society of Clinical Oncology, Working Group on Genetic Testing for Cancer Susceptibility. (2003). American Society of Clinical Oncology policy statement update: Genetic testing for cancer susceptibility. *Journal of Clinical Oncology, 21,* 1–10.

American Society of Human Genetics Social Issues Subcommittee on Family Disclosure. (1998). ASHG Statement: Professional disclosure of familial genetic information. *American Journal of Human Genetics, 62,* 474–483.

Clayton, E. W. (1998). What should the law say about disclosure of genetic information to relatives? *Journal of Health Care Law & Policy, 1,* 373–391.

Freedman, T. G. (1998). Genetic susceptibility testing: Ethical and social quandaries. *Health and Social Work, 23,* 214–222.

Health Insurance Portability And Accountability Act of 1996, Pub. L. No. 104-191 (1996).

Harper, P. S., Lim, C., & Craufurd, D. (2000). Ten years of presymptomatic testing for Huntington's Disease Prediction Consortium. *Journal of Medical Genetics, 37,* 567–571.

Institute of Medicine. (1994). *Assessing genetic risks: Implications for health and social policy.* Washington, DC: National Academy Press.

Liang, A. (1998). The argument against a physician's duty to warn for genetic diseases: The conflicts created by *Safer v. Estate of Pack. Journal of Health Care Law & Policy,* 437–453.

Lowden, J. A. (1992). Genetic discrimination and insurance underwriting. *American Journal of Human Genetics, 51,* 90–93.

Lynch, H. T., Severin, M. J., Mooney, M. J., & Lynch, J. (1995). Insurance adjudication favoring prophylactic surgery in hereditary breast-ovarian cancer syndrome. *Gynecologic Oncology, 57,* 23–26.

Patenaude, A. F., Schneider, K. A., Kieffer, S. A., Calzone, K. A., Stopfer, J. E., Basili, L. A., et al. (1996). Acceptance of invitations for *p53* and *BRCA1* predisposition testing: Factors influencing potential utilization of cancer genetic testing. *Psycho-Oncology, 5,* 241–250.

Peterson, E. A., Milliron, K. J., Lewis, K. E., Goold, S. D., & Merajver, S. D. (2002). Health insurance and discrimination concerns and BRCA1/2 testing in a clinic population. *Cancer Epidemiology, Biomarkers, & Prevention, 11,* 79–87.

President's Commission for the Study of Ethical Problems in Medicine and Biomedical and Behavioral Research. (1983). *Screening and counseling for genetic conditions: The ethical, social and legal implications of genetic screening, counseling and education programs* (Report 44). Washington, DC: U.S. Government Printing Office.

Rothenberg, K. H. (1997). Breast cancer, the genetic "quick fix," and the Jewish community. *Health Matrix: Journal of Law-Medicine, 7,* 97–124.

Safer v. Estate of Pack, 677A. 2nd 1188 (N.J Sup. Ct. App. Div 1996).

Wagner, T. M. U., & Ahner, R. (1998). Prenatal testing for late-onset diseases such as mutations in the breast cancer gene 1 *(BRCA1)*. *European Society for Human Reproduction, 13,* 1125–1128.

10

GENETICS AND SOCIAL CHANGE

Genetics is changing medicine. Changes in medicine change society. Changes in society require adjustment at the level of the individual, the family, and at the level of the laws that bind and define the society. Change, even change for the better, exacts an emotional cost. Therapists in a changing society are in a unique position to help those affected by the changes to weigh the personal costs and benefits of the new order.

Contemporary biology has been described as "genocentric" (Richards, 2001), and there are those who speak of the genes as "icons" for our time (Nelkin & Linde, 1995). President Clinton, borrowing a phrase from Francis Collins, director of the National Human Genome Research Institute, said that genes are "the language in which God created Man" (Richards, 2001). Some advise caution in not over-selling the ways in which genetics will change biology, medicine, or society. There are, however, portents that at all developmental stages our choices will be influenced in the near future by recent advances in genetic technology.

BEFORE BIRTH

Embryo selection with in vitro fertilization or prenatal diagnosis of inherited disease with the possibility of pregnancy termination is likely to be offered as an option to many who are found through genetic testing to be carriers of serious disease-predisposing mutations. Once thought to be in the realm of science fiction, it is now possible for those with the finances or (more rarely) the health insurance coverage to pay for in vitro fertilization to determine before birth if an embryo is free of a parent's deleterious mutation and to select that embryo for implantation. It is also possible to determine whether a fetus has a mutation in a gene that predisposes to serious illness and to give parents the choice of aborting that fetus. Neither option is much used today, partly because of prohibitions against prenatal diagnosis of adult-onset disease; partly because of the financial, emotional, and moral burdens of either approach; and partly because of the psychological issues implicit in deciding against the birth of a child on the basis of characteristics carried by one of their parents. It may be true that as the number of diseases for which these techniques can be applied increase, they will be more widely used. The availability of these options raises some difficult issues for parents who are known mutation carriers.

BIRTH

Birth marks a significant turning point in genetic testing policy. Current ethical policies accept the testing of children before birth for many late-onset disorders that are considered unethical to test for once the child is born.

CHILDHOOD

Children in increasing numbers will grow up with an awareness of the possibility that diseases which affect their parents and grandparents have a hereditary etiology and may affect them too. In some families, the children will learn they will have the option to decide if they want to determine their personal level of risk. In some rare families, children will be tested (as in familial adenomatous polyposis families) to determine whether they need to begin screening programs to detect or prevent cancers of a hereditary predisposition. Notions of health and illness will be taught differently, and the issue of personal responsibility (the child's, their parents', their providers) may become more complex.

There is also concern that parents in the not-too-distant future may use genetic technology to produce "designer children." The question of what is remediation of a medical problem and what is selecting traits to enhance one child's chances of success concerns many ethicists. Is small stature a remediable problem? Predisposition to adult-onset cancer? Mild mental retardation or even average intellectual skill? Weak eyesight? Concern is particularly acute because of the likely unequal social access to such genetic remediation.

ADOLESCENCE

Puberty may have different meanings for adolescent daughters who are worried about whether they will develop cancers of the breasts or ovaries that are known to be due to an inherited mutation in their family. The loss of a parent in adolescence to a disease of inherited etiology can have a profound effect on children, often generating motivation for radical prevention strategies, such as prophylactic mastectomy. Although current ethical policy precludes genetic testing in adolescence for adult-onset disorders, as testing becomes more available directly to the layperson, it may be that more adolescents are tested, either at their own request or because their parents are eager to know whether the familial genetic mutation has been passed on. If there are preventive measures that can reduce disease risk if started in adolescence, that, too, could increase the likelihood that adolescents would be tested for adult-onset disorders. As the inherited predisposition to lung cancer, for example, is clarified, the testing of adolescents for related genes could be advocated as part of antismoking campaigns. Many high school science curricula teach components on the New Genetics, spreading awareness of hereditary disease risks and the expectation of increased genetic knowledge of disease etiology in coming years.

YOUNG ADULT

Already in some cultures, genetic disease risk is being considered one of the qualities to be considered in choice of a mate. Among some groups of Orthodox Jews, findings from Tay–Sachs screening programs are considered in matching young people for marriage (Davis, 1998). The matching plan is a complex one with codes so that it may not be clear (unless both members of a couple are carriers) who is the carrier, only that the match is unsatisfactory. How such predispositions will figure in the mating behaviors of the larger population of future generations is unclear. Although it is likely that the perpetual optimism of young lovers will lead to their overlooking much about inherited disease risk, will those with "good" genes (in the medical rather than the social sense) be thought to have a social advantage? There also may be pressure on people who achieve the age of majority in families with known deleterious mutations to undergo genetic testing. Many may resist, especially until they are married and ready to begin a family.

Reproductive choices about inherited risk may complicate the choice to become parents for those who are mutation carriers.

Reproductive options to avoid the birth of a child who carries a familial mutation raises deep questions for parents who are known carriers about the value of their own life. Complex emotions arise as they contemplate that if their parents had made such a decision, they would never have been born.

ADULTHOOD

Adulthood is when preventive or screening practices are recommended for those with most inherited deleterious mutations or those unwilling to be tested. Much work remains to be done in motivating carriers or others who may be at risk to adhere to recommended prevention strategies.

Adults with young adult children may worry profoundly about their children's risks. In some families, this can be a difficult period when several generations experience illness of hereditary origin. When an adult is a carrier of a disease-predisposing mutation, this knowledge may also affect career choices and future planning. Feelings of helplessness or vulnerability may predominate, depending on the defenses and coping strategies of those at risk.

Adulthood is when many of the diseases for which genetic testing is available typically occur. We do not yet know the emotional burdens of having early knowledge of hereditary predisposition and then of waiting to see if, when, and in what form the disease occurs. Nor do we know much about the emotional impact of doing everything that was recommended to prevent disease but having it occur nonetheless.

CONCLUSION

Awareness of genetic disease risk will come much more profoundly and earlier to some families than others. Unlike single-gene disorders like Huntington's disease or *BRCA1/2*-caused brease or ovarian cancer, the genetics of most common diseases are multifactorial, caused by a complex combination of genes or through gene–environment interactions. As such combination effects are revealed, there will likely be greater confusion about individual risk and less clarity for many years to come about the extent to which preventive interventions are effective.

Genetic advances have most obviously affected changes among those diagnosed with cancers for which predisposing single genes have been cloned. All newly diagnosed cancer patients have (or should have) their family histories explored. Most will not have enough family history of cancer to raise concern, and treatment recommendations will proceed without much consideration of hereditary issues. Those with patterns of breast, ovarian, colon, or prostate cancer that suggest the presence of a hereditary mutation may opt for immediate genetic counseling and possibly testing. Among this group, those found to be mutation carriers will have some particular issues to think about in deciding which treatment they will choose. Taking BRCA1/2 mutation carriers as an example, they will learn that their risk for getting breast cancer in their other breast is much higher (in some cases up to an 85% chance) than for individuals who develop breast cancer who are not carriers of a predisposing gene This may lead someone who might otherwise opt for a lumpectomy to instead choose to have both breasts removed surgically (bilateral mastectomy). In addition, women with significant family history of breast cancer will learn that their risk is not just for contralateral breast cancer, but that they also face a much-increased risk of ovarian cancer, which may lead to a decision to undergo prophylactic oophorectomy. Providers will encourage patients to talk with relatives about the chances that they, too, carry the same mutation. Mothers in these families who are mutation carriers will worry about inherited risks passed to their children, especially their daughters. Instead of the general fear that individuals who have had cancer have that their children might, as a result, be at higher risk, these mothers will have specific knowledge that their children have a 50% risk of having inherited a cancer-predisposing mutation. Counseling and testing of additional family members may reveal other relatives who are positive, with new cascades of testing resulting from their testing and further consideration of preventive measures, including surgery, by those who are mutation positive. Similarly, when a man or woman is diagnosed at present with colon cancer, the family history is explored to discover whether there are any indications that the cancer might be part of a hereditary syndrome. If the family history is suggestive, counseling and testing are likely to be recommended. As a result, the first diagnosis of cancer in the current generation may be followed by a wave of medical exploration within the family, possibly resulting in colonoscopies and even colectomies (removal of part or all of the colon) preventively in those found to have many premalignant polyps upon colonoscopy.

The final number of patients found to be mutation carriers is likely to be in the range of 5% to 10% of the total population of breast, ovarian, and colon cancer patients. Nonetheless, it will be a far greater percentage who are made aware of the risk of hereditary disease through the process of family-history taking, and, for some, genetic counseling and testing. Given the considerable media coverage of hereditary cancers, especially breast and ovarian cancer, and increasingly colon cancer, many people believe that the risk of carrying a deleterious mutation in a cancer predisposition gene is much greater than it is. Many also believe that everyone can be informatively tested for such a mutation. Even among those who receive counseling, there is often the misperception that an uninformative negative result, a not-uncommon finding, is actually an exoneration of any possibility of carrying a deleterious mutation, rather than simply a statement that, with current methods having ruled out some of the more likely possibilities, there is no way of knowing whether a deleterious mutation is present.

There is much work underway to educate the public and health care professionals about genetic advances, their benefits, and their limitations. Efforts to educate professionals include the National Coalition of Health Professional Education in Genetics (NCHPEG) and the work of several groups developing projects to educate primary care providers about current knowledge in genetic disease (Burke & Emery, 2002; Greendale & Pyeritz, 2001; F. Walters, personal communication, January 29, 2003). The Genetic Alliance, Human Genome Education Model Project (HUGEM), and other groups are working similarly on public education. Programs to educate journalists and judges about genetics are also underway or in development.

Many professional groups are also preparing to fill the current gap in the provision of genetic counseling. The field of genetic counseling is growing, especially in the area of cancer genetic counseling. Nurses are being trained to prepare patients for genetic testing (Middleton, Dimond, Calzone, Davis, & Jenkins, 2002). Mediators have voiced an interest in helping families make decisions related to testing and helping with family disputes related to genetic issues (Gentry, 2000).

Some of the most important issues are how genetic advances in this new area will alter family life and whether the availability of genetic information will lead to improved health behaviors and a reduced burden of illness. How will families share risk information? What will happen as people try to integrate information about many risks? Will overload breed apathy? How will the inequities in the distribution of deleterious genes affect family relationships? How will cultures that already hold differing ideas of family expectation and obligation integrate the responsibilities connected to this new genetic knowledge? How will society legislate the handling of genetic information, the insuring of all people for their medical needs, whatever the etiology of their disease?

Much of what therapists deal with in psychotherapy practices concerns family relationships and illness. Psychotherapists are experts in human connectedness, in issues of personal identity and self-esteem, and in the way people cope with mortality. Psychotherapists are trained to help individuals weigh priorities, resolve conflicts, seek understanding, feel empowered, and achieve balance between self and society. Therapists are familiar with problems of conflicting goals, ambivalence, and the challenge of tolerating uncertainty. They are aware of the role of cultural and family traditions that sometimes govern "gut-level" reactions more than reasoned, intellectual argument. Such skills will be much needed by 21st-century patients as they adjust to the availability of new medical options and changing social dynamics brought about by the New Genetics.

Psychotherapists who, to at least a moderate degree, understand the basic parameters of the New Genetics, have a grasp of the basic concepts, and know the limitations inherent in our present level of knowledge can anticipate potential personal and family dilemmas much more competently than can someone with only a vague understanding. Knowledgeable psychotherapists will not be thrown by the issues, nor will they burden the patient by their need for explanation of basic concepts. A well-informed therapist will also be better able to pick out misconceptions or misunderstandings in the patient's construction of the situation. Therapists will, as always, learn a good deal from their patients about the particulars of the medical or familial circumstance that is affecting the person's psychological state, but it is hoped that these details will fall on the ears of a therapist with a sound basic knowledge of how the hereditary nature of familial cancer or other illness is determined, what can and can't typically be known, and the range of ways families typically cope with genetic predisposition. Knowledge of basic concepts will allow therapists to focus on patient-related specifics. Educated mental health professionals will know which genetic professionals can answer critical medical questions, enabling the patient to make better use of such consultations. Patients and therapists with particular interests in this area will also find useful the CD-ROMs and Web sites designed to offer relatively quick and often sophisticated knowledge of particular hereditary conditions.

The therapist's ability to anticipate family issues or possible conflicts related to genetic concerns will help the patient to feel understood. Therapists with an awareness of the ethical and legal ramifications of genetic information will help the patient to feel safe and encourage open communication. Mutually agreed-on plans for the storage of any resulting notes or other information will make it less likely that the handling of the genetic information brought up in the course of therapeutic sessions is misunderstood. Knowledge of the implications of genetic information for children, siblings, parents, spouses, and extended family members will hasten the discussion of emotional issues related to the sharing of genetic information within the family and may help in the prevention or resolution of intrafamilial conflict. Therapists who combine knowledge of health behavior change and genetics will likely be more successful in helping patients make choices from the growing range of preventive or risk-reducing options, many of which have as yet unproven efficacy. Therapists with experience in this area can help determine which patients are likely to prefer action to watchful waiting. Work with patients of both sorts may bring to light conflicts about prevention strategies related to the family experience of illness that may be interfering with optimal self-care.

Therapists and research psychologists who see patients from families affected by hereditary cancers or other serious, inherited illness will, in turn, be useful voices in advocating for patients and families in the formation of ethical and professional policy related to genetic advances. Many of our social norms are challenged by genetic advances. Is abortion legitimate when the fetus has a predisposition to childhood cancer? To an adult-onset cancer? A predisposition to short stature? Whose autonomy counts most?

Clinicians and researchers will also gather information relevant to genetic policymaking. There is much yet to be learned in this area. How do people cope with the foreknowledge that, in middle age, they will almost certainly develop a life-threatening illness? Who do they tell? What do they do differently as a result of this knowledge? How will people react when our genetic knowledge expands to the point where individuals receive multiple predictions about highly variable levels of risk for many diseases?

Much of what is presented in this book concerns clinically relevant knowledge about hereditary predisposition for cancer, but much of what readers learn here will be applicable in the near future to understanding those at risk for other diseases. The focus here has been on inherited disorders with classic dominant and recessive characteristics. There will be other cancer genes found in the future, as well as genes for cardiovascular disease, diabetes, and other illnesses that tend to cluster in families. Those disorders that follow Mendelian rules of inheritance will likely be found first, because it is easier to find families to study when genes are inherited in a Mendelian pattern. As more genes are cloned, more risks determined, and more families counseled, many of the same dilemmas will emerge. Education about the particulars will be easier to understand in light of what is understood about hereditary cancer predisposition. Also, there will be findings that link one cancer predisposition to another, or one nonmalignant condition to cancer predisposition. Life, in its most basic form, will become both simpler and more complex.

Over the next decades, more and more genes will also be found that follow other rules of inheritance. This will include genes that do not operate independently to control a disease predisposition, but interact with other genes or with environmental factors in much more variable patterns. There may well be differences in the ways people understand and react to these more complicated forms of inheritance. We can use knowledge gained from testing for hereditary predisposition to cancer and other conditions governed by Mendelian patterns of inheritance as a basis for comparison to cases in which the genetic knowledge offered to patients and families is more complex.

For every true "cancer family," there are dozens of others in which the presence of even one case of cancer makes family members fearful of hereditary consequences. For every patient who goes through genetic testing, there is one who opts not to, who is too fearful or skeptical or poor to be tested. For every woman deciding about prophylactic mastectomy or tamoxifen, there are family members—a husband, mother, father, daughter, son, sister, brother—who wonders whether they can help her and how? For every patient with a colon cancer of inherited etiology, there is a parent upset about having "given" the predisposition to his or her son or daughter. Doctors, nurses, genetic counselors, and other health professionals will have patients who need their help in understanding inherited disease predisposition, decoding complex information, and receiving undesirable test results that represent bad news not just for the patient, but potentially for many other family members as well. Health professionals will need advice about how to motivate patients to do what they can to avoid hereditary illness. Psychotherapists can help patients and health care professionals in understanding what works, what doesn't, and what may be worth trying, even in the absence of proof to try to neutralize or counter such inherited bad luck.

Eric Juengst, former head of the Ethical, Legal, and Social Implications Program of the U.S. Human Genome Project, has said, "If genetic testing and counseling are to be judged a success, it must be from the recipient's point of view, in terms of their ability to use results to enrich their lives" (Juengst, 1995, p. 24). The role of psychological factors in determining the "success" of the amazing work of the Human Genome Project scientists worldwide cannot be overestimated. Ultimately success in this field, as in psychotherapy, comes down to the individual case—not just in terms of mortality and morbidity but in the way illness is experienced. There is much work to do in spreading to the population at large and to those charged with the challenges of health care our awareness of both the simplicity and the complexity of inherited predisposition to illness. Knowledge is not always power, but preparation is usually the best treatment for fear. In that spirit, it is hoped that this book will empower its readers to feel better prepared for the journey ahead as we increasingly integrate and use knowledge of those aspects of our fate that are encoded at conception.

REFERENCES

Burke, W., & Emery J. (2002). Genetics education for primary-care providers. *Nature Reviews Genetics*, 3, 561–566.

Davis, D. S. (1998). Discovery of children's carrier status for recessive genetic disease: Some ethical issues. *Genetic Testing*, 2, 323–327.

Gentry, D. (2000). Genetic technology and family conflict. *Mediation Quarterly, 18*, 5–17.

Greendale, K., & Pyeritz, R. E. (2001). Empowering primary care health professionals in medical genetics: How soon? How fast? How far? *American Journal of Medical Genetics, 106*, 223–232.

Juengst, E. T. (1995). The ethics of prediction: Genetic risk and the physician–patient relationship. *Genome Science & Technology, 1*, 21–35.

Middleton, L., Dimond, E., Calzone, K., Davis, J., & Jenkins, J. (2002). The role of the nurse in cancer genetics. *Cancer Nursing, 25*, 196–206.

Nelkin, D., & Linde, M. S. (1995). *The DNA mystique: The gene as cultural icon.* New York: Freeman.

Richards, M. (2001). How distinctive is genetic information? *Studies in History and Philosophy of Biological and Biomedical Sciences, 32*, 663–687.

ADDITIONAL RESOURCES

RESOURCES ABOUT CANCER

The National Cancer Institute maintains and regularly updates information summaries about cancer treatment and prevention on its Web site in what are known as PDQs, Physician Data Query summaries. These summaries are created by boards of professional specialists who read and critique recent articles and write the summaries. Specialists write summaries for both health professionals and patients or other laypeople. These are excellent sources for updated descriptions of particular cancers, survival statistics, and information about available treatments. Links to information about open clinical trials can be found as well. In addition, the PDQ Screening summaries detail what is known about the risk factors for many cancers and about recommended forms of screening, along with data about the efficacy of screening. Information about the risks of screening is presented as well, for example, the possibility that the screening may not be sufficiently specific to differentiate cancers from nonmalignant conditions that could lead to unnecessary worry and medical intervention. These summaries can be accessed at http://cancer.gov/cancerinfo/pdq/.

A valuable source of statistics on cancer incidence, cancer deaths, and epidemiological factors in survivorship is the annual article published by the American Cancer Society. The most recent example is *Cancer Statistics, 2004* (Jemal et al., 2004). (See reference list for chap. 1 for full citation.)

A variety of valuable sources of information are available about the emotional aspects of cancer treatment and survivorship. Two journals focus exclusively on these topics, *Psycho-Oncology* (Wiley) and the *Journal of Psychosocial Oncology* (Haworth Press). Psychologists Jimmie Holland and Julia Rowland published the second edition of *Handbook of Psycho-oncology: Psychological Care of the Patient With Cancer* (Oxford University Press) in 1999. This edited book reviews major psychiatric reactions of cancer patients as well as suggested treatments. In addition, *Cancer and the Family* (Baider, Cooper, & Kaplan de Nour, 2000), also in its second edition, focuses on the impact of cancer on patients' families.

BREAST, OVARIAN, AND COLON CANCER RESOURCE WEB SITES

American Cancer Society

http://www.cancer.org

Cancer Net (National Cancer Institute)

http://www.cancernet.nci.nih.gov

Colon Cancer Alliance

http://www.ccalliance.org

Colorectal Cancer Alliance

http://www.colorectal-cancer.net

Hereditary Colon Cancer Association (HCCA)

http://www.hereditarycc.org

Living Beyond Breast Cancer

http://www.lbbc.org

Men Against Breast Cancer

http://www.menagainstbreastcancer.org

National Breast Cancer Coalition

http://www.natlbcc.org

National Ovarian Cancer Coalition

http://http://www.ovarian.org

Ovarian Cancer National Alliance

http://www.ovariancancer.org/

Susan B. Komen Breast Cancer Foundation

http://www.komen.org

Wellness Community

http://www.wellnesscommunity.org

Women's Cancer Network

http://www.wcn.org/

BOOKS ON CANCER GENETICS OR RELATED TOPICS

Cancer Genetics

Offit, K. (1998). *Clinical cancer genetics: Risk counseling and management.* New York: Wiley-Liss.

A highly readable, well-documented introduction to field of clinical cancer genetic counseling and testing. There are chapters on counseling and on psychosocial issues.

Schneider, K. (2002). *Counseling about cancer: Strategies for genetic counseling* (2nd ed.). New York: Wiley-Liss.

A wonderful sourcebook for background information about cancer and cancer genetics. Thorough descriptions of the characteristics of all major hereditary cancer syndromes. Much material on the work of cancer genetic counselors and on the process of testing, including the psychological aspects of cancer genetic counseling.

Related Topics

Clarke, A. (1998). *The genetic testing of children.* Oxford, England: BIOS Scientific Publishers.

A thorough consideration of ethical, legal, developmental, and practical considerations regarding the pros and cons of informing children and adolescents about hereditary risks they and other family members carry for serious diseases. An international group of authors considers clinical evidence and calls for increased research in this area.

Bennett, Robin L. (1999). *The practical guide to the genetic family history*. New York: Wiley-Liss.

Considerations in gathering family history and drawing and evaluating pedigrees for evaluation of hereditary disease risk. Helpful for learning to recognize patterns suggestive of hereditary illness and to record such information systematically and usefully. One chapter is devoted to hereditary cancer susceptibility syndromes; others consider mental illness, deafness and visual impairment, neurological disorders, and birth anomalies.

Marteau, T., & Richards, M. (Eds.). (1996). *The troubled helix: Social and psychological implications of the new human genetics*. Cambridge, England: Cambridge University Press.

An intelligent mélange of patient stories and essays on clinical issues including decision making, counseling and testing, testing of children, ethics and legal matters, and social impact of the new genetics. A classic in the field.

Love, S. (2000). *Susan Love's breast book* (3rd ed.). Cambridge, MA: Da Capo Press.

A book much used by breast cancer patients to guide them through the decisions involved in treatment for and adjustment to breast cancer. Chapters on genetics of breast cancer and genetic risk.

VIDEOS AND CD-ROMS ABOUT CANCER GENETICS

Green, M. (2001). *Breast cancer risk and genetic testing*. Niagara Falls, NY: Medical Audio Visual Communications; (800) 757-4868.

An interactive, multimedia decision aid for women making decisions about genetic testing for breast cancer susceptibility. Can be used by patients independently or with a health professional.

American Psychologcial Association (2002). Genetic Issues (with A. F. Patenaude). In *American Psychological Association Psychotherapy Videotape Series III: Behavioral Health and Health Counseling* [Video]. (Available from the American Psychological Association, 750 First Street, NE, Washington, DC 20002-4242)

Videotape using actual patient interview material to illustrate the issues involved in counseling patients whose family histories suggest hereditary illness.

National Action Plan on Breast Cancer. (n.d.). *Genetic testing for breast cancer risk: It's your choice*. Fairfax, VA: Author.

Videotape from the National Action Plan on Breast Cancer (http://www.napbc.org). Provides an introduction to genetic testing for breast cancer susceptibility and includes interviews with genetics providers.

Henderson, J. V. (n.d.). *Genetics in clinical practice: A team approach.* Available at http://www.acmg.net/resources/cd-rom-01/intro.asp

A CD-ROM developed by Dartmouth Medical School and the Centers for Disease Control. Offers didactic and interactive learning about clinically relevant topics in genetics.

PREDICT. Newton, MA: Inflexxion. Available at http://www.genetic-testing.com/

An interactive CD-ROM computer program that offers help in decision making about *BRCA1/2* genetic testing for women and men.

WEB-BASED RESOURCES ABOUT GENETICS, CANCER GENETICS, AND GENETIC TESTING

ASCO (American Society of Clinical Genetics)

http://www.asco.org

Features a CD-ROM cancer genetics curriculum with an impressive slide collection for teaching purposes.

Ethical, Legal, and Social Implications Program of the Human Genome Project (ELSI)

http://www.genome.gov/search.cfm?searchString=ELSI

Reports research on informed consent, ethical concerns, social-psychological research, and legal issues conducted under the auspices of ELSI, the branch of the National Human Genome Research Institute that deals with human implications of genetic science. Much of the research concerns individuals at increased hereditary risk for cancer.

FORCE (Facing Our Risk of Cancer Empowered)

http://www.facingourrisk.org/

A nonprofit organization providing information about genetic risk and options for women who are members of hereditary breast and ovarian cancer families. Offer support for the women and their family members.

GROW: Genetic Resources on the Web

http://www.kumc.edu/gec/grow.html

Search engine for genetic information. Includes links to many other Web-based genetics resources and organizations with genetic focus.

GeneTest

http://www.genetests.org/

Offers expert-written summaries of genetic diseases (under Gene Reviews) and related genetic information. Also offers listing of laboratories that perform particular genetic tests.

Genetic Alliance

http://www.geneticalliance.org/

A consumer organization offering information about pending legislation that affects families with genetic illnesses and names and locations of support groups for people with a wide range of hereditary disorders, including both rare and more common diseases.

HumGen

http://www.humgen.umontreal.ca/en/

A comprehensive international database on the legal, social, and ethical aspects of human genetics. A good source on the policy statements of various groups related to genetic information.

Myriad Genetics Laboratories, Inc.

http://www.myriad.com/med/

The company that does much of the laboratory genetic testing for full sequence *BRCA1/2* and for colon cancer genes provides information about the tests and about genetic counseling.

National Human Genome Research Institute

http://www.genome.gov/

Access to multimedia educational materials for teachers about human genetics. Also, a talking glossary of genetic definitions, some read by leaders in the field.

PDQ Cancer Genetics Summaries

http://www.cancer.gov/cancerinfo/prevention-genetics-causes/genetics

Summaries and updated critiques of the literature on the genetics of various cancers, cancer genetic counseling and testing, risk reduction and prevention options for mutation carriers, and summaries of recent literature on psychosocial aspects of cancer genetics.

HOW TO FIND A CANCER GENETIC COUNSELOR

National Association of Genetic Counselors

http://www.nsgc.org/resourcelink.asp.

National Cancer Institute

http://www.cancer.gov/search/geneticsservices

INDEX

285

testing for
    ethical and legal implications of,
        64
Breast cancer resources, 281, 282, 283
Breast cancer risk
    misunderstanding of personal risk *vs.*
        population risks and, 120
    models for estimating risk, 87
    overestimation of, 119–120
        death of parent from cancer and,
            119–120
        first-degree relative who had
            breast cancer and, 120
        and prophylactic mastectomy,
            178
    perception of, 119–120
    rate in *BRCA1/2* mutation carriers, 46
    reduction with prophylactic
        mastectomy, 176–177
Breast–ovarian cancer predisposition
    testing
    psychological outcomes of, 146–149
Breast self-examination
    compliance with, 130
Bush, G. W., 261

Cancer
    death rate from, 18, 19, 20
        decline in, 20
    distribution of, 18, 19
    familial *vs.* inherited, 24
    hereditary
        age of onset for, 18
        connections between, 18, 20
        predispositions for, 18, 20
    incidence by type, 18, 19
    overview of, 18–26
    risk for
        acquired, 20–22
    treatment and survivorship of
        journal and book information on,
            277–278
Cancer families
    duty to warn in
        benefit to branches unaware of
            hereditary risk, 252–253
    multi-generational experience in,
        111–112
    prenatal diagnosis for individuals
        from, 258

testing in, 5
    unresolved grief in, 110–111
Cancer family label
    impact on family members, 207–208
Cancer genetics
    books on, 280
    videos and CD-ROMs on, 280
Cancer patient, counseling and testing
    of, 271
Cancer phobia
    justification for prophylactic surgery,
        194
    in individuals at-risk for cancer,
        132–133
Cancer predisposing mutation
    selection of embryos negative for,
        217
Cancer prevention, 23, 25, 49, 51, 89, 91
Cancer syndromes
    rare
        information about, 61–62
Career choice
    genetic knowledge and, 270
Caregiving
    distress and, 115
Carriers
    insurability of, 260–261
    percentage in total population, 271
    reasons for failure to inform
        relatives, 255–256
    reluctance to inform relatives, 253
    reproductive choice and, 270
    spouse as, 219–220
CA-125 testing, for ovarian cancer, 185
Certificate of Confidentiality, 92
Chemoprevention, 45
    in *BRCA1/2* mutation carriers
        emotional and psychosexual
            impact of, 51
        risk reduction with, 49, 51
    counseling discussion of, 90
Childbearing
    decision to forego, 217
    and testing in lesbian relationship,
        222
Children
    with *APC* mutation-positive siblings
        anxiety of mutation-negative
            sibling, 245–246
    APC test results and
        parental depression and, 150

results-induced, 11
risk for with testing, 145–146
in seekers of testing, 110, 116–117
in women *vs.* in men, 114
Divorce, testing and genetic risk,
    220–221
DNA. *See* Deoxyribonucleic acid (DNA)
DNA-repair gene, 28, 29
Drazen, J. M., 8
DudokdeWit, A. D., *205, 223–224, 227*
Duty to warn
    Parents', 256–257
    Professionals', 252–256
        about future risk information,
            255
        American Society of Human
            Genetics policy statement on,
            252
        clinician disagreement with,
            254–255
        impact on family, 256
        negative consequences on
            doctor–patient relationship,
            253–254
        ownership of genetic information,
            252
        provider confidentiality limitation
            on, 255
        Safer v. Pack, 252
        when patient refuses to inform
            family member, 253

Education
    of public and health care
        professionals, about genetic
        advances, 272
Educational materials, National Human
    Genome Research Institute, 279
Ethical, Legal, and Social Implications
    (ELSI) program, 278
Ethical, legal, social aspects database,
    HumGen, 279
Ethical issues
    autonomy, 257–259
    duty to warn, 252–257
    and implications of testing, 64
    policy and, 274
    in preadoptive testing, 215–216
    privacy and discrimination, 259–263
    testing and adoption, 215–216

Ethnicity
    penetrance and, 35–36
    and testing, 43–44

Familial adenomatous polyposis (FAP)
    APC gene mutations in, 57, 58
    cancer risk in, 196
    cost of testing for, 93
    in father
        reaction in tested children, 245
    in mother
        reaction in tested children,
            244–245
    natural history and associated
        conditions, 58
    testing of children and, 243
    testing outcomes
        anxiety, 149–150
        parental depression, 150
Familial adenomatous polyposis (FAP)
    families
    prophylactic colectomy for individu-
        als who have polyps, 196
Familial adenomatous polyposis (FAP)
    mutation carriers
    prevention measures for, 58–59
    screening for noncolorectal condi-
        tions in, 59
Familial cancer, *vs.* inherited, 24
Family
    biological, 205
    communication in
        issues in lesbian relationship, 222
        men, 223–224
        problems in, 112
        psychotherapeutic intervention
            vs. physician mandate to
            inform, 256
        to parents, 216–221
        to obligate carriers, 217
        to marital partners, 219
    emotional conflicts in
        referral to psychotherapist for,
            207
    impact on
        of professionals' communication
            of information, 256
    interaction prior to testing, 207–209
    issues of couples and individuals in
        counseling, 221

Family, *continued*
    pressure related to testing in,
        210–212
    and psychological outcome of
        BRCA1/2 testing, 148–149
    separation in after disclosure, 159
    social-psychosocial meaning of, 205
    special relationships and issues
        adoptive child, 215–216
        siblings, 214–215
Family history
    accuracy of, 210
    collection for genetic counselor,
        209–210
    contact with relatives and, 79–80
    denial of, 209
    ethnicity and founder mutations
        in, 79
    in first counseling visit, 79–80
    gaps in, 210
    genetic, 280
    hazards of gathering information
        for, 97
    incomplete or distorted knowledge
        of, 209
    information previously unknown
        misassignment of paternity,
            212
        on pedigree, 81
        processing of, 97
    medical records verification in, 79
    precounseling, 76–77
    in ruling out hereditary cancer pre-
        disposition syndrome, 89
Fanos, J. H., 215–216, 228
Fear
    of cancer, 274–275
    of family member of families with
        rare cancer syndromes, 65
    of genetic information, 10
    of genetic testing, 4
    of insurance companies, adverse
        selection, 259–260
    of uninsurability
        in refusal of testing, 259
Fetus
    with deleterious mutation
        abortion of, 258
    prenatal diagnosis in, 267–268
    prenatal testing for mutation status,
        257–258

limitation on, 258–259
    problems resulting from, 258
First, M., *117, 136*
First-degree relative, definition, 85
Founder effect
    in Ashkenazi Jews, 143–144
    in ethnic groups, 43–44, 79
    in French Canadian and Icelandic
        populations, 79
    in Mormon community, 225
Friend
    at counseling session, 102
    presence at disclosure session
        feelings of, 102–103

Gail model of estimating risk of inherit-
        ing BRCA1/2 mutation, 87
Gelehrter, T. D., *12, 16*
Gender
    and marital status, 222–224
Genes
    for breast and ovarian cancer, 41–51
    cancer-causing types of, 28–29
    cancer-predisposing, 34–35
    definition of, 28
    destructive power of, 113
    dominant, 32, 33
    recessive, 32, 33–34
    transmission of, 33
GeneTest, 279
Gene therapy, 8
Genetic Alliance, 61–62
Genetic concepts
    chromosome, 29–31
    DNA (deoxyribonucleic acid),
        26–27
    gene, 28–29, 32–37
    linkage, 30–31
    mutation, 31–32
    penetrance, 34–36
Genetic counseling
    adherence to recommendations of,
        164
    aims of, 10
    assessment in
        of client motivations, goals, risks,
            77–78
        of emotional well-being and
            safety, 98–102
    autonomy in, 77–79

illness attribution and culture, 127
loss of from cancer
distress of high-risk women and,
116
mutation carrier
counseling and testing of children, 271
Motivator, advocate of family involvement in genetic counseling, testing, 211–212
MSH2/3/6, genes associated with hereditary nonpolyposis colon cancer, 52
Multiple endocrine neoplasia type 2A
(MEN2A)
psychological effects of, 60
RET mutation testing for, 59
risk for medullary thyroid cancer in, 59
somatization in carriers of, 150, 151
testing of children and, 243
thyroidectomy for, 59, 60
Munchausen syndrome in genetic testing, 194
Mutation
definition of, 31
germline, 31
point, 31, 32
Myriad Genetics Laboratories, Inc.
BRCA1/2 gene analysis patent of, 42
colorectal cancer gene testing, 53
testing by, 282

National Association of Genetic
Counselors, 75
finding a cancer genetic counselor, 75
pedigree standardization, 82
National Cancer Institute, directory of
cancer genetic counselors, 75
Physicians Desk Query (PDQ)
Cancer Genetic Summaries, 75
National Coalition of Health Professional
Education in Genetics, 272
National Human Genome Research Institute, (NHGRI), glossary of terms, 17
National Organization of Rare Diseases
Foundation, 62
Negative result, 95
in cancer patient, 142

depression following, 158–159
general population risk and, 12–13
guilt and, 154
known mutation in family and, 142
in people with cancer from cancer
families, 156–157
polymorphism of indeterminate significance and, 12
population risk for sporadic mutation
and, 154
reaction to in cancer families, 45
regret and, 160
reversion to unhealthy habits and, 155
surveillance and screening recommendations and, 154–155
uninformative, 272
Negative without known familial mutation, screening and surveillance
for, 157–158
New genetics
gene therapy and, 8–9
impact on treatment, 7
methods of, 7–8
Non-paternity, 212

Obligate carriers
definition of, 217
identical twin as, 217
Oncogene, 28–29
Oophorectomy, prophylactic, 185–193
acceptability to high-risk women, 188–189
BRCA1/2 positivity and, 163
childbearing prospects and, 192
costs of and insurance coverage, 188
decision for
overestimation of ovarian cancer
risk and, 188
description of, 185
experience of
dissatisfaction in, 190–191
in pre- and post-menopausal
women, 191
relief from worry, 190
and findings in histological examination of ovarian tissue, 187
hormone replacement for surgical
menopause following, 185–186
issues for younger women, 192

ABOUT THE AUTHOR

Andrea Farkas Patenaude, PhD, is a psychologist at the Dana-Farber Cancer Institute and the Children's Hospital of Boston and an assistant professor of psychology in the Department of Psychiatry at Harvard Medical School. She was chair of the American Psychological Association's Genetics Advisory Council and is active on a number of national organizations devoted to the education of professionals about genetics. She is both a psychosocial clinician and an active researcher in the field of cancer genetics and has lectured nationally and internationally on this and related topics.